Group Counseling and Physical Disability:

A Rehabilitation and Health Care Perspective

Robert G. Lasky, Ph. D.
Arthur E. Dell Orto, Ph. D.

Department of Rehabilitation Counseling
Sargent College of Allied Health Professions
Boston University

Duxbury Press
North Scituate,
Massachusetts

Group Counseling and Physical Disability: A Rehabilitation and Health Care Perspective *was edited and prepared for composition by Billie Bolton Dickerson. Interior design was provided by Dorothy Booth. The cover was designed by Elizabeth Spear.*

Duxbury Press
A Division of Wadsworth Publishing Company, Inc.

Library of Congress Cataloging in Publication Data
Main entry under title:

Group counseling and physical disability.

  Bibliography: p.
  1. Physically handicapped—Rehabilitation.
2. Physically handicapped—Psychology. 3. Group
counseling. I. Lasky, Robert G., 1941–
II. Dell Orto, Arthur E., 1943–
RD795.G78   362.4'01'9   78–12316
ISBN 0–87872–196–7

Printed in the United States of America
1 2 3 4 5 6 7 8 9 — 83 82 81 80 79

This book is dedicated to those persons who live the rehabilitation process.

Contents

FOREWORD

Group procedures were introduced into counseling and psychotherapeutic practice with the aim of serving a greater number of clients within available professional time. With use, however, it was discovered that group methods added new and unique elements which could contribute to successful counseling outcomes. Not the least of these elements is the client's awareness of and support by other individuals attempting to cope with similar problems. For the disabled and hospitalized, who are frequently put into isolated or inferior life situations, these considerations can be particularly significant. It is, therefore, with great satisfaction that I note the publication of this book devoted to the application of group procedures with such clients and their families. I am, of course, particularly pleased that the individuals who recognized the need for this book and undertook the task of editing it are both faculty members in the Department of Rehabilitation Counseling at Boston University, Sargent College of Allied Health Professions.

Drs. Lasky and Dell Orto have recognized that effective development of counseling skills requires experiential as well as intellectual learning. Therefore, their inclusion of personal awareness and group process exercises in each chapter constitutes a vital contribution to the full understanding of the excellent selection of papers which they have chosen. Finally, the presentation of the Structured Experiential Therapy model, developed by Drs. Lasky, Dell Orto and Marinelli, offers one innovative approach to the effective utilization of the group procedures with persons having various disabilities.

It may be pointed out that this book deserves the attention not only of counselors who work with clients with medical problems but also of counselors who work with any clients facing issues of social isolation, stigmatization, or institutionalization. Just as counseling with individuals facing medical conditions developed from work with the emotionally disturbed, so the issues and techniques identified in this book may be employed to improve the use of group techniques with a wide range of client populations.

David B. Hershenson, Ph. D.
Dean, Sargent College of Allied Health Professions
Boston University

PREFACE

Group counseling is emerging as a significant therapeutic modality in the effective delivery of rehabilitation and health care services. There is a growing body of literature on the subject and numerous rehabilitation and health care professionals employ group methods with physically disabled persons in hospitals, clinics, and rehabilitation agencies. As rehabilitation counselor educators in an allied health environment, the editors have become increasingly aware of the need for a text that would bring together articles covering group processes and procedures as used in the rehabilitation of physically disabled persons. This awareness led to the development of the present volume combining selected journal articles and editors' original material. The purpose of this book is to provide students and professionals in Rehabilitation Counseling, Social Work, Physical Therapy, Nursing, Clinical Medicine, Occupational Therapy, Counseling and Guidance, Psychology, and Psychiatry with a resource that presents the application of theory, research, and practice in the use of group counseling procedures with persons having a wide variety of physical disabilities.

Articles were selected primarily on their scholarly merits regarding humanistic and therapeutic insights, clinical procedures and/or empirical contributions. We have attempted to provide an overview of what has been published, covering as many disabilities as possible. The initial six chapters are each prefaced by brief introductions written by the editors to define the subject area for that chapter and give an overview of the articles within. Chapter seven, an original contribution by the editors and Robert P. Marinelli, is designed to acquaint the reader with a structured group approach that is adaptable to a variety of rehabilitation populations and settings.

Two unique features of this book are the personal awareness individual exercises and structured group experiences in disability at the ends of chapters 1–6. These exercises contain a variety of thought-provoking questions and challenges on the disabilities discussed in each chapter. They are designed to help the reader transcend the cognitive focus of the articles and become emotionally aware of the impact of physical disability. The personal awareness exercises may be used as homework assignments or discussion topics. The structured group experiences in disability enable the reader to participate in or lead small group experiences that are designed to heighten personal and interpersonal awareness of the impact of physical disability. These experiences have been systematically developed by the editors with a focus on major themes from each chapter. Opportunity for participants to receive systematic feedback from their peers and instructor on their group leadership skills is provided by the group leadership feedback guide in Appendix A.

The book focuses on three levels: *didactic,* the selected articles; *affective*, the personal awareness exercises; and *skills*, the structured experiences in disability. By combining these three levels it is hoped the reader will feel as well as know the material.

ACKNOWLEDGMENTS

Many persons have contributed to the actualization of this book. We would like to acknowledge those physically disabled persons who have been role models for us and who have shared their personal concerns to help us more clearly understand and appreciate what rehabilitation means. The encouragement and support of our colleagues in the Department of Rehabilitation Counseling at Boston University: Bill Anthony, Mike D'Amico, Paul Power, Don Shrey, and LeRoy Spaniol, and our former colleague, Bob Marinelli, have been of great value. The original suggestions of our academic reviewers, Sherilyn Cormier, University of West Virginia, Celeste Dye, University of California, San Francisco, and Chrisann Diprizio, Illinois Institute of Technology, were most helpful. We would also like to thank Iris Zavala and our doctoral students, Sally Rogers, Martha Bernad, and Roger Davis, who assisted in the library review for this project. We also wish to acknowledge the contributions of J. William Pfeiffer and John E. Jones, whose leadership and publications in the area of structured experiential learning provided much of the impetus in the development of Structured Experiential Therapy (SET) presented in Chapter 7. The suggestions of Ed Murphy of Duxbury Press and the expertise of Billie Dickerson in copyediting were invaluable. Further, we express our appreciation to our office staff, Edie Aronowitz, Donna Crawford, and Ellen Miller, for their efforts in the preparation of this manuscript. Lastly, we would like to express appreciation to our wives, Mary and Barbara, and children, Todd, Sean, and Kenneth, for their support and understanding when our writing tasks intruded on family time.

CHAPTER ONE

Group Approaches in Rehabilitation and Hospital Environments

Overview

A historical examination of the rehabilitation and health care literature indicates that persons with disabilities have often been islands unto themselves, impacted and eroded by both the actions and the decisions of others. This role of "victim" is a result of disabled persons having limited control of and participation in critical incidents which shape, determine, alter, or even deteriorate their lives. Fortunately, this situation has been gradually changed through increased awareness on the part of the disabled and nondisabled, meaningful education, relevant legislation, and advances in the scientific and therapeutic aspects of the rehabilitation process. Group counseling has had a role in this process by providing rehabilitating persons with a viable therapeutic resource which has unified their concerns and established a dimension of peer group support.

The impact of physical disability is often first realized in a hospital or rehabilitation center. In such a setting the person must often face the irrevocable fact of disability alone. As the following articles show, informal groups composed of persons sharing similar problems are useful in reducing loneliness and restoring confidence in self and the future.

A poignant presentation of the value of group counseling during the initial phases of rehabilitation is found in Owen's article, "Is Group Counseling Neglected?" As a paraplegic, Owen is convinced that if group counseling had been available in her rehabilitation program, her period of readjustment would have been shortened. Owen stresses the necessity of family involvement during the critical stages of rehabilitation. She alerts the reader to the many complexities of the group process and its application to rehabilitation and health care. In approaching the readjustment process from a systematic frame of reference, Owen challenges the false assumption that a disabled person must live in an isolated and dependent state. Life and living are the main themes of this personalized article, which includes both a futuristic and practically oriented rehabilitation perspective.

In their article "Peer Counseling in a General Hospital," Guggenheim and O'Hara explain the use of peer help in adaptation to disability. While not a presentation on group counseling per se, this article shows that in addition to the resources of the regular hospital staff, the knowledge and experiences of "veteran patients," who have learned to cope successfully with disability, can be of tremendous value to the newly disabled person.

The concept of peer support is expanded in Blandford's article "Peer Group Membership of Young Women with Cancer," in which the development of an informal group in a hospital setting is set forth. Blandford highlights the group's resources, stresses its role as an advocate body, and emphasizes its potential as a vehicle to ease the adaptation of cancer patients to their disease, the hospital, and themselves.

In "Group Discussions: A Therapeutic Tool in a Chronic Disease Hospital," Rosin addresses the adverse conditions of institutionalization that typically encourage patient passivity and accelerate deterioration. He suggests that institutional staff might lessen such passivity by becoming active participants in the rehabilitation process. In Rosin's experience, the use of group discussions that offered opportunities for sharing personal reactions and concerns related to disability proved beneficial to both patient and physician. Traditionally, medical emphasis has focused on patients' physical concerns with a lower priority placed on emotional concerns. Neglect of emotional concerns is most damaging for persons having chronic illnesses, and Rosin sees the need for more group work with such persons.

Physically disabled children have emotional concerns related to hospitalization and treatment that often go unrecognized in a typical hospital program. In their article "Theme-Focused Group Therapy on a Pediatric Ward," Cofer and Nir describe how they organized and conducted a children's discussion group. The effects of hospitalization on children and the need for children to communicate their perceptions of their illnesses in relation to hospitalization prompted a structured group model in this case. To help children verbalize their particular concerns, significant themes, such as factual information about their disabilities or separation anxiety, were employed in a focused group discussion. Unfortunately, such children's groups are rare. By not providing children with the opportunity to share their concerns about hospitalization, a situation is created which neglects the emotional issues directly related to the child's disability.

Stroke and its concommitant effects extend far beyond the physical disabilities that result. Oradei and Waite in "Group Psychotherapy with Stroke Patients During the Immediate Recovery Phase" are concerned about the weaknesses of a rehabilitation process that does not facilitate the stroke patient's verbalization and resolution of basic fears and concerns. In detailing the process of a person's reaction to stroke and the subsequent hospitalization, the authors explain the role and benefits of group counseling with stroke patients. By assessing and altering old coping patterns and by developing new ones, group members moved beyond the initial impact of the stroke to focus on the future.

In "Crisis Groups in Special Care Areas" by McClellan the theory of crisis intervention and its application to special care areas in a general hospital is presented. While their own program was employed with patients undergoing dialysis, the authors provide a detailed picture of group therapy that can be generally applied to other types of crisis care. A four phase model of initiation, sharing, problem solving, and termination was followed and the group was perceived as a valuable resource by patients, family, and nursing staff.

This chapter presents an introduction to the need for group approaches with persons having physical disabilities. The reader is encouraged to be aware of the critical issues that are often faced by persons who are disabled and the suggested group leadership skills which are presented in the articles. Going beyond the factual aspects of the articles, the reader is encouraged to raise questions concerning group leadership with persons having disabilities and to be alert to what further specific skills or knowledge the reader might need to lead such groups.

1

Is Group Counseling Neglected?
—SUZANNE M. OWEN

THE practice of the counseling art for the physically disabled is not nearly as advanced as it has every right to be. Awareness of the needs of the traumatically disabled individual has been with us for a long time. Effective counseling techniques have also been available. But the extent to which the techniques have been applied to meeting those needs has been microscopic.

The full impact of this hit me only recently, when I had occasion to visit one of the leading rehabilitation centers in our area. Nine years ago, when I became paraplegic from an auto accident, I became convinced that group therapy, non-existent where I was, would be a technique useful in shortening the necessary period of readjustment. Over the years since then I had assumed, with group counseling becoming such an accepted technique in other contexts, that it had also taken the place it deserves in the rehabilitation process. I find that this is not true, difficult through it is to understand.

PATIENT GROUP COUNSELING

A seriously injured person is subject to a complete array of negative feelings, some of which can be violent, disturbing and frightening. Realization in the earliest stages, that one is not alone in his destructive thoughts can be most comforting. A sharing of these feelings with fellow patients, under guidance, in the frank atmosphere that hospital life brings about, can have a beneficial effect on all involved. The chance to work out one's own angers, hatreds, frustrations and fears in an accepting and *non-judgmental* group session or in a one-to-one relationship is almost a must in any plan for a quick return to a productive life. Psychological therapy should be just as active a part of the rehabilitation program as physical therapy and something that the individual should undertake as a matter of course. It is perhaps better for the physician to prescribe it for the patient when he

Reprinted by permission from the *Journal of Rehabilitation* 38 (6): 12–15, 1972.

believes him to be ready than to leave it up to the individual.

The hospital setting is not the only possible place for this, it should be emphasized. Many times a perceptive family member, friend or minister can be just as, or more, helpful than a professional counselor.

Not only can group therapy help to lessen one's emotional problems but often can alleviate practical ones as well. The newly disabled person is filled with fears concerning his and his family's future. Every sort of question runs over and over through his too active mind. "How will my family manage financially while I am in the hospital? Will I be able to hold a job again? If I have to change jobs how can I find a suitable one? How can my wife take care of me? What will happen to our marriage? Can sex still be a part of our life?" One person's answers to these and similar questions may give help to another wrestling with the same problems.

Finances are usually the domain of the social worker, but here, too, they can bear group discussion. State and federal aid to the totally disabled, social security, welfare, unemployment compensation, veterans benefits, insurance both private and group, scholarships of various kinds, etc., all need to be clearly understood by each family.

A speedy return to *work*—to the individual's former job if possible — is much to be desired. If his former job is no longer possible, the best vocational counseling available is called for. A plan one can work on will divert the mind from the excessive anxieties and fears which plague it. For the housewife, the sooner she can once again take over her duties of mother and cook the better off she will be. No member of the family, through misplaced kindness, should shield her from any job that she is willing to tackle. The feeling of being of some use is of great benefit.

Sex is also an important topic. Couples can be encouraged to experiment and the possibility of pregnancy can be discussed. Paraplegic and otherwise injured mothers who have been successful in conceiving, bearing and raising children can be brought to the attention of the group.[1] A few of the more helpful articles on the subject should be part of a library available to this group.

Therapy groups should be small—not more than six to eight in a group will allow everyone a chance to be heard—and should include one or two individuals who have been successful in their return to a full, active life. The latter should not be present merely for their practical knowledge of how to cope with themselves and the outside world, but should also be there for the intangible strength they can impart to the group.

OUTSIDE ACTIVITIES

Group counseling does not have to be considered only a talking process. Social contacts outside the hospital are important too in paving the way back to good mental balance. Before leaving the hospital it is next to impossible for many to imagine taking an active part again in the everyday world. This is why it is so important for a rehabilitation center to have an ongoing program of outside contacts for all its patients. Each patient should get out to as wide a variety of events as he can, and as soon as he can—movies, ball games, lectures, plays, concerts, etc. This should not be a privilege but an expectation that includes prodding by the staff if necessary. When one has been in the hospital for a long time among those similarly recovering, it is frightening to think of facing the normal world outside. "What will they think?" "What will they say?" "They will be sorry for me." "I can't stand it." This is why it is so necessary for the hospital to provide for the initial contacts. To go as a group to a public event is probably much easier in the beginning than to be the only one (the feeling is) on whom all eyes are turned.

Those who leave the hospital without these outings are apt to find that they are very hesitant to make that first move into the outside world. Weekends at home are a bridge from hospital life to home life, but they fail to serve the purpose under discussion. They are of little value in introducing an individual once more to society. He is already used to his family members and close friends. It is contact with more casual friends and strangers that is important.

Usually at the time of leaving the hospital a person's total attention is focused on himself, a state somewhat like a teenager's acute self-consciousness. But, in addition, there is almost a sense of disgrace because of body impairment. He certainly doesn't accept himself and, therefore, sees no reason why other people should accept him. It may be a long time before he discovers that he and his body are not identical, that he himself has not changed, but is the same self-determining person as existed before the accident, with all his talents and capabilities (except physical) still intact.

FAMILY GROUP COUNSELING

Family members can benefit also from special sessions tailored to their needs. A time in the hospital just after evening visiting hours once a week can be set for informal group discussion. Since there will be a continuous turnover of participants, there will have to be considerable thought given to the structure of the discussion—perhaps an effort could be made to cover the field every six to eight weeks with specific topics brought up each time. Therefore, those who missed a session might catch the subject on the next round. Perhaps the first hour should be channeled and the second open to talk about anything on the individual's mind.

Attendance of the injured one's spouse should be insisted upon, and other adult family members should be encouraged to attend as well. If the doctor will personally explain to the husband or wife, mother or father, how important these discussions will be to the welfare of the whole family, I believe there would be a high percentage of attendance. The impersonality of a big hospital is very disheartening to the family as well as the patient. A little personal attention can do much to ensure the cooperation of the entire family.

Most people know nothing about severe disability. When a serious accident occurs to one of their family group it may seem like the end of the world. Fear may be so gripping that their overriding response is to run away. The doctor needs to spend some unhurried time with the spouse as soon after the accident as is possible. He cannot, of course, make promises that may not come true, but he can give support to a person in dire psychological need. If he will take the time to acquaint himself with the many successful handicapped people who are leading active, rewarding lives he will be in a better position to be constructive in these discussions. At this time, he can point out the great value of the group discussions to the family.

The following paragraphs give an outline of some of the major areas to be covered in family discussion. The subjects mentioned under patient group counseling are also applicable here.

TEMPORARY CHANGE

The family must understand that the disabled person, when he does return home, will not respond to others as he did before the accident. He may become more himself later, and this will largely depend on the people around him. At best, it may be a long time before he adjusts to his disability, at worst he may be quite unbearable. The perceptive counselor will have practical suggestions tailored to the individual to ease this transitional period. He should stress the extreme importance of the family at this time. The person lacking family support will find it much harder to regain his former outlook on life. Support is not meant to imply a sheltering of the individual. Rather it involves a full recognition of the individual as a person who lost none of his former personal attributes, and encouragement in every way possible for him to seek the mainstream of life again.

CARE AT HOME

The work involved in taking care of the disabled person is likely to seem overwhelming at first. It should be pointed out that he will gradually learn to do many things for himself, though this will be a very slow process. But he will need support and encouragement in order to want to do as much as possible.

Sources of help in the community should be clearly outlined, both for help within the home and on the outside. In addition to the usual sources of household help, neighborhood teenagers may be available for afternoon, evening, and weekend jobs. The activities of the Visiting Nurse Association should be explained. For outside needs such as emergency meals and occasional transportation to doctors, therapists, etc., volunteer agencies such as FISH, Meals on Wheels, and local agencies should be described. The American National Red Cross keeps a list of people who will drive for pay. The possibilities of therapy at home by students (physical therapy, pre-med, physical education majors, etc.) under the guidance of a registered physical therapist can be explored.

RECOVERY STAGES

The successive stages of recovery should be considered. Emphasis should be placed on understanding what takes place in a deeply depressed individual. For, unless the accident is seen by him as atonement for some past sin he will surely be depressed. Deep depression can lead not only to a *feeling* that one is not able, but to increased physical inability. The family should be aware of this factor, as well as the more obvious reason for not doing what it seems he should for himself, namely, that a great many activities are physically difficult and tiring to carry out.

At this point the will to live is in jeopardy, but the realization deep inside that one is truly needed by his family—even though there is no apparent place for him to fit—is something to which to hold. The important objective is to weather the depression, to get to the other side of the abyss. His family's dependence on him is at the same time both disheartening and strengthening. Its need is real, and those individuals who are saddled with it are far luckier than those without. This is a very important point for the family to realize. They must understand that their role, both active and passive, is vital. It is almost as important for the patient to know that he has a family who needs him as it is for the husband or wife to be active in helping him find his way to a new life.

As the deep depression finally slackens, there will probably be an extended time of just existing. The world is no longer black, but neither is there any spark to it. Then, for those who are fortunate, there comes a time when life once again becomes normal, interesting, even exciting, with the disability still there but relegated to its proper subordinate position.

FACTORS TO CONSIDER

Group discussion should also cover the subject of self-pity. This is the one emotion which is almost universally unacceptable to others, even though the majority of us have experienced it at some time in our lives. It needs to be pointed out that it is as normal an emotion as any other and that no one should be made to feel guilty because of it. In the course of a normal recovery, it will gradually fade away until it is lost in new activities and a new self-respect.

Overprotection is one of the biggest stumbling blocks to the rehabilitation process in families who are oversolicitous toward their member. There is a fine line to be drawn here, and no one except those concerned can do it. However, one general guide can be given. Always be alert to what the disabled person is willing to do for himself and never take over for him in this regard.

PATIENCE

For emphasis, I am including patience in the list of major areas for consideration. Patience is a necessity, and this goes for counselor, patient and family alike. Gains, large and small, are made over an extended period of time, and often it is only in looking back after six months, a year or longer that these become obvious. No one is born with patience; we have to learn it through living. The disabled person and his family have to realize that progress will be exceedingly and painfully slow, *but that it will be there.* It might help to write down all the areas of improvement every six months or so just to become aware of the forward movement.

Impatience can destroy those feelings of satisfaction over the little advances. The pleasure one gains from a minute accomplishment can be an incentive for the next small step forward but not if the intial feeling of joy is swallowed up in impatience, in thinking that one should be further along. A family who realizes this can be of much assistance.

FAMILY CONSIDERATIONS

The effect of a parent's catastrophic accident on his children will show through in a variety of ways. Children from a secure home may do well and actually rally to the support of the home front. The behavior of others will reveal that they are upset and frightened. The able parent needs sensible advice so that he is not misled into punishing behavior that has its cause in pure fright or fantasy. The counselor will do well to spend some time outlining listening techniques for parents.[2] To be sure that the child does not feel that he is in some way responsible for the accident is especially important. To reassure him that this is something that rarely happens, and that it is highly unlikely to happen to him, is important too.

The active spouse also needs attention. He needs sympathy, understanding and support. In the case of a wife, she needs to know the importance of finding some trustworthy person to take over while she gets away from home at least once a week, preferably oftener. She needs to be thoroughly instructed (by therapists, nurses, etc.) in all of her new duties before her husband leaves the hospital. If she is made aware of these, she can assume some of the respnsibility for seeing that they are taught to her. Husband or wife will have many worries that group discussion can help to alleviate. The realization that other wives and other husbands have identical problems is somehow reassuring. Talking them over can ease the feeling of loneliness and help one to put his problems in better perspective.

An extension of the family counseling group for those who have left the hospital but still have need of advice and support should be provided. No one really knows his individual problems until home life is actually tried. There will then be many more problems, seemingly unsolvable at home, that may have relatively easy solutions when threshed out in a group.

Most people respond to a challenge. If the family group discussion can lead its members to see that they have just as vital roles to play in the recovery as the doctor or the therapist or the psychologist, then I believe subsequent failure of the marriage will be less probable. If each family member can feel his or her importance as a full member of the rehabilitation team and the support that this would create, then he would regain the stability which the accident has destroyed.

COUNSELOR'S RESPONSIBILITY

The therapist who conducts the group counseling, both for the patients and for their families, has the responsibility of seeing that all the areas discussed, plus others he may have in mind, are covered for each individual. In order for him to be more effective, he should be well aware of the many disabled people successful in all walks of life and be able to point out examples that illustrate the point under discussion. More advantage will be gained by emphasizing the successes of ordinary people rather than those of such celebrities as Franklin Roosevelt or Helen Keller. The latter seem too far above most of us—at least to our limited way of thinking. The People-to-People Program has published one booklet giving short biographies of a number of successful disabled persons and is planning a series.[3] Follow-up studies in his own hospital would also give the counselor more knowledge on which to draw, and would be of some psychological benefit to former patients. There are a limited number of books, biographies and autobiographies that could be kept for the group to borrow and would be profitable reading for the families. (Upon request, a list may be obtained from the author.)

It is debatable, however, if such literature will be acceptable to the patient at this time. For a long time, the only thought the disabled person entertains is that of physical recovery. Success stories may be depressing if presented too early. Everyone is different, however.

PHYSICIAN'S ROLE

Physicians are going to have to play a much larger part in rehabilitation than they have generally done. Because of their excessively busy lives, day-to-day responsibility for most of the rehabilitation has fallen to the therapist and psychologist. The doctor, however, because of his social image as well as his professional skills is in a position to exert far more influence over the patient than anyone else. This means that the physician must be extremely careful of his judgments and never underestimate his patient's abilities, for many times the patient will go no farther than his doctor visualizes. It has been said that the physician tends to accept averages as his basis for expectation, yet the wise physician will always allow for the exception, and will strive to give just the right psychological impulse that will bring about the exceptional recovery.

If the physician would become acquainted himself with the many handicapped who are engaged in a great variety of productive activities, I think he would be in a naturally more optimistic frame of mind and would convey this feeling to his patient. Doctors understandably do not want to hold out false hopes. However, people respond to expectations. If the orthopedist knows that a certain level of achievement has frequently been reached, then his belief that this particular individual can also attain this level can be a powerful stimulus to accomplishment.

ENCOURAGEMENT

Encouragement need not necessarily be a time-consuming process. When I left the rehabilitation hospital, I went back in my wheelchair to visit the nurses in the hospital, where I spent the first three months. Later I went back on crutches to visit again. As I was leaving the office of Sister St. John, who by then had become hospital administrator and thus, sad to say, was removed from contact with the patients, she said, "Next time, one crutch!" Because she truly meant it, whether literally or figuratively does not matter, those four words have stood by me through the years.

REFERENCES

1. Epstein, June. *Mermaid on wheels.* Taplinger, 1969. (Biography of an Australian girl who, paraplegic, finishes college, travels widely, marries, has three children.)
2. Gordon, Thomas. *Parent effectiveness training.* New York: Peter H. Weiden, Inc., 1969. (Practical techniques that will help in dealing with worried children.)
3. President's Committee for Employment of the Handicapped. Successful Disabled Persons' International. *People-to-people,* Vol. 1, Washington, D.C. (Twenty-five, two-page biographies of handicapped people around the world.)

2

Peer Counseling in a General Hospital
—FREDERICK G. GUGGENHEIM, M.D.,
and SUZANNE O'HARA, R.N., M.S.

PEER help, organized outside the traditional health care framework, has been an important therapeutic modality for several decades.[1] Prominent self-help groups include Alcoholics Anonymous,[2] Recovery Incorporated (for patients with mental illness),[3] TOPS (for patients with obesity),[4,5] Ostamates (for patients with colostomies),[6] and Widow-to-Widow.[7]

Reprinted from the *American Journal of Psychiatry,* vol. 133, pp. 1197–1199, 1976. Copyright 1976, the American Psychiatric Association. Reprinted by permission.

In most general hospitals, patients often help each other on an informal basis—only rarely is such interaction arranged by the hospital caretaking teams. The following cases represent instances in which significant support was given in a planned therapeutic approach that brought together two patients with similar illnesses, one who had recovered from its major effects and the other who was in the initial stages of the illness.

CASE REPORTS

Case 1. Ms. A, a 53-year-old housewife and mother of four, was hit by a truck while touring with her family in a foreign country. She immediately sustained a traumatic above-knee amputation of her left leg and severe crush injury to her right leg. One week later, she was flown to Massachusetts General Hospital for treatment of gangrene that was developing in her right leg. Before the accident, Ms. A was a healthy, outgoing, independent, open person, involved in her community and devoted to her husband and children.

On admission to Massachusetts General, she appeared mildly depressed as she focused on details of her accident. She became seriously depressed over the next two months as multiple complications made it increasingly evident that she would lose her remaining leg. Despite active staff support and family encouragement, she became deeply enmeshed in self-pity and bitterness. She experienced sleeplessness, decreased appetite, and apathy. Administration of 150 mg/day of amitriptyline for the next 4 weeks did not produce an appreciable improvement; in fact, her depression increased. The psychiatric nurse clinician suggested peer counseling. Ms. A's physicians were reluctant initially, but the patient's progressive depression, without any other means of effective treatment, prompted them to allow a therapeutic trial.

On another unit there was a 36-year-old married accountant, Mr. B, who had sustained bilateral above-knee amputations 20 years earlier. He used his leg prostheses until an intercurrent illness forced him to use his wheelchair again. After learning from the psychiatric nurse clinician about Ms. A's predicament and needs, Mr. B agreed enthusiastically to the encounter. Ms. A agreed to the meeting.

The psychiatric nurse clinician introduced Ms. A to Mr. B and his wife. All four participants were tense as Ms. A opened the session by asking, "How do you manage to live in a wheelchair?" Mr. B responded by talking about the difficulty of his initial adjustments. He said that he had resented his condition until he began to think, "I'm better off like this than dead. It's all I have. I had better adjust if I want to live normally." He began to boost his own morale and acknowledge the help he received from his family, who were able to treat him as an individual and not a "china doll." Mr. B shared his feelings about encountering embarrassing situations and demonstrated his mobility in and out of the wheelchair.

Both patients related details of their accidents and phases of their adjustment, and genuine closeness evolved through humor and serious talk.

The psychiatric nurse clinician helped set the tone of the session and bridged communication gaps. She asked questions when the patient seemed hesitant to discuss certain issues that were important to her, e.g., how to minimize the financial drain and how to diminish social embarrassment.

In concluding the interview, Mr. B addressed Ms. A's discouragement by saying, "You're only as limited as you limit yourself. Naturally, I'd much rather have my own legs than be in a wheelchair but then again I'd rather be rich than poor." Ms. A said she would have to "learn to be an invalid in a wheelchair," and Mr. B quickly replied, "I'm not an invalid! I consider myself handicapped, living a normal life." Later they parted with a feeling of warmth that accompanies a shared, moving experience. Mr. B subsequently said he was grateful to have had this opportunity; he realized how much he had helped Ms. A. On follow-up Ms. A said, "I felt that it was extremely worthwhile to watch him and his wife's acceptance of him and to see him as a well-adjusted person even though he has no legs. I was amazed and would not have believed it if you had just told me. But I believe it because I saw him." During her lengthy rehabilitation, she often reflected on Mr. B's successful adaptation and said it increased her motivation to persevere.

Case 2. Mr. C, a hypochondriacal 56-year-old factory worker and physical fitness enthusiast, was hospitalized for infectious polyneuritis. His Guillain-Barré syndrome produced almost total paralysis, and he required assisted respiration for the first two weeks. Concomitantly, his depression increased from mild to severe. He wished for death as a way out of his predicament, but he was fearful of it. He asked repeatedly to be disconnected from the mechanical apparatus so he could die peacefully. As he began to recover, the staff was disconcerted to find that their encouraging comments about his potential for full recovery were greeted with mounting suspicion. He refused to be weaned from the respirator; he would not try to cough or cooperate in other aspects of his pulmonary care. He was convinced that he had a terminal illness because his brother had died recently with paralysis from metastases to the spinal cord.

Because of his rapidly mounting depression and unresponsiveness to staff interaction and psychoactive medication, the team thought that Mr. C might benefit from talking with someone else who had recovered recently from the same disease. The house officers were pessimistic about the usefulness of this procedure because of the depth of Mr. C's depression, but they agreed to have the psychiatric nurse clinician introduce him to a former Guillain-Barré patient. Mr. D, a 36-year-old married tradesman and jogger who had recovered fully from the disease, agreed to talk with the patient. Mr. C thought that such an encounter would be useless, but he did not protest. His wife was eager for the meeting.

The psychiatric nurse clinician summarized Mr. C's principal concerns and background for Mr. D and gave him an informal agenda. In the meeting she acted to facilitate communication, steering Mr. D's conversation away from herself and toward Mr. C, who was able to talk in limited amounts. Mr. D was the most active participant. He reflected on the unbearable length of time it had taken him to communicate, the impatience he and his family had felt as a result of the slowness of his recovery, the loneliness of being unable to express feelings or ideas, and the frequent frustrations and irritability. Mr. D pointed out how staff and family had helped him and mentioned how burdensome it was to realize that rehabilitation is really up to oneself.

Mr. C's immediate crisis was communication, and Mr. D discussed some of the techniques he had used to inform staff of his needs. He had learned to pantomime messages and feelings and to use cards when he could not talk or write. He also told Mr. C that there was no permanent damage from the disease and mentioned his increasing appreciation of life in the postrecovery phase, with the experience of real independence. The former patient told Mr. C that the illness had brought him closer to some friends he had not seen in years and had facilitated a new openness in family relationships. Mr. C and his wife asked questions about personal reactions to various events in the recovery phase, about posthospital financial difficulties that needed to be arranged, and about returning to the job.

At the end of the meeting, Mr. D gave the patient his telephone number and shook his hand. A warm feeling was generated by their sharing of important fears and desires.

There was a drastic change in Mr. C's attitudes and behavior within several hours after the encounter. He became more cooperative with staff during the painful respiratory therapy treatments and his pulmonary function studies showed dramatic improvement. He began to accept more responsibility for his role in his recovery. His depression lessened, although he still had brief episodes of despondency. After 5 months of hospitalization, Mr. C was discharged. He spontaneously emphasized the importance of peer counseling as a primary aid to recovery and offered to act as a "recovered" patient should the need arise. Mr. D was very pleased to have served as a resource person, and the two men have continued their relationship since Mr. C's discharge.

DISCUSSION

The prospects of disabling or disfiguring illness can fill a patient with dread and despair. We have observed that two particularly troublesome issues for many severely ill patients are fear of the unknown and the absence of any meaningful model for successful adaptation. The timely introduction of a patient who has traveled the rigorous, frightening pathways of disease may do much to facilitate coping, as the two case reports have illustrated.

At this point, several caveats should be mentioned. For a meaningful interaction between a newly disabled patient and a successfully coping "veteran," the staff must consider certain conditions.

1. *Agreement.* The patient must agree, even if halfheartedly, to see someone with his disease.

2. *Timing.* The patient must have moved beyond shock and denial. If he has entered into a state of marked perturbation or repudiation of help, his ability and desire to attend and absorb may be diminished.

3. *The "veteran."* The former patient has to be enthusiastic, articulate, and believable. Similarities in cultural, economic, and educational background as well as age and sex are helpful, although apparently not vital.

Previous clinical experience has indicated that patients whose personalities are dominated by passivity, stoicism, and lack of imagination[8] or who have premorbid extremes of schizoid, paranoid, unstable, or inadequate traits[9] are not good candidates for rehabilitation. The question of whether peer counseling can be effective among such subjects needs further investigation and is beyond the scope of these pilot observations.

The therapeutic task of the newly disabled individual is to contend with and develop some sense of mastery of his disability. Encountering a patient who has coped successfully can help the recently disabled patient to perceive himself as handicapped rather than as an invalid. Peer counseling, in certain instances, has the capacity to cut through overwhelming anxiety and move a patient from hopelessness to motivation and to shift his/her perspective from one of self-pity to self-improvement. As is the case with self-help groups, the emphasis is not on deep psychotherapy, but on faith, will-power, self-control, and day-to-day victories.[3]

Traditionally, medical personnel try to reassure the newly disabled, but their comments are often dismissed as irrelevant. Moreover, staff encouragement of the disabled person to "accept" his illness often falls short of the mark, as is shown in the following statement by a recently blinded woman.[10]

> I do not believe that an individual ever accepts blindness. Acceptance implies compliance and approval. However, adaptation to blindness is ongoing because the individual will continually meet unfamiliar situations. . . .
> I prefer the concept of "identity integration" to that of acceptance. I describe identity integration as a state of self-actualization in which the individual has learned to live with his disability, to acknowledge his limitations, to involve himself in a world outside of himself, and to return to the fulfillment of life goals. An individual who has achieved identity integration does not deny his feelings and expresses such feelings in constructive ways. Individuals who are self-actualizing, flexible, and spontaneous continue to grow. . . .

CONCLUSIONS

Questions and fears confront the recently disabled person as he faces uncharted pathways. Seemingly mundane but significant concerns can be responded to by the successful "veteran," who serves as a credible role model in the task of adjusting to a new identity.

Although variations of formal psychotherapy do have a place in the management of selected patients on medical-surgical wards,[11-15] many times it is best to use a friendly, familiar, here-and-now approach, dealing with reality issues and their interpretation. This paper describes peer counseling as an important technique that, in addition to traditional psychotherapy, hypnosis, drug therapy, and milieu management, can be used in an acute general hospital when staff motivation makes little impact on the patient. It can also be an adjunct to a successful rehabilitation effort.

REFERENCES

Dr. Guggenheim is Director, Private Psychiatric Consultation Service, Massachusetts General Hospital. He is also Assistant Professor of Psychiatry, Harvard Medical School. Ms. O'Hara is a Psychiatric Nurse Clinician at Massachusetts General Hospital.*

1. Dumont M. P.: Self-help treatment programs. *Am. J. Psychiatry* 131:631–635, 1974.
2. Trice H. M.: A study of the process of affiliation with Alcoholics Anonymous. *Q. J. Stud. Alcohol* 18:39–54, 1957.
3. Wechsler H.: The self-help organization in the mental health field: Recovery Inc., a case study. *J. Nerv. Ment. Dis.* 130:297–314, 1960.
4. Wagonfeld S., Wolowitz H.: Obesity and the self-help group: a look at TOPS. *Am. J. Psychiatry* 125:249–252, 1968.
5. Levitz L., Stunkard A.: A therapeutic coalition for obesity: behavior modification and patient self-help. *Am. J. Psychiatry* 131:423–427, 1974.
6. Lennenberg E., Rowbotham J. L.: *The Ileostomy Patient.* Springfield, Ill. Charles C. Thomas, 1974, pp 74–87.
7. Silverman P. R.: The widow as a caregiver in a program of preventive intervention with other widows. *Ment. Hyg.* 54:540–547, 1970.
8. McMahon A.: Psychiatric observations of vocational rehabilitation failures. Presented at the Symposium on The Heart in Industry, Boston, Tufts University and the Massachusetts Heart Association, Nov. 10, 1967.
9. Hyams D. E.: Psychological factors in rehabilitation of the elderly. *Gerontol. Clin.* 11:129–136, 1969.
10. Giarratana-Oehler J.: Personal and professional reactions to blindness from diabetic retinopathy. *New Outlook for the Blind* 70:237–239, 1976.
11. Hackett T. P., Weisman A. D.: Psychiatric management of operative syndromes: part I. *Psychosom. Med.* 22:267–282, 1960.
12. Hackett T. P., Weisman A. D.: Psychiatric management of operative syndromes: part 2. Ibid., pp. 356–372.
13. Stein E. H., Murdaugh J., MacLeod J. A.: Brief psychotherapy of psychiatric reactions to physical illness. *Am. J. Psychiatry* 125:1040–1047, 1969.
14. Sapira J. D.: What to say to symptomatic patients with benign diseases, *Ann. Intern. Med.* 77:603–604, 1972.
15. Norton J.: Treatment of a dying patient. *Psychoanal. Stud. Child* 18:541–560, 1963.

*Affiliation information given throughout this book places the authors of the articles at the time the articles were written.

3

Peer Group Membership of Young Women with Cancer —BELVIN R. BLANDFORD

T HE value of group support and sharing has long been recognized by colostomy clubs, parents of leukemic children, amputees, etc. Less attention has been paid to this phenomena among hospitalized cancer patients and others with potentially fatal diseases. The seriousness of these patients' conditions has often led to staff reluctance to accept or encourage group membership and activity. Here a patient group will be considered which formed naturally and was deliberately encouraged by the staff as an added resource to help patients cope with their illness. The advantages and disadvantages of group membership to individual patients have to be considered to know when it is necessary to reinforce, supplement, or negate group actions.

THE DISEASE

During the three and half year period from 1 November 1961 to 30 April 1965, one hundred women with gestational throphoblastic disease were treated on the Endocrine Service, National Cancer Institute. Eighty-one had a remission, 19 died. This was a heterogeneous group well informed about their disease and facing together the possibility of death or recovery.

Gestational throphoblastic disease is a rare tumour which follows pregnancy. The pregnancy itself may result in normal birth, an abortion, a still birth, or a hydatidiform mole. The disease includes the histological classification of hydatidiform mole, chorio-adenoma destreuns and chorio-carcinoma, each with or without metastases. The primary treatment, intense chemotherapy in intermittent courses, is not without hazards. Drug toxicity may last several weeks. At such times the patients generally develop panmucosal ulcerations, weight loss, falling hair and the tendency to hemorrhage and infection which comes with depression of the bone marrow.[1]

Although physical examination and serial X-rays were also used, the most important indicator of tumor regression was the measurement of the excretion of chorionic gonadotrophin in 24-hr urine specimens. This determination was commonly called the titer report. It was required that at least three of these at consecutive weekly intervals be in the normal range before a patient could be considered in remission. The patients quickly learned of

Reprinted with permission from the *Journal of Chronic Disease* 21: 315–322, 1968. Copyright 1968, Pergamon Press, Ltd.

the importance of these tests, and their results were awaited with anxiety and suspense.

At discharge patients were returned to their referring physicians. A strict home regimen was not prescribed. However, during the first year their chorionic gonadotrophin was frequently measured. Patients were advised to avoid pregnancy and each was readmitted to the hospital twice for examinations and tests. As of now there are no tests which precisely differentiate an early pregnancy from an inadequately treated, rapidly spreading malignancy of this type. After a year of remission no further admissions were thought necessary and patients were told that pregnancy could be safely undertaken. However, urinary gonadotrophin titers were determined regularly at 6–12 month intervals. These specimens were mailed to the hospital.

THE SETTING

These women were treated on a 26-bed research unit in the Clinical Center, National Institutes of Health, Bethesda, Maryland. At any one time, 6–14 of the beds were being used for this study. Like many other patients, the women were encouraged to be dressed and out of their rooms as much as possible. Religious, diversional and recreational services were provided, and passes were granted for sightseeing, shopping, and visiting.

The clinical social worker assigned to the unit knew each patient and usually her family. A part of the initial casework interview was an exploration of some of the aspects of the overwhelming anxiety which all new patients experienced. When the problems were well focused and the patient aware of them and mobilized, casework treatment began immediately. With patients whose anxiety was more diffuse and who were not able to avail themselves of services, the worker continued brief contacts two or three times a week so that when services could be used, her interest was known. Problems dealt with in individual treatment covered a range from concerns about health and adequacy, marital relationships, and death and dying to a host of environmental problems concerned with the patient's and the family's efforts to maintain equilibrium and family intactness during the patient's absence.

PATIENT CHARACTERISTICS

These one-hundred patients ranged in age from 16 to 49 yr with a median age of 25. They were predominantly in the middle income, white, Protestant group. Sixty-five were Protestant, twenty-eight Roman Catholic, four Jewish and three were of other religions. Ninety-two were white and eight were Negro. Ninety-three were married, six were single and one was divorced. Thirty-six of the patients developed this disease during a first pregnancy. At the time of admission they resided in thirty states, the District of Columbia, Puerto Rico and two foreign countries. Sixty-four had high school educations or above. Of these, nineteen had finished college and three had post-graduate degrees.

These women fell within the normal range of psychological functioning. One had had a previous hospitalization for psychiatric disorder and five others had had psychiatric treatment as outpatients. Thirty-five were employed outside their homes. One was receiving financial assistance from a local welfare department and another four were existing submarginally. The remaining ninety-five had adequate to very comfortable family incomes. In the families accustomed to the double salary of husband and wife this hospitalization meant a reduction in income as well as added child care expenses. The length of treatment ranged from 30 to 871 days with a median stay of 71 days.

BEGINNING TREATMENT

Some patients were told their diagnosis by their referring physicians. Others inquired immediately of their new doctors. A few tired not to hear it at all. But no matter when or where they were told they shared a feeling of doom. Many spoke as if "the bottom had dropped out" of their world and "nothing could be done about it." One fled hysterically from her doctor's office, exclaiming disbelief. Others attempting to deny the truth, challenged their doctors, "How can you be so sure!"

Most had never heard of the Clinical Center. No matter what they had been told at home they did not see it as a place of hope but only as a last resort. They tended to interpret their referral as rejection. "I thought my doctor was just trying to get rid of me," one recalled. Another said, "When he wanted to send me away I knew he had given up and didn't want the responsibility for my case any longer."

The move to a distant hospital on short notice posed many practical problems. Fifty-nine of the women had from one to ten children at home. In most instances a relative took responsibility for the children. Some families had to employ help or use day nurseries. Often these arrangements were not stable and had to be changed. All of this stirred up new anxieties in addition to the one the mother already had about her condition.

All had an overriding sense of urgency about admission and the beginning of treatment. Such fears, already severe, were often reinforced by their referring physicians and their families. Comments like the following were common: "When I heard I had cancer or might have a precancerous condition I pictured it racing all over me. Every hour counted." All had a great fear of cancer—some a cancer phobia of long duration. However, this group of women did not hold an image of themselves as being sick. They did not have visible congenital abnormalities or histories of chronic debilitating disease. To think of themselves as young and healthy and yet be told they had cancer was a perplexing and alien situation. Although all were worried, most felt relatively well on admission. Only ten were in critical or grave condition. This made it easy for the majority of them to try to deny disease and reinforce hope for an incorrect diagnosis. Although most were ambulatory at the time of admission, they envisioned a ward of dying patients. They were surprised to find others ambulatory too.

Most were accompanied to the hospital by husbands or parents or both. Even those from far away and those of limited finances wanted their families along for comfort and support or as means of escape if the treatment or surroundings proved intolerable. The few who arrived alone felt especially forlorn and isolated.

THE GROUP IN ACTION

The state of overwhelming intense anxiety was a matter of past, though recent, experience for those of like diagnosis who had been admitted earlier. Here they will be called The Group, as this is how they were known to each other and to the staff. In two's and three's they paid a newcomer a welcome visit within the first 24 hr. Thus began an interaction which would prove to be one of the strongest factors in a patient's adjustment to hospitalization. In retrospect many patients remained hazy about details of their first few days but all graphically remembered this welcome. The sight of women with heads almost bald or lips swollen and ulcerated was a shock. The mental image of being similarly stricken made the newcomer almost deaf to reassurance.

Most believed they were dying or, conversely, fantasied they could be cured in a couple of weeks. An extended illness was one of the most dreaded possibilities, and this fear was intensified when they learned how long some others had been hospitalized. Long-term patients would try to avoid this issue with the newly admitted one but she would quickly perceive the evasion.

It was usually not too long before the patient's negative reaction to prolonged hospitalizations was softened by meeting a member of The Group who was a returnee. Her presence was visible proof that patients did live through the treatment and its toxicity, the loneliness, and even the disease, and yet return looking and feeling well. Such reality yielded more hope than verbal reassurance given by the staff. As one patient said, "As much as I wanted to believe you, it kept gnawing at me that the staff, all of you, were paid to say those things."

As her initial anxiety abated, the new patient began to hear what was really being said to her. She opened to encouragement and was incorporated into the waiting peer group. She could accept the knowledge that this disease, more than many types of cancer, had proven responsive to treatment and that there was a reasonable hope for cure. A mother of three, who had arrived alone, now could look at pictures of her children and share them with others. Those with accompanying families could send them home, to visit again when convenient. Thirteen had someone, such as husband or mother, stay with them throughout hospitalization. Several more relatives found employment for a while in the area. Of those whose family member remained, the majority were either recently married and still trying to break parental ties or were special cases excluded from The Group.

When the new patient identified with The Group, she sought and was given "the word" on staff personalities, on rules to be obeyed and those to be ignored, on matters about which it was safe to complain and on matters sacrosanct. Her distortions, whenever possible, were pointed out and clarified. Racial, religious, regional, or economic differences were relinquished when facing their common enemy, the disease. There was little pairing off to the exclusion of The Group. Intra-group rivalries were minimal and the leadership fluctuated. In spite of its constantly changing membership because of admissions and discharges, The Group remained fluid and was aggressive in seeking new recruits. Thus it perpetuated the support its members mutually derived in their major aim in life, trying to get well.

The caseworker was not part of The Group structure, but because individual treatment was being maintained, the worker was aware of the stresses and the methods of coping of the patients. The physical arrangement of the unit also meant much group action was observable. The worker has access to The Group by invitation or on her own initiative but she did not attempt to exercise direction or control of daily group activities. The Group often served the same purpose a group therapy experience can provide in readying a patient for individual treatment. In these situations the worker encouraged and reinforced the patient's participation. In other situations it was necessary to neutralize negative or detrimental group actions, such as exclusion.

Two types of patients were not found in The Group: the unmarried and those who arrived gravely ill. The majority of The Group, albeit uncomfortable, did make some overtures to the unmarried patients. These overtures, however, were seldom accepted by these women, who were embarrassed, expected rejection, and feared involvement. They had not shared the common experience of marriage, homemaking, and child-rearing. Five of the six were still in their teens. All had pregnancies resulting in hydatidiform moles. A molar pregnancy would raise doubts in any patient about her ability to produce a normal child, but the unmarried patients did not propound the usual question, "Why did this happen to me?" They looked upon it as both a retribution for sin and, in a sense, as a gift in that they did not have to make plans for a full term infant. In order to disengage themselves as much as possible from painful reminders of their diagnosis and its antecedent they tended to associate with patients of their own age group whom they usually found on other hospital units.

The Group did not welcome very ill newcomers. They hesitated to "try to get close to them." This identification was too threatening. However, if one of their own members became gravely ill they took pride in "sticking with her." They visited less frequently but group support was tendered. To watch one with their own diagnosis deteriorate and yet continue to support her exerted a heavy emotional toll and added to their reluctance to take on a new patient whom they thought to be a "loser."

After the busy initial medical workup there was waiting, much waiting—for toxicity to subside, for titer reports, for treatment to begin again. There were questions, many questions—"Will it work?" "Will I need three courses or will I need ten?" In such a situation of chronic anxious expectancies, moods were rampant and contagious. Patients infected each other with encouragement and depression. When a member became too melancholy, The Group mobilized itself to help the depressed individual. However, if its ministrations by concern and support were not successful The Group felt the full backlash of the member's distress and turned outwards for assistance. The depressed one might be brought to the attention of the social worker. Such reporting was sometimes done with hostility as if to say, "You've let us down. Why haven't you noticed this before?" At such times The Group's need for a strong, dependable buffer was as evident as the depressed patient's need for more intensive treatment. Similarly, when a patient was very emotionally upset and The Group felt overwhelmed, members alerted the staff and pressed the patient into discussing her concerns individually.

One of the most important by-products of the group interaction was the development in each member of the capacity to share her hopes and despairs with others. Some found it easier to do this first in The Group. Others were freed by group discussion to pursue these concerns with the worker on an individual basis. The ideas of refusing treatment or of signing out against advice were discussed and occasionally serious threats were made to do these things. The fear of dying was also discussed. However, here The Group excluded the very sick member as they could not tolerate hearing her fears. Thus, to hear the voice of the dying was left for the staff and the family.

While there was a great deal of medical knowledge of the disease and of technical considerations in its treatment, the patients often coupled this with good luck pins, folklore and magical thinking. Some such as "Today is the day we wear our butterfly pins for luck," were left undisturbed as harmless creations. Others, such as, "You have to lose your hair and get an ulcerated mouth to get well," might require correction, especially if intended to awe a newcomer. One could, however, hardly contradict such a statement if it were made by a very toxic patient as a matter of self-consolation. Still others, such as a patient with a high titer saying, "I'll get by with only one more course of treatment," were so falsely hopeful and doomed for disappointment as to require direct reconsideration.

The Group, on occasion, offered its members protection and permission for regressive and infantile behavior of a type usually not acted out on an individual basis. For instance, in an episode where, to accommodate a very ill person, many room changes were necessary, a patient objected that her new bed faced East rather than West. The Group took up her cause and added their own complaints about the position of their beds and baths, about their lunch trays and the fact they had not been consulted before the changes were made. They quarrelled with all in authority and deplored a bureaucratic system which could deprive them of their "homes." The rational explanation of the life-threatening situation of the acutely ill patient was minimized or ignored. Individual case intervention was of little benefit because of the mass nature of the opposition. Direct confrontation with the leadership core of The Group was necessary to clarify the hospital's responsibility for the acutely ill person and the other patients' roles, rights, and responsibilities.

The anxiety level soared when a patient died, especially "one of our own." The Group expected the patients' husband or parents or both to be present during the terminal phase of the illness, and in most instances this occurred. In the few cases when it did not, The Group was upset and critical of the family. Their own fears of desertion had been reactivated. With the family present The Group felt that some of its responsibility for emotional support of the moribund patient was lessened. Nevertheless, all remained in close touch with the situation and were keenly reactive to each change in the dying patient.

This impending crisis was supplemented by special casework help for patients who lacked group support and/or acceptance. Others were also especially needful because of their closeness to the terminal patient. The atmosphere at such times was ripe for rumors and distortions. When all patients could not be seen the most influential group members were sought by the caseworker and given some interpretation and preparation for the expected occurrence.

After a death, patients experienced much of the sadness, guilt and ambivalence that is usual in the loss of a family member. "The good die young . . . Her children needed her . . . I wish I had visited her more often . . . It's not going to be the same without her." They would recall how she hadn't followed recommendations early in her disease or would label her doctor "no good." The inevitability of the death had to be denied by blaming someone, and the implication was voiced that by being good patients and having good doctors no such harm could befall them. The Group searched out detailed differences between themselves and the deceased. "She was six months post-partum and I was only two when treatment began . . . My titer was never as high." In this they were supported by the staff.

When one of The Group was discharged an intense ambivalent reaction ensued. Jealousy would be evident. It was a time not only for self-sorrow but also for well-wishes and self-examination. Discharges were especially hard on those in treatment for a long time. The magic of "number one in, number one out; number two in, number two out" had been broken again. Yet for all its negative aspects discharged was a good sign and gave all the opportunity for positive reinforcement. Group encouragement resulted.

In this sex-based disease a few patients arrived feeling frankly antisexual, but more appeared asexual. The unmarried patients expressed easily (usually during periods of drug toxicity) the feeling "This is the punishment for my sin." The reactions of the married women were mixed. Universally their husbands felt guilty. Some patients took advantage of this by railing directly and punitively at them "This is your fault!" Others accomplished similar ends by intimidation or by overdenying their resentments.

As patients felt better, their sexual feelings returned and often became the subject of jokes. Some worried about their husbands' infidelities during their separation. Others tried not to think about this. All were anxious to avoid pregnancy during the first year. Once the contraceptive method was accepted as prescribed, members could turn to deeper concerns about the influence of the near-catastrophy on their own and their husbands' attitudes toward making love. Members could share such feelings as, "He's more scared than I am," "I've told him I'm not sick anymore," "I'm going to have to take a course in seduction 'cause things aren't like they used to be!."

When the patient returned for the first check-up at the end of three months, it was a happy time. She had gained weight, her hair was growing and she looked healthy. Such an occasion was a rewarding experience for The Group as well as the staff and was reflected in a warm welcome by all. The patient in turn had "loved" being at home, doing the housework and taking care of her children. She reported renewed feelings of appreciation for everything and everyone at home as well as appreciation of life itself. "It's great to be alive!" With other patients she took a motherly role and was reassuring and encouraging.

With the last check-up at the end of twelve months there was separation anxiety. Normality had returned and much of the novelty of being a "cured cancer patient" had worn off. The hospital, which had been the authority, had also been security. One said, "After the many times I wanted only to get away from here and forget the whole thing, now I feel you're kicking me out. You don't love me anymore." Another said, "Now you're only going to be interested in the bottle of urine I send you." Sometimes mentioned but probably always present was the wish to continue the relationship as a magical guarantee against future malignancies.

Sixty-two of the surviving patients were left with child-bearing function intact. Medical permission to undertake future pregnancies brought them face to face with freedom. The great and protective "Thou shalt not" was gone. For those who lived through the treatment for gestational trophoblastic disease it was fearful to think of future pregnancies. All wondered "Will it happen to me again?" They also wondered if all the drugs they had taken would affect a new baby. Interpretation and reassurance were needed and given. The semi-annual urine check, done as part of the research design, also served to assure them that remission was continuing. Even those whose conflict about future pregnancies appeared most fully resolved were known to remark, "I'm going to try to get pregnant again quickly before I lose my nerve." A subsequent birth by a discharged member of The Group was a heralded event.

SUMMARY

Described here is the influence of peer group membership on the adaptive behavior of 100 women hospitalized with gestational trophoblastic disease. Little attempt was made to screen these patients from reality. They went where they wanted and saw what they wanted with few barriers. They were deliberately educated about their disease to insure their participation in its treatment. Although such an approach led in the long run to confidence in staff and cooperation in treatment, it was nevertheless at first shocking and overwhelming. Individual casework treatment was necessary especially when The Group was threatened by an individual's anxiety or an individual was threatened by The Group's anxiety. While The Group served as a supportive device and functioned well in reducing day by day stresses, it was not a problem-solving device and had to relinquish responsibility when treatment was needed. The support of The Group was consciously encouraged and utilized when it served as an added strength for the patient. The Group's limitations were recognized and its actions supplemented when necessary.

REFERENCES

Belvin Blandford is a clinical social worker, Cancer Social Work Section, Social Work Department, The Clinical Center, National Institutes of Health, Bethesda, Maryland.

1. Ross, G. T., Goldstein, D. P., Hertz, R., Lipsett, M. B. and Odell, W. D.: Sequential use of methotrexate and actinomycin D in the treatment of metastatic choriocarcinoma and related trophoblastic diseases in women. *Am. J. Obstet. Gynec.* 94, 223–229, 1965.

4

Group Discussions: A Therapeutic Tool in a Chronic Diseases Hospital
—ARNOLD J. ROSIN, M.B.

I N hospital treatment, the doctor often is cast as the active mover and the patient as the passive recipient on whom the benefits of medical knowledge should be bestowed. This passivity is sometimes reflected in the situation in which a patient does not know, has not been told, and has not thought of asking what illness he has had or what operation he has undergone. In a hospital for chronic diseases, however, persistent passivity often leads to significant deterioration. In addition to the psychologic reaction to chronic illness, the problems of living in an institution make further inroads into the patient's individuality and personality.

Institutional neurosis is a well-recognized entity, and Townsend[1] has

Reprinted from *Geriatrics* 1975 (August): 45–48. © 1975 by Harcourt, Brace Jovanovich, Inc.

painted dramatic pictures of the passivity that encumbers inhabitants of even well-appointed residential homes. In a long-term treatment program, the medical staff must live with the patients' problems. The roles of giver and taker are modified because patients can participate in the therapeutic program and thereby strengthen their motivation.

Harzfeld Hospital in Gedera, Israel, has 240 beds, about 60 designated for rehabilitation and the others for long-term medical and nursing care. The hospital does not admit psychotic patients. A large number of the patients have sustained strokes in the recent or distant past, and between 8 and 10 percent have advanced malignant disease. Approximately 70 percent of the patients are over age 70. Some of the younger ones have degenerative neuro-muscular disorders. The patients receive a thorough medical investigation and treatment, and active physiotherapy and occupational therapy programs are carried out.

Staff members at the hospital became interested in organizing regular discussions with a group of selected patients and in determining and evaluating the effect of these sessions on the patients' well-being. The observations presented here were made over a three year period during which the group met weekly.

SELECTING THE PATIENTS

The discussion group was organized with the help of a social worker and a ward nurse, who was responsible for coordinating the activity in the wards. The common denominator among the patients selected for the group was chronic disease that necessitated admission to the hospital. The group included (1) patients who had mood withdrawal but were not pathologically depressed, (2) patients who had become isolated from normal social contacts through confinement to their house or because of an advancing illness such as cancer, (3) some who were judged likely to remain in the hospital for the rest of their life and who needed an outlet for expression, and (4) some who were selected for assessment of their reaction to the stimulus of group conversation.

The principal diagnoses in the patients were cerebral ischemia and stroke, multiple sclerosis, motor neuron disease, paraplegia from trauma, and advanced cancer; some amputees were included. Although deafness and speech disorders were at first considered contra-indications to inclusion in the group, a few patients with such disorders were admitted to the discussions on a trial basis and gained obvious benefit. Patients with frank dementia were not included.

During the three year period, a total of 60 patients participated in the group discussions. They ranged in age from 38 to 85 years, with a mean age of 65.2 years. Twenty-seven of the patients were discharged after at least one period of treatment, and eight of these were readmitted.

The discussion group usually consisted of about 10 patients, although sometimes, illness reduced the number to five or new additions increased it to 15. I conducted the discussions and limited the sessions to 45 minutes.

GAINING INSIGHT INTO PATIENTS' PROBLEMS

The discussions generally assumed a pattern, characterized by emergence of one or more leaders and participants who agreed with or opposed them. Others in the group listened but rarely participated, and some appeared to take little notice or even went to sleep. However, appearances sometimes proved to be deceptive. Apparent inattention because of limited mental capacity or indifference sometimes was contradicted by a follow-up report from the patient's relative.

Topics Discussed. Newcomers to the group were told that the purpose of the meetings was to give them an opportunity to talk about themselves, their interests, their illness, problems that worried them, and the hospital. Many of the patients touched on their personal symptomatology, in spite of the avowal at more than one group meeting that raising such matters was improper.

Hope. During the very first meeting of patients drawn from a number of different wards, a discussion about hope developed. Hope was described as a quality that springs from the patient, and the group observed that doctors should never suppress it by words, deeds, or lack of attention. The patients ventilated their feelings about some of the strictures of medical authority that they considered harmful to them.

Other discussion sessions brought out the patients' attitudes toward their illnesses, which varied from despair at the necessity of entering the hospital to frustration at the nonrealization of the higher hopes that they had nurtured at the time of their admission. Confrontation of opposing views sometimes was salutary to the patients expressing them, even without my intervening in the discussion.

Complaints. Many discussions centered around daily matters that caused patients personal discomforts. Nurses, being nearest to the patients' daily routine, received a grat deal of criticism, but closer evaluation of the patients' remarks often revealed that they reflected the patients' own physical and psychologic difficulties. For example, a retired 69 year old teacher who had extensive paralysis caused by motor neuron disease found it demoralizing to have to be fed and attended by young people who were not of his own family. This was the first time he had been in the hospital, and he reacted bitterly. His bitterness also reflected the fact that he had only a short time to live.

Other participants dwelt on the importance of education and culture among nursing attendants, pointing out that physical help is not the only contribution to be made even by unqualified staff members. Such complaints frequently were rebutted by other patients, who mentioned the difficulties involved when there are too few staff members for the number of calls. Indeed, some cited the egoism of sick people as a factor leading to certain dissatisfaction by patients toward the staff.

Dependence.   In discussions about old age, dependence was stressed as the aspect that hurt most. Patients referred to the difficulty of mobility and the loss of sensory function, especially poor eyesight. With their adaptation to long-term illness, the patients voiced little regret about the loss of past abilities and achievements, but rather the hope that they would be able to manage the basic activities of daily living with less help from others.

A 76 year old paraplegic who had been in a negativistic, morose mood for a period of months touched on the quality of patience. He told how he had learned patience when, as a farmer many years previously, he had ploughed with a team of oxen. His doggedness stood him in good stead when he came to making emotional and physical efforts to get back on his feet.

The patients occasionally spoke of death in relation to their illnesses, sometimes in the context of faith in another life and sometimes as a form of release from suffering.

Relationships Between Patients.   The patients in the discussion group expressed varying attitudes toward other patients. Some felt revulsion at the sight of others who were sicker than themselves, while some expressed relief at not having to face the problems of everyday life outside the hospital. Others voiced the opinion that meeting other sick people served as a salutary shock to their preoccupation with self. The oft-proclaimed egoism of the sick person was clearly evident in some group members, while others in the group exhibited a feeling of mutual responsibility and tolerance toward other demanding or disturbing patients.

Discussion group members agreed that organized entertainment could create an atmosphere of conviviality among patients and allow them to forget their individual troubles. Pain, however, was the exceptional symptom that did not respond to such "social" treatments.

The Hospital's Role.   Time after time, the group members indicated they regarded physiotherapy as the hospital's main contribution to their well-being. Even among patients whose indoor mobility was not greatly restricted, physiotherapy occupied a central place. One patient even compared his faith in it with his faith in God. Possibly because it provides obvious physical activity, physiotherapy displaced occupational therapy or even medical treatment as a topic of discussion. Members of the group, even those who had no prospect of leaving the hospital, criticized the hospital's inability to supply physiotherapy frequently enough during holidays or times of staff shortage.

More than once, group members compared the hospital with a prison. This allowed me to explore with them the limitations that illness imposes on freedom and to enlarge on methods by which they could regain a more independent outlook through the therapeutic and social medium of the hospital.

An 86 year old woman who eventually became a long-term patient because of general infirmity, failing vision, heart failure, and depressive tendencies that had resulted in two previous attempts at suicide considered the hospital as a new way of life. She compared her hospital day with a day in a factory, indicating a tight program with "work" in the occupational therapy department, group activities, and some physiotherapy amply filling the time between meals and rest periods.

Attitudes Toward "The Doctor."   The patients sometimes brought the role of the doctor into the discussion. In parallel sessions conducted by the social worker, patients said that the group was "different" when the doctor attended. The patients would ask questions on such matters that they considered to be within a doctor's control, such as the attitude of other staff members, medical treatment, arrangement of hospital social activities, seating of patients in the dining room, visiting hours, and other matters pertaining to daily hospital life.

Even if I did not seek to influence discussion about my role, my presence apparently served as a means of legitimizing a group discussion on intimate clinical topics, although patients obviously sometimes said what they thought I wanted to hear rather than what they really felt. In this respect, the group as a whole could react by more vigorously proclaiming the patient's point of view. For example, they often presented conflicting opinions on how to bear long-term illness—whether to accept it or to fight it—especially if positive results of hospital treatment were not apparent.

DISCUSSION

Therapeutic group discussions are well known as part of the treatment of psychiatric illness. In our hospital, the factors common to the participants were physical illness; admission to the hospital for weeks, months, or years; and the possibility or reality of social isolation and withdrawal. Physical illness occasionally precluded patients' participation in the group; however, the activity was viewed as one of the few benefits the hospital could provide patients who had an intractable illness.

Certain indirect findings from our study supported our belief that patients benefited from participation in the group. Patients who seldom or never spoke at the meetings reported the discussions to their relatives, who relayed their impressions to me at subsequent interviews. Some patients who at first were reluctant to attend the sessions later appeared as a matter of course. Some participants even prepared in advance what they wanted to say at the meeting. Furthermore, when it was necessary to suspend the sessions because of staff shortages or holidays, patients requested that they be resumed.

During the three years of this study, we often asked ourselves whether the discussion sessions served a therapeutic purpose, were a means of assessing patients, or served as a platform for social conversation. The topics discussed indicated that the project was somewhat successful in all these areas.

The group discussions could not be called formal psychotherapy, because the patients were not, on the whole, psychiatrically ill and had not been referred for psychiatric treatment. However, the group dynamics engendered tensions, conflicts, and catharses and also brought out various psychologic features in the patients—phobias, uncertainties, disappointments, or euphoria. The sessions allowed some patients to grapple with their emotional difficulties in the group setting and facilitated individual response to a difficult emotional situation.[2] Even though the opportunity that the group sessions afforded for a social get-together was deliberately played down, the meetings undoubtedly served as an important social outlet for some of the participants.

Burnside[3] observed that withdrawal was a prominent feature in a discussion group in an old people's home, especially at the beginning of the group activity. However, we felt that such a forum might be the only opportunity for patients to express their opinions about their doctor, the nurses, the hospital, and how life appears inside hospital walls. Goodacre,[4] who worked with a similar group, has confirmed our observations. Grauer[5] noted that in group discussions in an old-age home, a frequent theme was anger and complaints as an expression of fear of helplessness. Our group was conceived and acted as a positive means of dealing with such problems and helping the patient to overcome the suppression of his identity in a large hospital in which he might see himself as merely a number among 240 patients.

The group discussion provided an opportunity for me to learn a great deal about the background of the patients' illnesses, their families, and their environmental problems preceding their admission to the hospital. Much emerged about their ideas on their diseases, the treatment they were receiving, and their expectations. This knowledge not infrequently influenced rehabilitation assessment and prognosis. Although the patients often claimed that they came to learn about their illnesses from me, I must agree with Isaacs[6] that the reverse was often more true.

The doctor-patient relationship that emerged was somewhat different from the conventional one because of the community of interest expressed by the participation in the group. This allowed me to hear the patients at close hand and to listen to their viewpoint.[7] What the patients said about themselves was partly a reflection of reality and partly an expression of loss,[8] as well as a symptomatic reaction to the illness itself. The group setting allowed me to combine the leadership the patients expected with the opportunity to listen to them on an equal footing.

CONCLUSIONS

The content of the discussions, the extent of participation, and the patients' reactions showed that this group activity was an outlet for self-expression and a point of close contact with the doctor. Although the troublesome aspects of life in the wards were recurring themes in the discussions, the patients often came to deal with their attitudes toward their illness and their surroundings. As a result of learning about the individual patients, their social interaction, lucidity, and moods, it was possible to help them solve some of their material and emotional problems.

Patients who were in the group only temporarily found that it was a social stimulus, and the permanent members retained their group relationships as leaders, counterleaders, or more passive members.

The group discussions played an important part in the rehabilitation and reintegration program in geriatric and chronic diseases and added a further dimension to the treatment program.

REFERENCES

Dr. Rosin is medical director of the Harzfeld Hospital for Chronic Diseases, Gedera, Israel.

The author wishes to thank Dr. Arye Latz, psychologist, for helpful discussions; Sara Jacobowicz, social worker, for help and participation; and the nurses of Harzfeld Hospital for their cooperation.

1. Townsend P.: *The Last Refuge.* London, Russell & Kegan Paul, 1964.
2. Parloff M. B.: Group dynamics and group psychotherapy—the state of the union. *Int. J. Group Psychother.* 13: 393, 1963.
3. Burnside I. M.: Long-term group work with hospitalized aged. *Gerontologist* 11:213, 1971.
4. Goodacre D.: Experiences of group work in a rehabilitation unit. *Gerontol. Clin.* 15:352, 1973.
5. Grauer H.: Institutions for the aged—therapeutic communities. *J. Am. Geriatr. Soc.* 19:687, 1971.
6. Isaacs B.: Group therapy in the geriatric unit. *Gerontol. Clin.* 9:21, 1967.
7. The patient's view. *Br. Med. J.* 3:5, 1973.
8. Burnside I. M.: Loss: A constant theme in group work with the aged. *Hosp. Community Psychiatry* 21:173, 1970.

5

Theme-Focused Group Therapy on a Pediatric Ward —DORCAS H. COFER, Ph.D, and YEHUDA NIR, M.D.

IT is generally assumed that illness and hospital experience are often traumatic for children, sometimes with long-range sequelae.[1-8] It is also generally accepted that preventative measures are useful in helping children cope with hospitalization and illness. Neither of these assumptions has been rigorously investigated.[9]

When psychiatric and pediatric literature first began to reflect interest

Reprinted by permission from the *International Journal of Psychiatry in Medicine* 6 (4): 541–550, 1976. © 1976, Baywood Publishing Co., Inc.

in the effects of hospitalization on children, and children's perception of hospitalization, the focus was clearly on the separation experience. Spitz' description of the hospitalism response became the prototype of the deleterious effect of maternal separation.[10] Only gradually, following Bowlby's report,[11] was the contribution of other variables to adverse hospitalization reactions explored and better delineated by Robertson[12] and others.

Solnit, relating to aspects of hospitalization other than separation,[13] points out that the newest knowledge and technologies have tended to dehumanize the care of the child faster than we have been able to understand and cope with the psychological and social problems experienced by the child.[14] As a result of medical progress, children are exposed to more interventions than ever before, and they are more often subjected to uncomfortable diagnostic procedures which lack a sense of emergency and therefore are difficult for the child to rationalize.

Additional problems facing the hospitalized child are the unfamiliarity of the hospital setting, sensory-motor restrictions, and the effects of the illness itself, such as pain and immobilization. These traumatic experiences may result in moderate to severe depression and evoke various degrees of anxiety which is often clinically manifested in regression, withdrawal, lack of cooperation, and aggressive and disruptive behavior. Additional symptoms may be increased somatization and sleep disturbances.

Among the above symptoms, regression seems to be particularly disturbing. The child who has recently acquired sphincter control or perhaps the ability to bathe and care for himself may be frightened and confused by his temporary regression.[13] The loss of either well-established or newly-achieved ego functions often triggers retreat to even less adaptive levels of functioning.[15]

Clinical attempts to deal with reactions to hospitalization have employed general supportive methods such as rooming-in of mothers, volunteer-staffed ward playrooms, and psychiatric treatment such as play therapy in order to encourage an expression of fantasies, fears and anxieties aroused by hospitalization.[16-18] By encouraging the child to perform operations on a doll, the attempt is made to reverse the child's passivity into a more active mastery of the situation, basically an identification with the aggressor. Becker[19] advances the usefulness of Gardner's Mutual Story-Telling Technique as a principal method of therapeutic communication with the hospitalized child.[20] Schowalter reports the utilization of patients' meetings on an adolescent ward to provide a forum where patients can participate in making ward decisions, socialize with each other, and discharge affect in times of stress.[21, 22]

With adult patients who, like children, often tend to experience a regression in ego functioning as a result of hospitalization,[23, 24] approaches to anxiety reduction in hospital settings have included theme-centered group therapy sessions[25] and preparatory communications.[26] Janis, exploring the factors which appear to be related to tolerance for postoperative pain and distress, found that a group of adult surgical patients, given accurate prior warning of the pain and discomfort they might expect as a result of surgery, showed better adjustment to the stresses of the postoperative period than a matched group of patients given no special preparatory communications.

Even in the more extreme situations of terminal illness in either adults or children, the beneficial effect of more open communication has been described. Kubler-Ross found that dying patients are often reassured and less anxious when staff and family are able to adopt more open attitudes toward their illness and approaching death, thus permitting the patient to verbalize his own thoughts about dying.[27] Vernick and Karon report that when adults provide an atmosphere in which seriously ill children can feel completely free to express their concerns, the children are able to function better and the withdrawal and depression so often observed in gravely ill children occur only infrequently and transiently.[28]

THE PROGRAM

Against this background the department of Psychiatry conjointly with the department of Pediatrics at Beth Israel Medical Center in New York introduced a program of group intervention aimed at ameliorating negative effects of hospitalization in children.

Children from Puerto Rican and Black families receiving welfare assistance comprise the majority of Beth Israel pediatric patients. Inpatient facilities include approximately thirty-four beds for general medical patients and twelve beds for surgical patients. Ages range from early childhood through adolescence. The pediatric staff includes a child psychiatrist and a child psychologist who participate in pediatric rounds, conduct weekly psychiatric seminars for pediatric residents and weekly conferences for staff nurses in addition to individual consultations. As a result, the mental health consultants have been considered an integral part of the pediatric staff rather than specialists called only to evaluate selected cases. This productive liaison between pediatrics and child psychiatry is dependent on the continued support and encouragement of the chief of pediatrics.

Theme-centered group sessions are held three times a week on the pediatric ward with two therapists present. The number of participants varies from three to ten; a session lasts thirty minutes. Due to the fact that children of various ages are concerned with different developmental tasks, it is necessary that there not be too wide a range of ages in the group.[29] Occasionally, we have to exclude a child who is significantly older or younger than the mean age of the group. In practice, most ambulatory children are included with the exception of those who are markedly intellectually retarded or emotionally disturbed to the extent that their behavior or verbalizations would be disruptive. The average child attends three or four groups during his hospital stay. Sessions are optimally held in one of the patient's rooms. If a child is in traction or on complete bed rest, the group will gather around his bed.

Participation is voluntary but children are strongly urged to take part.

In view of the continuously changing population, the purpose of the group is explained at the beginning of each session. Following this, discussion ensues. Issues most commonly introduced by children are concerns about medical procedures. The therapists invite answers and explanations from group members before they attempt to correct distortions and misconceptions. A distortion common to many chldren is that the frequent blood-taking procedures will seriously deplete their blood supply. An unusual distortion was one girl's concern that the metal plate in her head following a skull operation would attract lightning if she stood near a window during a storm.

It is our impression that lack of factual information intensifies the children's fears and allows for pathological distortions. These diminish significantly in their intensity when facts are known. Persisting distortions may reflect various aspects of a psychological conflict or a defense constellation of a particular child. They are dealt with by referral for individual brief therapy when they interfere seriously with the functioning or the medical management of the patient.

The issue of illness itself is more difficult for children to discuss. In the group meetings, it is not unusual for a young child to deny knowing why he is in the hospital. Often, denial is specifically related to the child's developmental stage. In the five-year-old the threat of illness might be perceived as an interference with phallic pursuits and denial will be expressed in intensified motor activity making bed rest and medical procedures intolerable. Castration anxiety might be the motivating factor behind the denial of illness in the pre-oedipal and oedipal child while the threat of passivity and dependency might fuel the development of this defense mechanism in the adolescent. As in Schowalter's experience, we find that the group is particularly effective in dealing with this problem since, on the one hand, it explores the denial while on the other, due to the fact that all the children are ill, it does not force the issue "allowing everyone to reach their own acceptable level of denial."[22]

The following case history exemplifies the group's ability to deal with denial and distortion. Albert, an eleven-year-old with diabetes mellitus, was intelligent, friendly, cooperative and well-related. He appeared somewhat depressed and passive with a tendency to deny feelings. The hospitalization, which was his first, was for the purpose of confirming the diagnosis and regulating his diet and insulin dosage. This proved to be extremely difficult because Albert, unknown to the doctors, was cheating on his diet. He also refused to self-administer insulin. In group Albert showed much denial regarding his disease and did not mention his cheating until the group confronted him with it based on their own observations.

Once denial was broached, the issue of self-administration of insulin came to the fore when one of the children called Albert a "junkie." This turned out to be Albert's own perception of himself. The ensuing discussion of licit and illicit injections clarified the issue for him and enabled him to give himself daily insulin.

Separation anxiety, although perhaps the most pervasive concern of all children, is often inferred in the derivative forms of oral concerns, regressive behavior and heightened dependency needs. As Schowalter also found on an adolescent ward, we see complaints about food, quality of nursing, and boredom as directly related to separation anxiety and we confine our efforts to solving specific problems rather than interpreting latent meaning.[22]

In our experience young children, like Schowalter's adolescents,[22] displace their more basic fears and anxieties about separation to other less threatening topics. For example, Bridget, age twelve, hospitalized with recurrent stomach pain, angrily bit off the plastic hospital identification bracelet, insisted on wearing street clothes and talked threateningly of "walking out of this place." However, in group she only complained that she missed her friends and thought the hospital should provide more recreational facilities. The group accepted her complaints and sympathized with her feelings of isolation and boredom. Bridget never did address herself to her fears or the undiagnosed pain. However, after the group session she befriended another patient and began to attend hospital school regularly. In subsequent groups she did not repeat her complaints. The group did not tamper with her defenses but rather provided support to help her contain her anxiety. We are continuously aware of the fact that the groups are short-term and that a child may be discharged following any particular group meeting. Therefore, we are careful to promote closure at the end of each meeting.

The central themes of our groups—separation anxiety, fear of procedures, and concern about the illness—suggest a parallel with the observations of Natterson and Knudson who reported that a group of fatally ill children in hospital manifested behavioral changes in response to three environmental factors; separation from mother, traumatic procedures, and deaths of other children.[30] Natterson and Knudson found that the fully developed forms of these fears were age-dependent with separation fear most clearly present in the younger children, mutilation fear most present in school-age children, and death fear occurring later. Our groups are most frequently made up of latency age children which may account for the fact that the most common group theme concerns fear of procedures. Death fear does not often appear overtly in the children with whom we work. In those cases where we have seen it manifested, the children were severely ill—as were the children observed by Natterson and Knudson.

Sexual concerns are frequently raised. This probably reflects the fact that the groups are coeducational. We have found that discussion of sexual topics in a coed latency age or preadolescent group generates a great deal of anxiety. Since it is our practice to avoid areas that tend to increase the children's anxiety, we try to refocus the discussion on a topic related to the theme of the group unless the sexual concerns arise from specific medical conditions, such as hypospadias or cryptorchidism.

For example, at a recent session four boys had the following exchange.

Juan (9 years old): "I had my appendix out last week" (revealing his scar). Herman (11 years old): "So did I—see?" (pointing to a scar considerably below the appendix level).

Then there were cries of protest from Alberto (12 years old) who was still bedridden after a second operation for hypospadias. Alberto: "No he didn't. He's got two scars because something's wrong with his penis." Herman (sheepishly, but also with pride): "Yeah, that's right. They brought my testicles down."

There followed a general discussion about undescended testicles including the disclosure that Herman had volunteered for the operation himself, that his parents were afraid to send him to the hospital before for fear that he didn't have any testicles to descend and that he was thrilled with the outcome because now he felt "like the other boys and could have a girlfriend."

DISCUSSION

This group has characteristics of both counseling and guidance groups. The guidance aspect is reflected in our attempt to expose attitudes and feelings related to the hospital experience, bringing to awareness those repressed feelings which are responsible for impaired functioning.[31] When the group focuses on realistic difficulties, counseling techniques are utilized.

Group meetings are also theme-focused. The theme aspect is not unlike Cohn's formulation of a group which shares a common interest and in which the reactions to this theme are dealt with therapeutically.[32] Our theme is the hospital experience, and it has two components:

1. lack of, or distortion of, factual information and
2. fantasies, fears, and anxieties related to hospitalization.

Doubts have been expressed whether group therapy can be effective with children who are of latency age. Latency has been traditionally considered not amenable to verbal therapies. Bornstein concluded, based on the psychoanalysis of children, that the latency age child tended to resist treatment measures based on verbal communication because attempts at promoting introspection constitute a massive threat to the latency age child's strong need to maintain newly-gained ego organization.[33]

In recent years there are a growing number of reports of successful intervention with latency children on the group level.[34-38] It is our impression that the reason for the success of those groups is that they rely primarily on ego supportive, rather than introspective, techniques.

In our group the therapists encourage group interaction by stating precisely the purpose of the group meeting. This reduces initial anxiety by defining the role of group members and the level of interaction. Once the "rules of the game" are established, the therapists' roles become supportive by accepting the children's complaints and criticisms of their parents and the hospital personnel. In addition, the therapists attempt to reduce anxiety by eliciting peer support and encouraging reality testing.

An additional task for the therapist is modeling. Sometimes children are reluctant to admit to fears or concerns about their experiences. When appropriate a therapist will verbalize the child's feelings for him, pointing out how many children have also felt the same way and how even the therapist would have those feelings if he were in a similar situation. This kind of intervention provides reality testing and models a recognition of tolerance for negative feelings.

Occasionally the therapist will resort to providing specific information as to the nature of illnesses and procedures. This takes place only when the group itself cannot respond to the child's need.

On the level of group dynamics we feel that the group offers the children opportunity for cathartic expression of fears, complaints, worries, and grudges in an atmosphere of mutual emotional support. Children are usually quick to test reality through interchange of both factual information and distortions on a peer level. Some information provided by a peer is more cogent for the child than the same information coming from an authority figure. For example, a group member who has already gone for an operation and "survived" anesthesia becomes the most valid source of reassurance to those children who are still waiting for operations to take place. Naturally, in view of the short term nature of our group not all of the above dynamics are operant in all of the groups.

Two additional factors have allowed us to operate in group. One, the children are in a state of crisis, with resultant heightened sensitivity to therapeutic intervention. During the period of disorganization normally associated with crisis, old conflicts symbolically linked with present problems are revived and hence become accessible to intervention.[39] A person in crisis becomes more susceptible to the influence of "significant others" in the environment and the degree of activity of the helping person does not have to be high.[40]

Another factor which facilities our therapeutic intervention is the fact that the children live together on the ward. This allows for the development of bonds and mutual understanding that carry over into group sessions and can be counted on to foster quicker interaction than would be possible among strangers.

While the main purpose of the group is attenuation of negative effects of illness and hospitalization, its impact on the pediatric ward is more extensive. We see three advantages to using group. They are:

1. The group as a diagnostic tool. According to Stocking's finding, there is a high incidents of psycho-pathology among children admitted to a pediatric ward.[41] Group provides an opportunity to assess degree of pathology by observing the child's reaction to illness and hospitalization, the quality of the separation experience from the mother, peer interaction, and behavior within the therapeutic situation. If indicated, on the basis of our group observations, we refer children to outpatient child psychiatry for a more complete diagnostic workup. Otherwise, we provide the outpatient department pediatrician with a summary of our observations alerting him to watch certain areas of a child's development.

Our understanding of Albert and his psychological makeup proved useful when, several months following discharge, Albert, a non-athletic boy, attempted for the first time in his life to jump a bus. He fell off and was admitted to the hospital with multiple scalp lacerations and cerebral concussion. We were able then in a few short-term therapy sessions to help him understand the counterphobic nature of this behavior.

2. The existence of a therapeutic group on a pediatric ward raises consciousness to mental health problems among medical and nursing personnel by providing information in the areas of child development and psychological functioning that is usually not readily available to the staff. The group allows mental health consultants to become integrated into the service and offers an educational opportunity to pediatric residents in areas not often covered in training curriculae.

3. The group improves the daily functioning of the ward by reducing children's anxiety and eliminating a great deal of hyperactivity, aggressive behavior and reluctance to cooperate in treatment procedures. By offering the medical and nursing staffs more intimate knowledge of the children, the group helps them to manage the ward more effectively. Ideally a well run group can make the pediatric ward a total therapeutic milieu. In summary we feel that the group, due to its therapeutic, diagnostic, and educational aspects, can be seen as a psychiatric intervention which uses to maximum advantage the context of the pediatric ward setting.

REFERENCES

Dr. Cofer is a psychologist with the Child and Adolescent Psychiatric Services, Department of Psychiatry, Beth Israel Medical Center. Dr. Nir is Assistant Chief of Child and Adolescent Psychiatric Services, Beth Israel Medical Center. He is also Assistant Clinical Professor of Psychiatry, Mt. Sinai School of Medicine.

1. L. Jessner, G. E. Blom and S. Waldfogel, Emotional implications of tonsillectomy and adenoidectomy in children, *Psychoanal. Stud. Child,* International Universities Press, New York, 7, pp. 126–159, 1952.
2. D. Levy, Psychic trauma of operations in children, *Amer. J. Dis. Children, 69,* pp. 7–25, 1945.
3. S. D. Lipton, On the psychology of childhood tonsillectomy, *Psychoanalytic Study of the Child,* International Universities Press, New York, 17, pp. 363–417, 1962.
4. E. Mason, The hospitalized child–his emotional needs, *N. E. J. Medicine, 272,* pp. 406–424, 1965.
5. G. Pearson, Effect of operative procedure on the emotional life of the child, *Amer. J. Dis. Children, 62,* pp. 716–729, 1941.
6. D. Prugh, E. Staub, H. Sands, R. Kirschbaum and E. Lenihan, A study of the emotional reactions of children and families to hospitalization and illness, *Amer. J. Orthopsychiat., 23,* pp. 76–106, 1953.
7. H. R. Schaffer and W. M. Callender, Psychological effects of hospitalization in infancy, *Pediatrics, 24,* pp. 528–539, 1959.
8. D. T. A. Vernon, J. M. Foley, R. R. Sepowicz and J. L. Schulman,

Psychological Responses of Children to Hospitalization and Illness, Charles C. Thomas, Springfield, Illinois, 1965.

9. L. J. Yarrow, Separation from parents during early childhood, in *Review of Child Development Research,* M. L. Hoffman and L. W. Hoffman, (eds.), Russell Sage Foundation, New York, pp. 89–136, 1964.

10. R. Spitz, Hospitalism, An inquiry into the genesis of psychiatric conditions in early childhood, *Psychoanal. Stud. Child,* International Universities Press, New York, *1,* pp. 53–74, 1945.

11. J. Bowlby, Maternal care and mental health, *Bulletin of the World Health Organization, 3,* pp. 355–534, 1951.

12. J. Robertson, *Young Children in Hospitals,* Basic Books, New York, 1958.

13. A. J. Solnit, Hospitalization, An aid to physical and psychological health in childhood, *J. Dis. Child., 99,* pp. 155–163, 1960.

14. E. K. Oremland and J. D. Oremland, *The Effects of Hospitalization on Children,* Charles C. Thomas, Springfield, 1973.

15. A. Freud, The role of bodily illness in the mental life of children, *Psychoanal. Stud. Child,* International Universities Press, New York, *7,* pp. 69–81, 1952.

16. S. Cassell, The effect of brief puppet therapy upon the emotional responses of children undergoing cardiac catheterization, *J. Consult. Psychol., 29,* pp. 1–8, 1965.

17. M. Petrillo and S. Sanger, *Emotional Care of Hospitalized Children: An Environmental Approach,* Lippencott, Philadelphia, 1972.

18. J. Shaw, Volunteers prepare children for surgery via puppet therapy, *Mod. Hosp., 114,* pp. 126–127, 1970.

19. R. D. Becker, Therapeutic approaches to psychopathological reactions to hospitalization, *Int. J. Child Psychotherapy, 10,* pp. 65–97, 1972.

20. R. A. Gardner, *Therapeutic Communication with Children: The Mutual Storytelling Technique,* Science House, New York, 1971.

21. J. E. Schowalter and R. D. Lord, Admission to an adolescent ward, *Pediatrics, 44,* pp. 1009–1011, 1969.

22. J. E. Schowalter and R. D. Lord, Utilization of patient meetings on an adolescent ward, *Int. J. Psychiat. in Med., 1,* pp. 197–206, 1970.

23. K. A. Menninger, Polysurgery and polysurgical addiction, *Psychoanal. Quart., 3,* pp. 173–199, 1934.

24. H. Deutsch, Some psychoanalytic observations in surgery, *Psychosom. Med., 4,* pp. 105–115, 1942.

25. A. Stein, Group interaction and group psychotherapy in a general hospital, *Mt. Sinai J. Med.,* N.Y., *38,* pp. 89–100, 1971.

26. I. L. Janis, G. F. Mahl, J. Kagan and R. Holt, *Personality: Dynamics, Development and Assessment,* Harcourt, Brace and World, New York, 1969.

27. E. Kubler-Ross, *On Death and Dying,* Macmillan, New York, 1969.

28. J. Vernick and M. Karon, Who's afraid of death on a leukemia ward?, *Amer. J. Dis. Child., 109,* pp. 393–397, 1965.

29. J. Piaget, *The Psychology of Intelligence,* Harcourt, Brace, New York, 1950.

30. J. M. Natterson and A. G. Knudson, Observations concerning fear of death in fatally ill children and their mothers, *Psychosom. Med., 22,* pp. 456–465, 1960.

31. S. R. Slavson, *A Textbook in Analytic Group Psychotherapy,* International Universities Press, New York, 1964.

32. R. Cohn, The theme-centered interactional method, unpublished manuscript, 1963.

33. B. Bornstein, On latency, *Psychoanal. Stud. Child,* International Universities Press, New York, *6,* pp. 279–285, 1951.

34. A. Barcai and E. H. Robinson, Conventional group therapy with preadolescent children, *Int. J. Group Psychotherapy, 19,* pp. 334–345, 1969.

35. S. Rhodes, Short-term groups of latency age children in a school setting, *Int. J. Group Psychotherapy, 23,* pp. 204–216, 1973.

36. R. Sands and S. Golub, Breaking the bonds of tradition: a reassessment of group treatment of latency-age children, *Amer. J. Psychiatry, 131*, pp. 662–665, 1974.
37. S. Scheidlinger, Experimental group treatment of severely deprived latency-age children, *Amer. J. of Orthopsychiatry, 30*, pp. 356–368, 1960.
38. M. Sugar, Interpretive group psychotherapy with latency children, *Amer. J. Child Psychiatry, 13*, pp. 648–666, 1974.
39. H. J. Parad, *Crisis Intervention*, Family Service Association of America, New York, 1965.
40. J. S. Tyhurst, Role of transition states—including disasters—in mental illness, Symposium on Preventative and Social Psychiatry, Walter Reed Army Institute of Research, Washington, D.C., 1957.
41. M. Stocking, W. Rothney, G. Grosser and R. Goodwin, Psychopathology in the pediatric hospital—implications for community health, *Amer. J. Public Health, 62*, pp. 551–556, 1972.

6

Group Psychotherapy with Stroke Patients During the Immediate Recovery Phase

—DONNA M. ORADEI, M.S.N., and
NANCY S. WAITE, M.S.W.

THE psychosocial impact of a stroke upon its victims is well documented.[3,4] The stroke poses a threat to the patient's life style and to his normal control over his environment. The person's response to his disability may result in feelings of anxiety, depression, hopelessness, helplessness, and guilt. Interpersonal relationships and family functioning are disrupted. Forced reliance upon others may arouse unconscious desires to be cared for and to be removed from competitive struggles, thus intensifying the dependence manifested by the patient.[3] It is important that a program designed to care for stroke patients include an opportunity for patients to discuss these problems. This helps to relieve anxiety and to create an environment that treats each patient as an adult with the goal of independent functioning.[1]

Little has been written, however, about the use of psychotherapeutic groups in dealing with these emotional needs. Emphasis in the professional literature during the past ten years has focused upon the use of physical medicine and rehabilitative approaches and activity-oriented groups. In one rehabilitation facility, however, a social worker observed that a program whose major focus was physical activity could serve as a "screen" to pre-

Reprinted from the *American Journal of Orthopsychiatry* 44 (3): 386–395, 1974, by Donna Oradei and Nancy S. Waite. Copyright © 1974 the American Orthopsychiatric Association, Inc. Reproduced by permission.

vent psychological problems from being dealt with, and subsequently these unresolved issues could interfere with rehabilitation. In order to help patients resolve these problems, a "non-activity" group was recommended.[7] Shapiro and McMahon[8] recognized that patients' psychological difficulties can create a "stalemate," which may interfere with rehabilitation and in patient-staff cooperation. They observed that when patients were directly confronted with the extent of their disabilities early in their treatment, they were initially upset but began to work toward an acceptance of the disability. Within supportive relationships, patients were able to accept loss, to grieve, and to move on. Excessive and false reassurance served only to reinforce denial and dependency.

Hospitalization for the treatment of any acute illness, such as a stroke, constitutes a life crisis for the individual involved. According to Caplan, a life crisis begins with the occurrence of a hazardous event, *e.g.,* illness, death, birth, or the beginning of a developmental phase, which results in acute psychological upset as the individual attempts to utilize old coping patterns to deal with a new situation. The precipitating event usually involves: 1) loss of basic supplies (physical, psychosocial, or sociocultural); 2) threat of such a loss; and 3) a challenge involving the possibility of increased supplies but at a greater cost. The period of upset which ensues and which usually lasts from one to five weeks is characterized by intense feelings of anxiety, fear, guilt, and shame. The individual's usual functioning is disrupted, and this is associated with a feeling of helplessness and ineffectuality in the face of the insoluble problem. Resolution of the crisis occurs when the individual is able to establish new coping patterns to deal with his stressful situation.[2]

Crisis intervention by professional staff with the affected individual involves the following steps:

1. Helping the individual to identify the nature of the crisis.
2. Assisting the person to express his feelings about the crisis. Some of the feelings might not be immediately accessible even to the individual involved.
3. Exploring possible new coping mechanisms with the individual.
4. Assisting the person with re-entrance into the social world.[8]

Patient discussion groups were developed by the authors as a group crisis intervention approach to assist stroke patients at a Veterans' Administration hospital in their adjustment to a variety of physical disabilities and changes in their social environment. Purposes of the group included assistance with the four areas described above, and provided a forum for expanding the understanding and skills of staff members in dealing with stroke patients' varied concerns. Patients experiencing some degree of difficulty with verbal communication or a decreased level of mental clarity were also invited to attend meetings, even though it was recognized that their participation would be limited.

GROUP FORMAT AND COMPOSITION

Patients involved in the ongoing groups were those who had been transferred from the intensive care unit of the Stroke Unit* to the subacute ward. When the groups were in progress, all subacute patients participated. The groups met five days a week and lasted for thirty minutes each day. Originally, the meetings had been proposed for seven days per week, but the unit nursing staff did not continue the meetings on weekends. All nursing staff were encouraged to attend and participate in the leadership along with the authors. Twelve staff members, including the authors, were involved in the groups. The number of staff members per meeting ranged from one to four. At the majority of meetings there were only two staff members present. Following each meeting, staff members met together to discuss the content and the process of the meeting, as well as the level and types of staff intervention. A summary of each meeting was also recorded.

The two groups used as a basis for this paper were held several months apart. The minimum requirements for group composition were four patients who were capable of some degree of verbal communication. The subacute ward population did not always meet these requirements, which resulted in the time lapse between the two series of group meetings. A total of twenty-two patients was seen in the two series of open-ended groups. In the first series, ten patients attended fifteen meetings. There were three women and seven men, with an age range of 53 to 82 and a median age of 66. The second series consisted of twelve patients attending eleven meetings. There were eleven men and one woman ranging in age from 48 to 79, and a median age of 59. The difference in age was reflected in some of the specific areas of concerns presented by the patients, as will be discussed in the development of the groups.

GROUP PROCESS AND DEVELOPMENT

INTRODUCTORY PHASE

The beginning of the groups (first and second meetings) was characterized by a general "getting acquainted atmosphere." Patients introduced themselves to each other, talked about their particular entrance into the hospital, and began to share their disabilities with each other. This comparison stimulated questions regarding the different causes and effects of strokes. This discussion was probably based partly on the patients' real

---

*The Stroke Unit is a four-bed intensive care unit where persons with symptoms of an acute stroke are admitted and cared for. A post-acute stroke unit consisting of twelve beds is adjacent to the intensive care unit. Persons admitted to the Stroke Intensive Care Unit might remain there for a period of five to seven days, during which time they are kept on bed rest and receive continuous EEG and cardiac monitoring. When transferred to the subacute area, patients are mobilized to develop and utilize their capabilities for independent functioning. Continued emphasis is placed upon family involvement in the emotional and social aspects of treatment, rehabilitation, and discharge planning.

desire for additional factual information, but also served to avoid discussion of some of the feelings associated with their condition. Misconceptions about strokes were rectified by the staff when they became apparent, and this discussion sometimes provided important insights into the concerns of individual patients. For example, one patient (who had a mitral stenosis and a complicated cardiac condition for several years) casually mentioned that he was glad that only the right side of his body was affected by his stroke, because a stroke affecting the left side "would make your heart stop working." Staff discussed with the patient and the group why this was not so, but interpreted to him that his concern and his misconception were understandable in view of his longstanding worries about his heart.

Patients began to discuss their anxieties about the unknown future, and posed questions such as, "Will I have another stroke?", "What can I do to prevent another stroke?", and "Will I ever be able to use my hand again?" to illustrate their concerns. Patients also began talking about discharge plans in very unrealistic ways. One female patient who had a dense hemiplegia was convinced that immediate discharge to her home would pose no problem because her son-in-law was a "big, strong man who can stay at home during the day to carry me around." Staff members, with some assistance from patient group members, gently pointed out some of the more obvious reality factors that were being ignored in these situations. No attempt was made to force patients to abandon their denial.

Staff interventions were primarily supportive and clarifying. After giving a general introduction to the group, staff provided some concrete information regarding strokes upon request and encouraged group members to verbalize their varied concerns. Initial ambivalence about attending the group was interpreted by the staff as an understandable desire to avoid some of the anxieties associated with discussing their concerns. This approach proved successful because, in spite of anxieties, few patients actually missed entire group meetings. They usually made an attempt to attend at least part of the meeting, even if another appointment had caused them to be late.

MIDDLE PHASE

As patients came to know and trust each other and the staff, they began to share their seemingly endless amount of anxiety, despair, and feelings of helplessness. Fear of further disabilities and the threat of loss of control over their lives was a common worry. Patients talked about "getting close to death" and "being near the end." Previous life styles were often now impractical, and adjusting to physical as well as social losses was a task confronting most patients. Patients acknowledged this task in their discussion, and expressed the helplessness they felt in attempting such an adjustment. Patients were grieving not only over lost body function but also over the loss of independence which resulted. During meetings in which the helplessness theme predominated, there was much talking about wanting the staff (or someone!) to make them better again. Requests for further rehabilitative therapies were frequently made, and a patient's lack of progress was seen by other patients as evidence of a lack of adequate effort on the part of the staff. Group members' anger about this situation sometimes focused on the staff. It took the form of patients refusing to talk in the meetings, coming late for meetings, or, on some occasions, voicing a direct expression of anger at the staff responsible for their care. At times, the patients' anger was mixed with envy for the youth and health of the staff. In their search for a reason for their slow or non-existent progress, patients sometimes held themselves responsible for not recovering faster. There was a tendency to believe that "if you just set your mind to it, you can do it." Patients felt sad and guilty when such an attitude did not seem to result in a speedier recovery.

With occasional exceptions, this venting of anger and despair gradually gave way to realistic thinking about discharge and its inherent problems. Older patients were concerned that they might not be useful any longer to their families. Younger patients discussed some of their concerns about sexual functioning after discharge, and also talked about the feasibility of returning to former employment. All patients were concerned that their disabilities would make them a "burden to the family" or would necessitate such major household changes that the family would feel that continued care would best take place in a convalescent home.

As patients faced these issues, there continued to be some reworking of their earlier grieving over lost independence. This was shown by their occasional reversion to denial of the illness and tearful depression over their loss. As time elapsed, patients were confronted with the fact that many of their fantasies about near-total recovery by discharge would not be realized and that it was time to begin coming to terms with assuming an altered role in the family and community. During this phase of group development, staff intervention consisted of allowing the patients to vent their anger and frustration about the issues and conflicts that the illness has produced for them and their families. Most staff comments to the patients were ego-supportive in nature, and attempted to encourage self-reliance in those areas of functioning in which it was realistic. Patients often required assistance in identifying new methods of coping with their current situation. Alternative methods of dealing with the stress were often available but were not always immediately apparent to the patients involved.

TERMINATION PHASE

The ending process, which took place in the last three or four meetings of both groups, was prompted by the granting of trial weekend visits at home and the actual discharges of patients from hospital care. These meetings were marked by feelings of confusion, ambivalence, and apprehension.

As patients planned for their discharges and changes in plans were necessary, they reiterated their feelings of confusion and anger with the staff. Their occasional confusion about external situations was seen by staff as reflecting a resurgence of earlier internal confusion, uncertainty, and lack of control. The prospect of discharge elicited patients' concern and questions about the staff members' actual interest in them and possible rejection of them. Staff members continued to allow the expression of anger, which was diminishing, and attempted to clarify and interpret patients' true feelings about leaving the hospital.

In both groups, the patients attempted to retain memories and hopes of better days. In one group, the members reminisced about the "good old days"; in the other group, the patients talked about famous people who had recovered from similar illnesses. Staff responded to this as the patients' need for drawing upon times of success and hope in order to feel more optimistic about their impending discharges.

Although there was generally a developing realistic awareness of their illness and prognosis on the part of the patients, they verbalized anxiety and frustration about their present functioning, and uncertainty about the future. Patients who had been home on weekend passes gave vivid descriptions about their failures and accomplishments. Several patients wondered how they would be viewed and accepted by "well" people when they left the hospital. The group was unified by their mutual apprehension about the future, and their motivation to resume functioning at home and in the community. Throughout these discussions, the staff provided support of patients' progress, empathized with their concern, and helped to clarify their feelings and the realities about their leaving.

Final decision to terminate both groups evolved as most patients left the hospital within a few days of each other. Although the decision was a gradual one made by both staff and patients, the ultimate decision was made by the staff.

PATIENTS' EVALUATION

In order to evaluate the patients' feelings about their participation in the group, and the impact of these meetings, the authors sent them a brief questionnaire. The questionnaire consisted of fifteen true/false statements, two multiple choice questions, and one open-ended question containing a request for suggestions. Twenty-one questionnaires were mailed out, and eight were returned and completed. One was returned uncompleted by the patient and one was returned because the patient had recently died. Eleven were not accounted for. Since the questionnaires were anonymous and not coded, it was not possible to get a more complete return through further follow-up.

Of the eight questionnaires returned, the responses were generally positive with regard to the helpfulness of the group (six). Patients felt that the group discussion helped them to understand their illness (six), to ask questions about the illness (six) and its effects, and to accept their illness and its limitations (six). The patients also agreed that the group meetings

helped them to feel more comfortable in the hospital (six), including helping them to feel less alone and providing a means of occupying their time
(six). They further concluded that group meetings were a good way to meet
people during their hospitalization (six).

Although some respondents did not concur, the majority of patients
agreed that the group helped them to cope with their feelings of depression
(five), and assisted them in knowing what to expect in the future with
regard to their illness and functioning (five).

Group members were divided in their opinions (four–four) as to
whether or not the group meetings had 1) aided them in making plans for
their future, and 2) given them an opportunity to express any feelings of
anger that they may have had.

One aspect of the group in which all patients agreed was its helpfulness
in learning that other patients had similar concerns and feelings about their
illness, hospitalization, and the future (eight).

STAFF'S EVALUATION

In an attempt to assess Stroke Unit nursing staff's reaction to the
patient discussion groups, a brief anonymous questionnaire consisting of
true/false, multiple choice, and one open-ended question was administered
to those staff who had actually participated in the groups at some time. The
authors were interested not only in personal reaction of the staff to the
groups, but also their perception of the impact of the group meetings upon
patients. Out of a total of nine nurses, nine returned questionnaires. Nurses
characterized their reactions to the group as "comfortable" (eight), but also
"thoughtful" (four), and "helpful" (four). There was general agreement
among the staff members' responses that the groups were helpful both to
patients and to staff alike (six). Anxiety and depression were perceived by
the nursing staff as concomitants of group attendance for the patients
(eight). Five staff members felt that participation in the groups had been
"anxiety provoking" for them; three respondents found them "depressing."
Most staff members (seven) felt that the meetings had "helped them to increase their understanding of the feelings of stroke patients."

When asked for their recommendations for continuing or changing the
meetings, nursing staff indicated that they would like to "center them more
around specific patient teaching" (seven), "include more talking by staff"
(four), and "make the groups available for outpatients" (five).

IMPACT ON PATIENTS

It was the authors' observation that the group members developed an
awareness of their identity as a group and a sense of cohesion early in the
group's formation. Within the first few meetings, patients began to
recognize members' absences or departures, and progress or lack of it in
their rehabilitation. They were united in numerous ways, and this was evident as they described themselves as a patient group in contrast to healthy

staff members, and as people who shared an experience—a sudden illness, dependence, and disability. Their cohesion provided them with feelings of security and acceptance. This enabled them to express intense and intimate feelings of hopelessness and despair, frequently accompanied by tears. The expression of some difficult feelings, including anger, to each other and to staff members reflected the patients' feelings of trust and safety. Patients were able to express and act out anger, not only individually but also as a group, and to deliberately plan to control group interaction. Within this supportive framework, the patients were able to begin as a group to accept their losses and changes in life style, and to plan for resumption of functioning. Likewise, the mixed emotional response of the group to the discharge of each member, and the disorganization and resistance that occurred with the introduction of new members reflected the strong cohesive quality of the group.

The formation of the discussion group was also responsible for increased interaction outside the group. It was evident that when groups were not in operation on the wards, patients remained more isolated. They confined socializing to their roommates and were silently aware of one another. With the formal recognition in the group of one another as people who had similar experiences and feelings, the patients continued to share their thoughts and plans with each other outside the group. At times, it was obvious that subgroups had formed in which patients continued discussion or comment on the larger group interaction. In addition, informal socializing increased among patients, which occasionally resulted in interaction among families as they visited the patients.

The nature of the group discussion, the group cohesion, and increased interaction resulted in patients' intimate feelings being more apparent within the ward community than when there was no group in existence. The groups provided an opportunity for patients to recognize and react openly to issues such as dependency, loss of function, and even death. This display of intense emotion was evident outside of group meetings also. Events such as patient's lack of progress, recurrence of one's symptoms or a patient's discharge were responded to freely by patients with one another as well as with staff. Whether prompted by the confrontation and ventilation of emotions within the group or by the support and acceptance fostered in the group, increased expressions of emotions in the entire ward community were evident simultaneously with the group experience.

Although the authors have given considerable attention to verbal interaction and expression within the group in this paper, it is their belief that the group meetings were also helpful to patients who were unable to verbalize. There were eight patients with speaking impairments who were involved and accepted in the two groups. The group experience gave these patients an opportunity to hear thoughts similar to their own verbalized, and to express their own feelings through laughter, crying, gestures, and even humming. Verbal patients expressed interest in the aphasic members, and learned to recognize and understand their nonverbal communication. This experience enhanced all of the patients' understanding and appreciation of others as well as their own capabilities and limitations.

IMPACT ON STAFF

Participation as well as tangential contact with the group meetings aroused a variety of intense feelings in nursing staff. The anxiety that patients began to verbalize early in the meetings succeeded in producing similar anxiety in the nursing staff. When patients talked about the many areas of their lives that would require restructuring and the great anxiety they felt in facing so many "unknowns," nursing staff had a difficult time listening to the discussion. Their "helping role" to the patients was perceived by them as dictating that they provide concrete answers and reassurance to the questions and feelings that patients were expressing. There were many discussions after the meetings that the group would be "more helpful for the patients" if they were reorganized by staff to be centered around specific teaching and lectures. Since the same staff was already involved in active individual patient teaching on the ward, this feeling on their part was judged to be a reaction to the patients' expressed anxiety rather than to the existence of any real lack of adequate patient instruction.

Two other major group themes posed problems for the staff. These were the issues of depression and anger. At the point in group development when the patients were feeling very hopeless and depressed, these feelings seemed to become more apparent in their everyday behavior on the ward. Nursing staff also became depressed and began to suggest ways in which the group meeting times could be used "to cheer everybody up." Discussion of depression in the meetings eventually gave way to the general feelings of anger. Patients gradually became very verbal about the hostilities they felt towards the fact of their illness and hospitalization. Initially, this feeling took the form of diffuse anger at the ward staff for a variety of seemingly trivial events and policies. The response of nursing staff present in the meeting was to become defensive about the events in question. It was difficult for the authors to assist them in objectively assessing the source of the patients' complaints rather than to continue personalizing them.

When structuring the meetings initially, the authors felt strongly that there should be "a meeting after the meeting" with staff to discuss the content of the discussion and staff's reaction to it. During these sessions, it became apparent that the group meetings were confronting nursing staff with their personal feelings about very potent issues (for example, death, despair, dependency, anger, and changes in family relationships). Nurses began to discuss their reactions to individual and group issues in terms of their own life experiences. The nursing staff who attended the group discussions most frequently had more opportunity to begin dealing with their own feelings. These staff, in the authors' opinion, eventually became the most successful in being able to support the patients in their efforts to talk about their concerns. In retrospect, the authors feel that it was unwise to have structured the group to permit the intermittent attendance of a number of nursing staff. A fixed group structure in terms of staff attendance would have been preferable. This would have allowed for the more adequate discussion of related personal issues on the part of nursing staff. It was the authors' opinion that this process was a necessary prerequisite to professional growth.

In spite of some of the difficulties encountered in the utilization of unit nursing staff in the patient discussions, the authors did feel that this participation resulted in their greater understanding of the process of emotional adjustment to an acute and potentially chronic illness. It was also the impression of the authors that during the periods when patient discussion groups were being held, there was more involvement of the nursing staff with the patients and a greater awareness of the individual issues facing patients during the course of their hospitalization.

IMPACT ON AUTHORS

The authors shared many of the common reactions to the group experiences that have been described in the preceding paragraphs. In addition, the provision of leadership for the group meetings and the overall community-staff struggle with the issues involved was time-consuming and frustrating, but challenging. Many times, the feelings of helplessness and anger were focused on the authors by both patients and staff. Mutual support and frequent collaboration proved to be essential in sustaining the authors in this endeavor.

CONCLUSIONS AND RECOMMENDATIONS

Participation by stroke patients in daily ward discussion groups had several positive outcomes. Patients became acquainted with each other in the group meetings, and subsequent socialization on the ward was enhanced as a result. A sense of community developed rather quickly, and more frequent interactions among patients, families, and ward nursing staff were observed.

The supportive group meetings provided patients with a regular outlet for the ventilation of feelings of depression, anger, and gradual acceptance of their losses. Group members received assistance from each other and from the group leaders in clarifying the nature of the social and psychological issues confronting them. These processes were a necessary prerequisite to successful grieving.

Alternative methods of coping with disabilities were discussed and patients often had the opportunity to "try out" new behaviors at home on weekend passes before their actual discharge from the hospital had occurred. The sharing of experiences by patients, made possible by the group setting, encouraged more realistic thinking about discharge and its implications.

Patients indicated that the group helped them to understand their illness, cope with feelings of depression, and feel less alone by learning that other patients had similar concerns and feelings.

Patient group discussions provided important insights into the staff's emotional responses to the catastrophic nature of stroke illness. Participation in the meetings confronted nursing staff with their own feelings about dependence, aging, and death, and resulted in discussion of group issues in terms of their own experiences and relationships. Staff also expressed discomfort with the use of an unstructured group approach. For these reasons, it is recommended that, in similar groups, there be a fixed assignment of staff who would attend regularly, and have an opportunity to participate in the development of group process and "work through" their own emotional responses.

It was the authors' observation that while patient group meetings were being held, staff-patient interaction increased, and staff involvement with patients' expressions of intense emotion, independent of the meetings, was more frequent. Likewise, staff members discussed more readily the emotional aspects of stroke illness and its implications for patient care. Overall treatment and discharge planning were enhanced by the information and understanding gleaned from patient group meetings.

Because of the quantity and quality of emotional expression by patients and staff in these groups, the use of co-leaders is recommended. This involves constant collaboration and cooperation but provides the support and understanding essential for both the nursing staff and the group leaders.

REFERENCES

Donna Oradei and Nancy Waite are both affiliated with the Veterans Administration Hospital, West Haven, Conn.

1. Borden, W. 1962. Psychological aspects of stroke: patients and family. *Ann. Inter. Med.* 57(Oct.):689–692.
2. Caplan, G. 1964. *Principles of Preventive Psychiatry.* Basic Books, New York.
3. Fisher, S. 1961. Psychiatric considerations of cerebral vascular disease. *Amer. J. Cardiol.* 7(March):379–385.
4. Hartshorn, A. 1967. Psychosocial aspects of stroke illness. *Med. Soc. Wk.* 18(March): 323–329.
5. McClellan, M. 1972. Crisis groups in special care areas. *Nursing Clinics of America* 7(June):363–371.
6. Morley, W., Messick, J. and Aguilera, D. 1967. Crisis with paradigms of interventions. *J. Psychiat. Nursing* 5(Nov.-Dec.): 531–544.
7. Richards, L. 1966. Group therapy in a rehabilitation center. *Canad. J. Occupational Therapy* 33(Winter):141–147.
8. Shapiro, L. and McMahon, A. 1966. Rehabilitation stalemate. *Arch. Gen. Psychiat.* 15(Aug.): 173–177.

7

Crisis Groups in Special Care Areas
—MURIEL S. McCLELLAN, M.N.

When a patient requires the services of a specialized care area of a general hospital, he and his family experience various stresses and obstacles. When these obstacles cannot be removed by usual coping devices, an acute psychologic upset occurs. This upset, which is not indicative of a mental disorder, but is rather a sign of adjustment to the stress, creates a high level of tension, and the person is considered to be in a crisis.

At this point the need for crisis intervention is great, and measures to facilitate psychologic adaptation should be a vital process in the care of these patients. Mental health specialists are becoming more aware of this need, and are becoming increasingly involved in the management of these patients.[1]

This paper will discuss the use of a crisis group as one approach to the management of the crises patients encounter in special care areas. This will be done by considering the theoretical aspects of crisis intervention, the group approach in psychotherapy, and the characteristics of a crisis group. To facilitate understanding, examples of direct and indirect crisis groups will be given.

THEORETICAL ASPECTS OF CRISIS INTERVENTION

A crisis is said to have occurred when a critical event or situation cannot be met by usual methods of problem-solving. Some crises are part of the usual course of normal growth and development, such as birth, death, marriage, and adolescence, while other may follow stressful external or environmental events, such as physical illness, surgical operations, or disasters.

Each crisis that an individual encounters is precipitated by a hazardous event, followed by a period of acute psychologic upset, and ends in resolution. Hazardous events usually include either (1) loss of basic supplies, (2) threat of loss, or (3) challenge. The period of upset, which usually lasts from one to four or five weeks, is characterized by feelings of anxiety, fear, guilt, or shame, along with some disorganization of function. Resolution of the crisis occurs when the individual establishes a new pattern of coping with the situation. This new pattern of coping should be at the same level or

Reprinted by permission from *Nursing Clinics of North America* 7 (2): 363–371, 1972, W.B. Saunders Company, Philadelphia, Pa.

a higher level of functioning than the individual's pre-crisis state, but may be at a lower level.[2]

Crisis intervention is a type of psychotherapy in which activities are directed toward assisting the individual to a healthy resolution of his crisis. Various steps in crisis intervention have been identified in the literature. Rapoport identifies them as follows: (1) clarifying the problem that leads to the call for help, (2) accepting the expression of feelings, and (3) arousing interpersonal and institutional resources.[3] Similarly, Morley and associates have identified the steps in crisis intervention as including: (1) helping the individual gain an understanding of the crisis, (2) helping the individual to bring into the open his present feelings, (3) exploring the coping mechanisms by examining the alternatives, and (4) reopening the social world, perhaps through new relations.[4]

Crisis intervention can involve either dealing directly with the individuals and their families during crisis, or personal contact with the caregivers, who in turn intervene in the crisis situation. These two methods have been called the direct approach and the indirect approach, respectively.[5] In the direct approach, Caplan advocates that the mental health specialist gain access to a population of individuals in crisis, and screen this population to identify those who are having difficulty in dealing with the crisis. A follow-up of individuals with crisis behavior is made in order to assist them toward resolution of the crisis. Caplan states that his approach was first used by Lindemann in 1944 in helping bereaved people in their grief work. He cites response to surgical operations, birth of a premature baby, entry into kindergarten, difficulties of nursing training, marital problems, and urban relocation as other areas in which the direct approach has been utilized.

In the indirect approach, Caplan advocates a more economical approach in terms of the mental health specialist's time and effort. The role of the mental health specialist in this approach would be to study the crisis situation, communicate this knowledge to the caregiver who will have direct contact with the individual in crisis, and support the caregiver when he is dealing with the individual in crisis. Knowledge of the crisis can be obtained by the mental health specialist's collecting data himself, or by his deriving data from the work of others. Communicating this knowledge can be done through group or individual instruction of the caregivers. However, support of the caregivers is the crucial aspect of the indirect approach. Support is fundamental to keep the caregiver from becoming discouraged, and additional learning can be accomplished during sessions regarding difficult patients.

THE GROUP APPROACH IN PSYCHOTHERAPY

Despite variations in technique and emphasis, most types of therapy take one of two forms, either a group focus or an individual focus. The individual method is accomplished in a one-to-one relationship, while the group method involves a group setting of two or more individuals. Apparently, the group method of therapy has been used since the beginning of time. Dreikurs and Sonstegard report that Socrates used a form of group counseling with youths.[6] However, group therapy as we know it today is a product of the twentieth century, with definite advances and acceleration around the time of World War II.

Agreement to an actual definition of group therapy does not appear in the literature. Slavson states that group therapy must meet the following criteria: (1) small group size of approximately eight people; (2) permissive or catalytic type of group leadership, rather than authoritative or didactic; and (3) grouping of patients based on diagnostic classification, rather than an indiscriminate collection.[7] Gaza states that Slavson has made a strong case, but he points out that practitioners who work with groups larger than eight people, are authoritarian or didactic in their leadership, or use few or no criteria for selection are often considered group therapists.[8] Sullivan describes group work, which includes many of the ingredients frequently reported in definitions, in the following manner:

> Group work stresses programs evolved by the group itself, in consultation with the leader who guides toward socially desirable ends. Creative activities are encouraged to provide legitimate channels of self-expression and to relieve emotional stress. Competition for its own sake is minimized and the group members learn from situations where cooperation brings rich satisfaction. The trained leader arranges for leadership practice by group members, individual responsibility and group responsibility grow as the group takes on new functions. The atmosphere is friendly, informal, and democratic.[9]

CHARACTERISTICS OF A CRISIS GROUP

Crisis intervention, like other forms of therapy, often utilizes a group focus. The overall goal of a crisis group is to help the individual group members resolve their crises so that they function at a pre-crisis level or higher. The major focus is on problem-solving, rather than long-term therapy. Consistent with the theoretical concept that a crisis is resolved, for better or worse, in four to six weeks, each group member is limited to six weekly group sessions. If by that time the person has not been able to resolve his crisis, other types of long-term treatment modalities are considered.

The membership of a crisis group can vary. Some groups are composed of people in different types of crises, others, of people who are in similar types of crises. Aguilera et al. have pointed out the advantages of grouping people with similar types of crises together.[10]

Certain individuals often have been excluded from crisis groups. They include persons who are severely suicidal or homicidal and require intense individual therapy, and those who have some impaired ability to communicate in a group setting.

Most crisis groups have been conducted on an ongoing basis, whereby group members are added as crises occur and other group members terminate as the crisis is resolved. Therefore, patients within the group represent individuals at various stages of crisis resolution, which is helpful, since those close to termination can serve as role models. Additional helpful characteristics of a crisis group include the rapidly occurring cohesion, which is perhaps a result of the universal feeling of crisis, and the support and appropriate suggestions which group members who "understand" can give.

The role of the therapist in a crisis group is to facilitate the group sessions. His primary responsibility is to keep the group on the task of problem-solving, rather than on irrelevant topics. The therapist may also suggest appropriate alternatives or offer support to group members. In doing so, he usually follows specific steps of crisis intervention in the group setting.

Strickler and Allgeyer have identified three steps in group crisis intervention.[11] The first step, which occurs prior to the group sessions, includes provision for the therapist to meet with the individual to explore his crisis situation with him. This would involve identification of the precipitating stressful event, the previous coping behavior, and the impasse brought about by the failure of the present inadequate coping mechanisms to deal with his particular emotional hazard. With this accomplished, the individual should have a noticeable lowering of tension, a regained sense of problem-solving, and potential for entering the group situation. In the second step, the group is used to help the individual attempt to solve his problem. This would involve group members or the therapist offering new ways or solutions to the problem, or encouraging the individual to identify these himself. In the third step, the group reinforces and helps sustain the individual's new way of coping. When more adaptive behaviors have been maintained, the individual is ready for termination from the group.

Only a few reports on crisis groups have appeared in the literature. Strickler and Allgeyer studied one short-term group of people in crisis and evaluated its performance over a six-month period.[12] The group consisted of 30 patients who were seeking help from a crisis-oriented clinic and were experiencing various types of crises. The size of each group session varied from four to eight members and fluctuated owing to the open-ended structure of the group. Each patient was limited to six weekly group sessions. Strickler and Allgeyer reported that the majority of patients made obvious and dramatic progress, as evidenced by the following: (1) quick welding of the group into a working group because of the universal feelings of crisis; (2) the group functioned to assist the person into awareness that his coping needed to change; (3) group support for changes in coping; (4) open and enthusiastic support by the therapist for the patient's efforts; and (5) a general atmosphere of hope and trust.

Morley and Brown also studied the use of crisis groups with similar patients; however, the results that they reported were not as optimistic.[12,13] They found that analysis of the group process had to be sacrificed since the group was problem-centered and short-term, attention was placed on individual problems, and the group interaction was dealt with only on a superficial basis. They also reported a lack of spontaneity because the therapist frequently had to utilize the technique of "going around."

Aguilera also conducted a crisis group with the same format with the exception that selected group members were in crisis with a specific and similar problem.[10] The study group consisted of parents who were having problems with young adult children. These crisis groups were reported to be extremely effective because of the limited focus on one problem area and the high interaction of group members. Support from group members in decision-making regarding their problems, and the exploration of alternative ways of coping, were reported.

Allgeyer studied the use of crisis groups with the disadvantaged, and she also supports the use of crisis groups as beneficial.[13] Her work was with six disadvantaged women who were suffering from loneliness and feelings of low self-esteem. She found that by clustering the women into treatment groups they were able to empathetically and practically aid one another in coping with problems.

EXAMPLES OF CRISIS GROUPS IN SPECIAL CARE AREAS

Although most of the work on crisis groups has been done within the area of general mental health work, the relevance to special care areas of a general hospital is pertinent. Patients in special care areas experience various stresses and obstacles, and the potential for crises to occur is great. A special care area which exemplifies this concept is the dialysis or kidney center which promotes a home maintenance dialysis program. Such a program consists of training patients and their families in the technique of hemodialysis. Once training has been completed, the patient and his family administer dialysis in their own home without direct supervision.

Frequent reports have appeared in the literature regarding the stresses of the home maintenance dialysis patient.[14,15,16] Cummings has identified economic stress, toxic factors, social role disturbances, and dependency as particular salient stress factors among kidney patients. Economic stress starts long before the patient and his family are involved in a home program. From the onset of renal disease, medical care is extensive and costly. Once on the program, financial strain is increased by the initial cost of equipment and supplies, the ongoing expenses each year, and the possible necessity of new housing, an extra room, or remodeling to house the equipment. Toxic factors, which are caused by rising levels of waste products in the patient's system, impair the basic mechanisms of attention and concentration, and higher intellectual functions cannot be effectively executed. The rigors of kidney disease and the nature of hemodialysis, as in other chronic illnesses, tends to place the patient in a dependent situation and causes social role disturbances. If the dependency and the role change run counter to the patient's values, the situation can be extremely disturbing to the patient.

Assisting the dialysis patient to deal effectively with the stresses of a home program often indicates the need for crisis intervention. A crisis intervention approach was utilized at the Kidney Center of Good Samaritan Hospital in Phoenix, where a home maintenance dialysis program was in existence. The approach utilized this author as a mental health nursing specialist to work with patients, their families, and the Kidney Center nursing staff in direct and indirect crisis groups.

The crisis groups that had the direct focus consisted of group meetings with patients and their families while they were undergoing the training program to prepare them for home dialysis. The major focus of the groups was on problem-solving related to the stressful events and initial anxiety of a training program, current feelings about dialysis treatment, and concerns of preparing to administer dialysis at home without direct supervision.

The size of each group varied from four to ten patients and family members. Group sessions were held weekly for about one hour, and were open-ended. Patients entered and left the group as they entered and terminated from the training program; therefore, the group represented patients at various stages of their training. Each patient and family member attended an average of six sessions. This author functioned as therapist to facilitate the movement of the group. A member of the Kidney Center's nursing staff acted as co-therapist. The co-therapist was fundamental in offering solutions to the group members, as well as being in a position to gain more knowledge about crisis intervention.

The process of each group meeting centered around four phases: (1) initial, (2) sharing, (3) problem-solving, and (4) termination. The initial phase included introductions and statements of the purpose of the meeting. The sharing phase encouraged discussion of current stressful events, and feelings surrounding these events. The sharing phase was essential in order to reduce tension enough to proceed to the problem-solving phase. Problem-solving was accomplished by alternative solutions to problems being presented by other group members and the co-therapist, or encouraging the individual to identify his own solutions. Termination included a summary of what had been discussed during the session. In doing so, support was frequently given to the progress that each group member was making.

The group sessions were identifed as valuable by patients, family members, and the nursing staff. Items that were noted as most beneficial included: (1) rapidly developing cohesion of group members; (2) support by other patients and family members that "you are not alone," which extended outside the group meetings; (3) practical suggestions of solutions to problems by other group members and the co-therapist; and (4) general reduction of tension and anxiety.

The crisis groups that had the indirect focus consisted of group meetings with the nursing staff of the Kidney Center. The primary goal of these group meetings was to assist the nursing staff in their ability to intervene in the crises encountered by dialysis patients and their family members. However, a secondary goal of assisting the nursing staff to deal with their own crises associated with working in a dialysis center was a part of these group meetings. This is not unusual, since the stressful conditions of working in a dialysis center have been frequently cited in the literature.[17]

Group sessions were held weekly for about one hour and included the total nursing staff. This author functioned as the therapist to facilitate group movement. The process of each meeting was flexible depending upon the needs of the group, but was always centered on either the primary or secondary goal. When the group was centered on the primary goal of assisting the nursing staff to deal with patients' and families' crises, the group sessions accomplished the following tasks: (1) a study of particular crisis situations currently affecting patients, including presentation of content by the therapist and mutual analysis of the problem; (2) considering the alternative actions that the nursing staff could take in providing care to the patient, again including presentation of content by the therapist; and (3) supporting the approaches taken by the nursing staff.

When the group was centered on the secondary goal of dealing with their own crises associated with working in a dialysis center, the group session accomplished the following tasks; (1) discussion of current stressful events, and the feelings associated with the events, such as the death of a patient; (2) support by other group members who had at one time dealt with similar feelings; and (3) active problem-solving regarding the stressful situations.

These group sessions were also identified as valuable by the nursing staff. Items that were noted to be most beneficial included; (1) increased staff knowledge about the emotional aspects of dialysis care; (2) increased staff involvement in the amount of crisis intervention offered to patients and their families; and (3) decreased involvement of the mental health specialist's time in dealing directly with patients and their families.

SUMMARY

This paper has identified the use of crisis groups as one approach to the management of crises patients encounter in special care areas of general hospitals. The theoretical aspects of crisis intervention, the group approach in psychotherapy, and the characteristics of crisis groups were discussed to facilitate the understanding of crisis groups. Examples of direct and indirect crisis groups in a dialysis center were presented; however, the same process could be utilized in many of the other special care areas of a general hospital.

REFERENCES

Muriel McClellan is a clinical specialist, Good Samaritan Hospital, Phoenix, Arizona. She is also Assistant Professor of Nursing, Arizona State University, Tempe.

1. Barton, David, and Kelso, Margaret: The nurse as a psychiatric consultation team member. *Psychiatry in Medicine,* 2:108, April, 1971.
2. Caplan, Gerald: *Principles of preventive psychiatry.* New York, Basic Books, Inc., 1964, pp. 26–54.
3. Rapoport, Lydia: The state of crisis: Some theoretical considerations. *Social Service Review,* 36:No. 2, 1962.
4. Morley, W. E., Messick, Janice M., and Aguilera, Donna C.: Crisis: Paradigms

of intervention. *J. Psychiat. Nursing*, 5:531–544, Nov.–Dec., 1967.

5. Caplan. op. cit., pp. 83–88.

6. Dreikurs, Rudolf, and Sonstegard, Manford: The Adlerian or teleoanalytic approach. In *Basic approaches to group psychotherapy and group counseling*. Ed. by G. M. Gaza, Springfield, Ill., Charles C. Thomas, 1968, p. 197.

7. Slavson, S. R.: Parallelisms in the development of group psychotherapy, *Internat. J. Group Psychotherapy*, V. 9:451, 1959.

8. Gaza, G. M.: Group psychotherapy and group counseling: Definition and heritage. In *Basic approaches to group psychotherapy and group counseling*. Ed. by G. M. Gaza, Springfield, Ill., Charles C. Thomas, pp. 3–26.

9. Sullivan, Dorthea: *Readings in group work*. New York, Associated Press, 1952, p. 189.

10. Aguilera, Donna C., Messick, Janice M., and Farrell, Marlene: *Crisis intervention. theory and methodology*. St. Louis, C. V. Mosby Co., 1970, p. 29.

11. Strickler, M., and Allgeyer, Jean: The crisis group: A new application of crisis theory. *Social Work*, 12:28–32, July, 1967.

12. Morley, W. E., and Brown, V. B.: The crisis intervention group: A natural mating or a marriage of convenience. *Psychotherapy: Theory, Res., Prac.*, 6:30–36, Winter, 1968.

13. Allgeyer, Jean: The crisis group: Its unique usefulness to the disadvantaged. *Internat. J. Group Psychotherapy*, 2:235–240, April, 1970.

14. Brand, Lucy, and Komorita, Nori: Adapting to long-term dialysis. *Am. J. Nursing*, 66:1778, Aug., 1966.

15. Shambaugh, P. W., et al.: Hemodialysis in the home: Emotional impact on the spouse. *Trans. Am. Soc. Artif. Internal Organs*, 13:41–45, 1967.

16. Cummings, J. W.: Hemodialysis—feelings, facts, and fantasies: The pressures and how patients respond. *Am. J. Nursing*, 70:68–76, Jan., 1970.

17. Abram, Harry: The psychiatrist, the treatment of chronic renal failure, and the prolongation of life: II. *Am. J. Psychiatry*, 126:157–167, Aug., 1969.

Personal Awareness: Individual Exercises

1. Contact your local chapter of the National Paraplegic Association and explore the possibility of attending their meetings, conferences, or social events.

2. It is easier to read about the problems of the disabled than to witness and react to them first hand. Your task is to spend four weekends at a rehabilitation facility as a volunteer. Try to experience contact with those disabled persons you might find most difficult to work with.

3. Conduct a survey in your community of all hospitals and rehabilitation facilities providing direct patient care to find out whether group counseling procedures are used. Describe the kinds of group counseling approaches used, summarize your experience, and state implications from your findings.

4. Suppose that you have been hospitalized with a disabling illness. A counselor visits you with an invitation to participate in group discussions where you and others could share reflections and projections concerning your disability and hospitalization. Would you participate? Discuss your reasons.

Structured Group Experience in Disability
—Welcome Back*

The following exercise is designed to sensitize participants to the impact of a disabling condition.

GOALS

1. To raise the awareness of participants to the qualitative dimensions of interpersonal relationships.

2. To enable participants to evaluate the differential impact of a disabling condition upon their interpersonal relationships.

3. To explore with participants the most helpful approaches in dealing with disability.

4. To list the most devastating disabilities that could occur in participants' lives.

5. To consider how participants' lives would be altered if a traumatic disability occured early or later in life, i.e., age 5, 10, 15, 20, 30, 40, 50, 60, 70.

PRELIMINARY CONSIDERATIONS

1. *Level of Intensity:* Moderate to high

2. *Group Size:* Groups of six to ten participants

3. *Time Required:* 3 hours

4. *Materials:* Paper and pencil for each participant

5. *Physical Setting:* Comfortable room with moveable chairs

---

*See Appendices A and B for detailed information on use of the structured group experiences in disability.

PROCEDURE

1. The group leader introduces the exercise by giving a brief talk concerning the impact of physical disability, focusing on the above goals.

2. Participants are asked to list the three most important people in their lives.

3. Each member is asked to list three specific disabilities that he or she would *least* want to experience personally.

4. Participants write a brief statement about each disability focusing on why they would not want it.

5. The leader then asks the group members to take the most undesirable disability and list five specific ways in which it would affect their relationship with each person listed if they were hospitalized and away from that person for one year.

6. The group leader asks the participants to verbalize their feelings and discuss what they have written.

7. The leader focuses on who would be most supportive and why and who would be least supportive and why.

8. The leader asks group members what would be most helpful to facilitate their integration back into the community.

9. Group is asked to select the age they would prefer the disability to occur.

10. Leader stresses the point that disability can occur any time and there is limited control of it.

LEADERSHIP SUGGESTIONS

1. The leader should be sensitive to the limited social relationships particular group members may have. If such issues surface, both the leader and group should be prepared to deal with them.

2. Group members may not have a complete understanding of the impact of a specific disability. The leader may want to introduce specific learning units to familiarize the member with more in-

depth information or assign group members to prepare such learning units for subsequent meetings.

VARIATIONS

1. Focus on a specific group—family, work, or social—for all participants.

2. Have participants pick the key person in their life and focus on the impact of specific disabilities.

3. Direct participants to focus on the adjustments a person would have to make in their aspirations and activities.

4. As an additional task ask participants to rank three ages at least ten years apart when they would least like to be disabled.

CHAPTER TWO

Group Approaches with Persons Having Various Disabilities

Overview

In this chapter selected articles provide the reader with examples of group work with a variety of physical disability populations. The articles selected for inclusion in this chapter help to provide a better perspective on the potential for group work for disability populations that might not otherwise be considered for such intervention. Further, the reader is presented with a broadened knowledge perspective on how certain disabilities may necessitate specific factual information and specialized group interventions prior to the beginning of group counseling.

In "Personal Adjustment Training for the Spinal Cord Injured," Roessler, Milligan, and Ohlson present their experience and insights in applying Personal Achievement Skills (PAS) to a group of spinal cord injured persons. This article offers the reader an excellent overview of the use of goal setting related to the needs of spinal cord injured persons. Additionally, valuable insights are provided into conducting groups with this population. Of particular relevance is the emphasis upon the whole person as reflected in the highlighting of the independent living, recreational, vocational, and physical needs of the spinal cord injured.

"Group Psychotherapy with a Paraplegic Group, with an Emphasis on Specific Problems of Sexuality" by Banik and Mendelson stresses the need to integrate the psychological and emotional needs of patients into treatment and rehabilitation programs. Responding to the expressed needs of a group of paraplegic and quadriplegic patients, the authors present a group program which focuses upon sexual needs and related issues of persons with spinal cord injuries. The reader is encouraged to be aware of how the group leaders helped to establish rapport with group members.

The focus of Sussman's article, "Group Therapy with Severely Handicapped," is on group procedures used with deaf young adults having multiple physical and social disabilities. Sussman found that use of a rudimentary form of sign language was necessary for the deaf adolescents to communicate in the group. He further suggests that group therapy with deaf persons may help to prevent later problems due to limited auditory contact with the hearing world. The reader is urged to be attentive to the necessity for creative leadership with difficult group problems.

Schwartz and Cahill, in "Psychopathology Associated with Myasthenia Gravis and its Treatment in Psychotherapeutically Oriented Group Counseling," present empirical findings of their study involving seventeen patients. The cumulative effect of isolation, fear of death, and self-consciousness are real issues for persons with myasthenia gravis; a group approach is presented as an additional technique which can be employed to reduce the negative impact of these factors and facilitate more effective coping strategies.

In "Social Group Work as a Treatment Modality for Hospitalized People with Rheumatoid Arthritis," Henkle suggests that disabled rheumatoid arthritis patients can benefit from group experiences, particularly as these experiences relate to the emotional concerns frequently associated with the disease. Henkle's insights into the problems of the environmental constraints of a hospital setting and of open group membership provide the reader with a better understanding of the difficulties in conducting groups in this setting. Evidence is cited that arthritic patients may experience psychosocial difficulties related to the sporadic nature of the disease and the necessity for continual medication. Henkle also discusses the importance of clarifying the purpose of group work with arthritic patients, especially in the context of the environmental strain of a hospital and role changes related to being disabled.

In "Group Rehabilitation of Vascular Surgery Patients," Lipp and Malone discuss the effort to establish group sessions in a Veterans Hospital setting. While not a traditional psychotherapy group, their group evolved into a vehicle for interpersonal support, encouragement, and development of coping skills. The impact of this group transcended the direct benefits to its members by creating within the staff a greater awareness of the relevant concerns of disabled persons and by having a direct impact upon ward management. Lipp and Malone found that members were encouraged by the gains of others and were motivated by the realization that they were not alone in their efforts.

Power and Rogers in "Group Counseling for Multiple Sclerosis Patients" relate their counseling experiences in an outpatient Veterans Administration Clinic. The authors feel that in group work with this population specific emphasis should be placed on the role of the family and on occupational considerations, both of critical concern to many neurologically disabled persons.

In a timely article entitled "Group Therapy with the Terminally Ill," Yalom and Greaves describe their experiences with a group of cancer patients. Living, rather than dying is the group's main theme. Meetings provide support, hope, and encouragement to members. Stressing the dying patient's intense need for others, the authors portray the group experience as a source of inner strength.

After completing this chapter the reader should have a better understanding concerning the need for specialized skills and knowledge in group work with persons having different disabilities. Certain topics that may be important for group members may necessitate the leader's value clarification (e.g. sexual issues, use of street language) if the group is to succeed. The opportunity for such exploration and understanding may present itself when the reader reflects on the personal awareness exercises and structured group experience which follow the articles in chapter 2.

8

Personal Adjustment Training for the Spinal Cord Injured
—RICHARD ROESSLER, TIM MILLIGAN, and ANN OHLSON

S PINAL cord injury is a catastrophic disability having distressing physical, psychological, and social effects. As a result of the wide-ranging effects of the disability, effective treatment must bring together a comprehensive network of services for the client (Margolin 1971).

Needs of the spinal cord injured client have been discussed extensively in the literature, which includes a clear outline of the medical or physical implications of spinal cord injury, spinal shock, spasticity, management of elimination, decubiti, cardiac and pulmonary complications, and the like (Bors 1956; O'Connor & Leitner 1971). The literature has also shown an emphasis on the significance of the psychological aspects of the disability, noting such issues as social atrophy, acceptance, and depression.

Obviously, effective therapy for the spinal cord injured must reflect an understanding of the physical and psychological aspects of the disability. Abramson (1967) has discussed the need for holistic, comprehensive, and flexible approaches for the spinal cord injured, stressing that this concept of treatment was, unfortunately, a viewpoint and not an actuality. According to Abramson, neither the knowledge of the "biology of paraplegia" nor the "sociologic and psychologic principles" involved have been integrated into rehabilitation of the spinal cord injured.

In order to expand and intensify services for the spinal cord injured, an experimental treatment project (SCI) was started in 1974 by the Arkansas Rehabilitation Services at the Central Baptist Hospital, Little Rock, Arkansas, and the Hot Springs Rehabilitation Center, Hot Springs, Arkansas. The project integrates intermediate hospital care, personal and vocational evaluation and training, individual counseling services, physical and occupational therapy, group, sexual, and family counseling services, and follow-along services. Additional services in the home and community are provided by SCI project field personnel.

Reprinted from *Rehabilitation Counseling Bulletin* 19 (4): 544–550, 1976. © 1976 by American Personnel and Guidance Association. Reprinted with permission from the publisher and authors.

PERSONAL ACHIEVEMENT SKILLS

As one part of their comprehensive treatment program, five paraplegics and five quadriplegics participated in Personal Achievement Skills (PAS), a personal adjustment program developed by the Arkansas Rehabilitation Research and Training Center. PAS was selected because it emphasizes experiences that reinforce client motivation for recovery from a severe disability (Rabinowitz 1961).

PAS is a structured group counseling program that focuses on an individual's personal awareness in terms of values, capacities, and acceptance of others (i.e., other spinal cord injured) and their needs and on skills in crucial functioning areas, such as communication, problem and goal definition, and constructive action. Since this program focuses on personal functioning, goal identification, and goal achievement within a group setting, PAS can contribute to realism and clarity in aspirations and to the identification of possible alternatives for one's life, both of which have been related to adjustment to paralysis (Kemp & Wetmore 1969–1970; Rabinowitz 1961).

EXPERIENCE WITH PAS

Ten clients in the spinal cord project were randomly assigned to PAS and ten to a control group. Self-report measures of psychological adjustment were administered at the beginning of the project and scheduled for readministration at the end. However, the program evaluation was never completed due to the high rate of attrition in both the experimental and control groups (60% to 80%). Despite the incompletion of the experimental study, the personal adjustment staff gained a deeper insight into the PAS program itself and into the problems in conducting personal adjustment training with the spinal cord injured and the needs of the spinal cord injured in a comprehensive rehabilitation program.

For example, the two students who regularly attended PAS achieved significant goals and improved in rated current adjustment. Each of the participants wrote and completed a goal program. One 20-year-old male, impaired since age 15, developed an independent living goal that included the following phases: (a) find out what I need to do to prepare myself physically, (b) learn the skill I will need to live on my own, (c) practice budgeting and banking, (d) develop friendships away from the Center, (e) move from the Center, and live independently.

Each phase was broken down into specific behavioral steps. For example, in the first phase (find out what I need to do to prepare myself physically), the client listed three steps: (a) talk with four other paraplegics now living independently, (b) talk with physical therapists at the Center to find out if they think I am physically ready, and (c) complete any physical therapy necessary to become physically ready.

Participation in PAS may have only been the catalyst for the client to act on a strong drive toward independence, but that in itself is important for the spinal cord injured. The client registered other changes. He became active in an effort to establish independent living training as part of the regular Center curriculum. His counselor noted a marked drop in minor disciplinary problems and reported that the client was currently living independently in the community.

The other client, injured at age 20, was 23 when he participated in PAS. He had had a history of disdaining "school-type" activities but later realized that he needed to make specific plans for his future. His goal program was a comprehensive one, including the following seven phases: (a) identify available jobs that pay adequately, (b) obtain General Education Diploma certificate, (c) obtain driver's license, (d) enroll in data processing, (e) improve study habits, (f) develop independent living skills, and (g) get a job.

The client received his driver's license and is now enrolled in the GED (General Education Diploma) program and in data processing training. He is also preparing to move into the community.

Although only two clients actually completed the goal-setting phase of the program, eight of the ten involved students requested further group counseling. Those working with the clients in the group session felt that PAS stimulated a need in the clients to share experiences in a meaningful way.

Admittedly, the minimal results regarding the PAS program pertain only to those who completed the program. Furthermore, the goal programs of the two individuals who completed the program may say more about the individuals themselves or about their situation than about the effectiveness of PAS. However, observed changes in personal adjustment and achievement of significant goals in realistic ways reflect an important outcome from these individuals.

IMPLICATIONS FOR PERSONAL
ADJUSTMENT TRAINING

Attendance.   Poor attendance diminishes the impact of any personal adjustment program, particularly one such as PAS, which builds on sequential experiences. Participants in the program missed a number of sessions, mainly for medical reasons. Clients should be screened to ensure that they are medically able to participate in the program.

Student attendance in personal adjustment training also depends on staff commitment to get students to the program on time. The staff must understand the role of personal adjustment training and be convinced of its merit. Attendance is also affected by outside issues, such as family pressures to return home and other family problems. These family problems could be mediated by staff members until the clients complete their facility program.

Personal Adjustment Training.   Dropping out of PAS occurred when students completed other center programs, such as physical therapy or occupational therapy, and left for home. In several cases, the students had not completed the PAS program, which required at least six weeks of participation. Again, involvement in personal adjustment training requires facility-wide commitment to it as an integral treatment element.

Group Cohesion. In any group counseling program, the importance of group cohesion cannot be minimized. Barriers to group cohesion for spinal cord injured clients occur at both psychological and physical levels. The group leader can at least eliminate physical barriers to cohesion early in the group by moving clients from wheelchairs onto comfortable chairs or couches, where they would not have to be overly concerned about what would happen if, for example, a leg bag should break. It is important to keep the wheelchairs convenient to the group training area and to have equipment nearby for problems such as leg bag leaks. Naturally, moving clients from wheelchairs requires someone trained in transferring individuals with different types of spinal cord injury.

Group Composition. In the PAS groups, homogeneity can be a problem. All participants of this group were males of approximately the same age. Group leaders felt that females could have contributed considerably to the group, particularly in the discussions of problems of sexuality. There is also a need for individuals of varied ages, with varying lengths of disability, who could provide insights into the adjustment problems ahead. Heterogeneity regarding age, sex, length of disability, and type of adjustment would provide enriched feedback for group members.

Leader Participation. The leader needs to have (a) leadership abilities in group counseling programs, (b) knowledge of spinal cord injury (e.g., on the effects of different levels of injury), and (c) the ability to recognize and deal with emergency medical situations. Medical assistance should be sought immediately when the leader sees such symptoms as sweating, dizziness, slurred speech, loss of facial color, fainting, and so on.

Screening Interview. At least one screening interview is suggested for discussing purposes and expectations of the group. In the screening interview, the leader can determine the client's interest in a group counseling experience that focuses on communication and goal-setting skills. Clients must be ready to take a realistic look at their capacities and desires so that they can begin to make concrete plans for the future. The screening interview might also determine whether there are any outstanding problems, such as family difficulties, that would make the client's participation unfeasible at the current time.

Program Demands. PAS requires a minimum IQ of 70 to 80 and the ability to read and write. Writing can be a real problem, particularly for quadriplegics. Quadriplegics might tape record their responses to exercises and have these tapes transcribed at the end of the session. Of course, the participants must be assured of confidentiality.

Length of Session.   Since the recommended length of PAS is two to two and one-half hours, the fatigue factor for spinal cord injured clients must be considered. Sessions need to be scheduled after either a morning break or lunch. Conflicts such as those with medical services must be considered in scheduling.

OTHER NEEDS OF THE SPINAL CORD INJURED

Implementing recommendations for improving personal adjustment training for the spinal cord injured can make a significant contribution to the effectiveness of the training. In addition, the following other psychosocial needs of spinal cord injured clients are apparent.

Orientation.   An orientation program for newly admitted spinal cord injured patients might feature a videotape of an individual with a spinal cord injury relating experiences in adjusting to the handicap and in completing a rehabilitation program. The taped presentation might be followed by a group discussion led by a trained leader. Another feature of the orientation program might be a self-help peer counseling approach in which new clients receive orientation and support from clients who have been at the facility for a longer period of time.

Family Counseling.   Family counseling should begin the very first day that the client enters the facility. Immediate family members will need information about the individual's medical needs, some insight into how to communicate effectively, and orientation as to how they can help the individual deal with his or her disability. The clients and their spouses also need sexual counseling and training. Facility staff need to recognize that family counseling is not a "one-shot" contact but rather requires continual attention to the client and the family throughout the rehabilitation process.

Sequence of Counseling Experience.   The effect of a sequence of counseling experiences might be investigated with the spinal cord injured. The initial experience might be one of involving PAS with a group that is homogeneous as to disability. The homogeneity of the group might allow participants to establish a sense of common bond and group identity. After completion of the PAS group, participants might move to a group counseling experience involving individuals with a variety of disabilities. The mixed group experience would enable individuals with the spinal cord injury to deal with attitudes toward themselves, attitudes toward others, and perceived reactions of others. It is essential that individuals preparing to depart from the center work with an individual counselor on applying the techniques of goal setting to life situations beyond the facility.

Independent Living Training.   Clients obviously need instruction in the area of independent living, which involves such problems as judging an apartment's suitability, budgeting, home safety, self-care, community resources, architectural barriers, driver's training, and the like.

Vocational Training Opportunities. There is a desperate need for additional vocational training opportunities for the spinal cord injured. In many cases, identifying appropriate vocational opportunities may require facility personnel to visit work sites in order to investigate jobs suitable for the spinal cord injured. Personnel might then return to the facility and modify existing training programs to prepare the client for such jobs. Vocational training should (a) establish on-the-job training as much as possible and (b) try to return the individual to an occupation similar to the pre-injury type of work.

Recreation and Leisure Time Training. Clients need help in identifying satisfying and creative ways to use the period during the day when they are not working or sleeping. Developing habits of creative use of leisure time requires reinforcement of participation in facility activities as well as assistance to the individual after leaving the facility.

Physical Fitness Training. Staff members also noted that several clients requested access to physical fitness equipment in the evenings in order to include additional physical conditioning in their recreational programs. Such clients might profit from a systematic physical fitness program described by Bolton and Milligan (1976) that is currently being adapted for the spinal cord injured by Milligan.

CONCLUSION

In essense, personal adjustment training for the spinal cord injured requires a sound approach to building an acceptance of the disability and to developing a goal-oriented approach to life. PAS is one such training approach; it attempts to teach clients communication and goal-setting skills in the context of group counseling.

But in order for PAS or any personal adjustment training to be successful, it must be implemented with due care given to such issues as group cohesion, attendance, screening, staff commitment, leader training, and the like. A properly developed training experience coupled with necessary support services, such as family counseling, leisure time, and vocational and fitness training, can increase the likelihood of successful rehabilitation.

REFERENCES

Richard Roessler is Associate Professor and Tim Milligan is a training assistant, both at the Arkansas Rehabilitation Research and Training Center, University of Arkansas, Fayetteville. Ann Ohlson is a counselor in the Spinal Cord Injured Project, Hot Springs Rehabilitation Center, Hot Springs, Arkansas.

Abramson, A. S. Modern concepts of management of the patient with spinal cord injury. *Archives of Physical Medicine and Rehabilitation,* 1967, *48,* 113–121.

Bolton, B., and Milligan, T. The effects of a systematic physical fitness program on clients in a comprehensive rehabilitation center. *American Corrective Therapy Journal,* 1976, March-April.

Bors, E. The challenge of quadriplegia. *Bulletin of the Los Angeles Neurological Society,* 1956, *21,* 105–123.

Kemp, B., and Wetmore, C. Adjustment factors among spinal cord injury patients: A follow-up study. University of Southern California Rehabilitation Research and Training Center Research Report, Los Angeles, 1969–1970.

Margolin, R. J. Motivational problems and resolutions in the rehabilitation of paraplegics and quadriplegics, *American Archives of Rehabilitation Therapy,* 1971, *20,* 95–103.

O'Connor, J. R., and Leitner, L. A. Traumatic quadriplegia: A comprehensive review. *Journal of Rehabilitation,* 1971, *37,* 14–20.

Rabinowitz, H. Motivation for recovery: Four social-psychologic aspects. *Archives of Physical Medicine and Rehabilitation,* 1961, *42,* 799–807.

9

Group Psychotherapy with a Paraplegic Group, with an Emphasis on Specific Problems of Sexuality

SAMBHU N. BANIK, Ph.D., and MARTIN A. MENDELSON, Ph.D.

IN August, 1974, the mental health division of Glenn Dale Hospital, a chronic disease hospital under the District of Columbia Department of Human Resources, was requested to provide some form of psychotherapy to a group of young paraplegic and quadriplegic patients. The average age of the patients was 24 years, in contrast to the majority of patients at Glenn Dale Hospital whose average age is approximately 50 years. This meant that this group of patients had lost the use of their limbs at an early age, often as adolescents or young adults, which drastically cut them off from ever experiencing the satisfaction of "normal" sexual, social, and economic lifestyles and arrested them in midstream in the kinds of activities leading to social and emotional maturation. Unlike some of the older patients who had experienced to some degree life's satisfactions and gratifications, the

Reprinted by permission of the American Group Psychotherapy Association from the *International Journal of Group Psychotherapy* 28 (1): 123–128, 1978.

young paraplegic group had been severely limited in the opportunity to gain such experiences. The younger paraplegic patient's frustration at being confined in a hospital, immobile at an age when able-bodied young adults are actively coping with the problems of life, had given rise to frequent conflicts with staff and peers. Although the medical treatment was up-to-date and relevant and the physical rehabilitative services provided were comprehensive and effective, it was clear that the psychological and emotional needs of the young paraplegic patients were not being met since the young paraplegic group engaged in considerable "acting-out" behavior, involving aggression, hostility, and anger, on the wards. Interested nurses and medical personnel consequently requested that staff of the Mental Health Division intervene to provide psychotherapy, group or individual, and to develop an effective therapeutic milieu for resolving these burgeoning disorders. It was hoped that a treatment program specifically designed for these patients would have the following benefits:

1. Development of more mature and adaptive modes of behavior on the part of the patients, considering the nature of their handicapping physical disorders.
2. Instillation in the patients of a desire to cope with institutional life in a more realistic and mature manner, which could perhaps then combat feelings of acute depression, anxiety, isolation, and insecurity.
3. Motivation of patients to take full advantage of the rehabilitation facilities available and set realistic goals of recovery in relation to the nature of their spinal cord injuries.
4. Increase communication between hospital staff and patient, thus avoiding conflicts arising out of misperceptions and omissions of items of information.

DESCRIPTION OF SUBJECTS

The average age of the 17 patients in this group was 24 years, with the range extending between 17 and 40 years. All but one of the patients, a female, were black. Of the 17 patients, three were currently married, eight were single, and six had been married but were either separated or divorced. All of the patients were confined to wheelchairs and had varying use of their upper bodies and arms. Some could engage in tasks requiring gross motor functions, while others were capable of performing tasks requiring fine motor functions as well. The group initially consisted of five females and 12 males. Most of the patients were able to manipulate their wheelchairs with their arms; however, several of the patients, particularly one male and one female, had wheelchairs equipped with small, electrically powered engines. One other patient stood out from the group as being so severely handicapped that he was confined virtually all of the time to a Stryker frame and required repositioning of his body from time to time to avoid bedsores. Virtually all of the patients were from a deprived socioeconomic background.

ESTABLISHMENT OF A PROGRAM OF
GROUP PSYCHOTHERAPY

One of the major concerns expressed by the patient group to the nurses was their inability to engage in sexual relations. Up to this time the patients had received very little in the way of information about this crucial area. The nurses requested, therefore, that initially the Mental Health Division staff conduct discussions about human sexuality relevant to the special problems of cord-injured patients. A review of the literature was initiated through the National Institute of Health library. Needless to say, the amount of material uncovered was quite sparse; nevertheless, the authors of this study were able to develop a comprehensive set of instructional materials for discussion with the group.

The group met once a week on Thursday afternoons in the auditorium of the hospital. Each session lasted for approximately two hours. The wheelchairs were arranged by the patients in a circle, with the staff members of the hospital making up a part of the circle. This arrangement seemed to be most productive and stimulated group interaction and communication.

The first problem tackled by the group was the election of patients to serve as "officers" of the group. A chairman, vice-chairman, secretary-treasurer, and sergeant-at-arms were elected from among the group in a democratic fashion. The second problem was the choice of a name for the group; it was overwhelmingly decided by the group to designate themselves as the "Action on Wheels Group."

At this first meeting the authors briefed the patients about their functions as staff members, emphasizing that they intended to work with the group on psychological and emotional problems that might arise during their stay at the hospital and, in addition, would assist them in preparing to adjust to the outside world prior to their discharge from the hospital. Several of the patients raised issues about procuring money through the establishment of small businesses in the hospital itself; unfortunately, District of Columbia regulations did not permit this kind of activity on the part of hospital patients. Other matters taken up by the group during the first session concerned a lack of appropriate recreational facilities, the availability of good and current movies, and, the most important problem of all, the lack of information on the sexuality of the typical paraplegic or cord-injured patient. It became clear, as the session went on, that some of the older paraplegic patients had attempted to educate the younger patients about sexual matters in general and that the older patients were deriving tremendous ego satisfaction from acting as "experts" in the area of sexuality. Although such interaction was mutually beneficial, a substantial amount of misinformation was being communicated. For example, one of the erroneous generalizations dealt with the use of various kinds of aphrodisiacs guaranteed to enable the male paraplegic to achieve erection and intercourse.

The authors were able to establish very good rapport with the group as a whole. Street language describing various kinds of sexual activities was encouraged rather than the usual Latin terminology, and every attempt was made to create an atmosphere of free expression. Presentations were made relating to the psychophysiology of sex, with an emphasis on individual differences. The authors translated the technical terms found in the professional journals into comprehensible terms to promote group understanding, and several filmstrips about normal human sexuality involving cord-injured patients were shown to the group. The members were encouraged to express their own feelings and emotions in relation to their being handicapped sexually. Their concerns can be exemplified in the statement made by one member that six months after his injury he still was not able to have an erection and, furthermore, that he did not have any kinesthetic sensation while urinating. This patient raised the question of how he would derive sexual satisfaction from ejaculation when he did not experience any sensation in his penis from urination. Discussion centered around the question of how one could have satisfactory intercourse without being able to ejaculate or experience orgasm. The group also explored among themselves various alternative means of sexual satisfaction besides "normal" and "acceptable" sexual behavior, e.g., fellatio, cunnilingus, etc. The patient group, under the guidance of the cotherapists, arrived at the concensus that the quality of the relationship between sexual partners was of great importance in adjusting to other modes of sexual behavior. It was emphasized that empathic understanding on the part of the spouse or friend played a vital role in the nature of any sexual relationship and that this was even more so when one or both parties were physically handicapped. Some group members expressed intense fears that they would be rejected by their spouses if they could not function satisfactorily, thus making them feel their inadequacy even more acutely than they already did. Several members felt that sexual relations with a prostitute should be considered as a means of improving their sexual abilities, with the hope that any improvement would carry over to the future spouse or girl friend.

The female members of the group, in contrast to the male, were reluctant to discuss their sexual problems, if any. They exhibited a tendency to hold back and feel uncomfortable when sexual matters were discussed, as evidenced by the fact that they rarely used street language during the discussion. One female member hinted that she was having no problem in sexual intercourse and that she was hoping to conceive a child. Another female member indicated that, other than a minor adjustment in previous sexual positions, she did not have any problem. It might have been that the female members were inhibited because of cultural stereotypes about sex (e.g., It's not "ladylike") or they might have been afraid to express themselves freely for fear it would be taken as an indication that they were readily available for casual sexual encounters. In any event, sex seemed to be primarily a male problem in this group of severely handicapped patients since sexual intercourse requires a penile erection and penetration whereas the female generally plays a "receptive" role.

Through presentation and discussion of sex-related movies and technical materials, many misgivings and fallacies about sexual habits and behaviors were resolved and positive changes in behavior, such as less anxiety, less conflict, etc., were noted on the ward. Nursing personnel, in informal discussions with the authors, commented on the improvement in their relationships with the patients. There was a reduction in chronic tension and anxiety, and significant improvement in communication between nursing staff and patients was observed.

The authors feel that sex education among such groups as the chronically ill or elderly should be part of any successful therapeutic program in a hospital or institution. Unfortunately, sexual behavior in any form is considered to be taboo in many hospitals, but turning away from discussion of such a vital area as human sexuality only serves to exacerbate the anxiety or maladjustment of the patient.

Dr. Mendelson is Chief and Dr. Banik, Assistant Chief, Mental Health Division, Glendale Hospital, Glendale, Maryland.

10

Group Therapy with Severely Handicapped
—ALLEN E. SUSSMAN, Ph.D.

WHILE at the Community Mental Health Center in New York City, several counseling and therapy groups were initiated. Among these, a pilot, and highly experimental, group therapy program was set up and geared to a special group of eight deaf individuals.

CLIENT CHARACTERISTICS

This particular group was made up of the so-called multiply-handicapped, extremely low-verbal, and socially disadvantaged late adolescents and young adults. The age range was 18–23. Some were diagnosed as having minimal brain dysfunction (MBD) with attendant behavior disorders, serious interpersonal relationship problems and overall poor life adjustment patterns. All had extremely poor communication skills and limited facility with the sign language.

This group comprised six males and two females. Three were Puerto Ricans with practically no formal education; they resided in "El Barrio," or what is known as Spanish Harlem in New York City. One was black, and came from a large fatherless family living in a tenement building located in

Reprinted by permission of the Professional Rehabilitation Workers with Adult Deaf, from the *Journal of Rehabilitation of the Deaf* 8: 122–126, 1974.

an East Bronx ghetto area. The remaining five were caucasians, with families representing the poor to lower middle class socioeconomic ranges.

Among five clients, the following physical disabilities were represented: retinitis pigmentosa, cerebral palsy, epilepsy, and borderline mental retardation. The remaining three had no physical disability other than early profound deafness. At one time or other five clients were seen by psychiatrists at other psychiatric facilities and put on medication, the regimen of which was not adhered to.

Three clients had poor work histories; at that time not one was able to hold onto a job for more than four weeks. Three were in "extended evaluation" or P.A.T. programs at different rehabilitation centers. One had "bombed out" from a sheltered workshop facility due to behavior problems. In all, five clients had had no prior actual work history. Collectively, they were considered by the DVR as not being feasible for rehabilitation services other than prolonged and protracted "evaluation."

In essence, these deaf individuals were rehabilitation rejects. One might say that referral to the Community Mental Health Center was a last gasp effort.

ORGANIZING THE GROUP

After individual interviewing and diagnostic sessions with each client, and at times, with family members, the eight clients were selected for the experimental group from a list of eighteen potential candidates.

At the very outset, a brief orientation as to the purposes of the group was given to each client. It was also made clear to each that attendance was voluntary, and that one was free to withdraw if he so desired. Much time was given to explaining direction and use of public transportation to and from the Center. For some of the clients, independent traveling was a new, strange, and oftentimes frightening, experience. Compounding the problem was resistance from parents, social workers and rehabilitation counselors who felt that some of the clients were unable to learn to use public transportation on an independent basis. Further, they wanted attendance to be on a mandatory basis, and that clients be accompanied while traveling to and from the Center. A compromise was effected in that clients not used to traveling independently be accompanied to the first session only. Voluntary attendance was agreed upon only after the need for each client not to be coerced was fully elaborated.

The group met once weekly. However, it was during the very first session that the clients were given the opportunity to decide the length of each session. They decided on one hour. The group met for 28 sessions, spanning 30 weeks.

THE FIRST FOUR SESSIONS

Admittedly, the group got off to an inauspicious start. There were so many idiosyncratic personalities; petulant and truculent behavior had to be contended with; explosive outbursts had to be handled carefully; stark apathy called for patient and gentle prodding; irrelevant and incoherent chatter impeded movement; diverse esoteric, arcanic and culturally-based communication styles did not make for meaningful group communication, not to mention a host of other difficulties.

The therapist did not want the group to become unwieldy "meeting sessions" that is characteristic of a get-together, with each client functioning as an isolate. He wanted it to be an interacting, ventilating, listening, learning, anxiety-reducing, constructive, and supportive group. In short, he wanted it to be a therapeutic group in which behavior and attitude change could occur. He also wanted the group to communicate with one another and to interact *meaningfully.* Above all, he desired for each member to fully understand *why* they were there and what the therapist was trying to do.

DEVELOPMENTS

After much experimentation, it devolved that very rudimentary sign language, liberally interspersed with pantomime, gestures, gesticulations, and subtle nuances in nonverbal language were quite effective in establishing intra-group communication.

With time, the group afforded each member, including the therapist, the opportunity to learn from one another's own communication styles, including home-made sign language. After some initial resistance and ridicule, each client came to readily accept and use sign language and other communication modes others were most comfortable with. (At this juncture Dr. Sussman gave a graphic demonstration of some of the signs and nonverbal language used within this group.)

It was found that *psychodrama,* involving considerable *role-playing* and *reverse role-playing,* was most effective in the gaining of understanding and insight, and in bringing about perceptual, attitude and behavior change.

Acting out of thoughts and feelings proved to be efficacious compensation for verbal expression on both intellectual and affective levels. For example, when a client could not express his feelings "verbally," he would put to use what he had by then learned, namely, to act out his feelings, giving a very lucid and illustrative demonstration of how he was feeling at the moment, or how he had felt during a certain past experience. (Dr. Sussman then proceeded to demonstrate, giving examples of feelings as were acted out by the group members.)

During the early stages of the group experience, however, certain clients evinced difficulty in acting out their feelings, whereupon the therapist, borrowing techniques from "Graffiti Therapy," in drawing on the portable blackboard simple faces, each depicting an emotion, e.g., happy, joyous, angry, sad, nonchalant, puzzlement. Each face is relatively simple to draw in that the circle is the head, two dots the eyes, a slash in the middle the nose; horizontal line the mouth — the type one sees on "Happy Buttons."

The client would point out to the face on the blackboard that most accurately reflects his feelings. In later sessions, the client himself would draw "feeling faces" to show how he was feeling at the moment or how he felt under particular past circumstances. Eventually, the clients themselves added variations such as the lifted eyebrow or gnashing teeth, thus broadening the spectrum of feelings and reactions. (Dr. Sussman turned to the blackboard and drew such feeling faces in way of illustration.)

The blackboard faces greatly facilitated the group's movement onto the affective level. Subsequently, all clients were able to dispense with the blackboard faces for, by then they were able to rely exclusively on themselves to identify and describe their feelings through the sign language, nonverbal and subverbal channels.

A most significant development was each client's understanding of the sign for "feeling," and consequently were able to respond to the highly abstract question "How do you feel. . . ?" This alone was a tremendous development in that the group was then able to discuss, and analyze feelings as expressed by self and others.

It was only until after such breakthroughs were achieved that the group began to "jell" in that it began to function as a therapeutic group. Corollary to this, interaction intensified: individual clients became less destructive and more constructive and supporting; give-and-take relationships increased; spontaneity accelerated. And, best of all, the clients were beginning to enjoy themselves.

CONTENT AND TOPICS

The sessions dealt largely with hypothetical as well as real-life, everyday situations, with clients having a go at demonstrating what they thought they actually did and what they should have done. There was considerable re-enactment of "scenes" in which clients acted out their roles and corresponding thought and feelings.

Through the mechanism of reverse role-playing or role switches, clients could learn from one another how they could have behaved differently. There was ample opportunity for the various corresponding reactions or consequences to be demonstrated. Thus the concept of *relationship* could be introduced, that is, a client then was able to perceive the association between his behavior and the elicited consequences. With the help of the "cast," the client would be permitted to test old response patterns against newer ones suggested by the group, and to compare differential results. A lively *analytical* discussion would usually follow, with an increasing number of constructive alternate behaviors thrown in for good measure. Thus, one could witness a growing repertoire of social skills that could be employed in actual situations outside the group. From time to time, a group member, through role-playing, would report back to the group the results of his attempt to apply what he had learned in the group to actual situations. If the client was unsuccessful, the group would empathize with him, support his efforts and make further suggestions. Should he succeed, he would receive praise and encouragement.

It is pertinent to point out that the therapist remained non-judgmental at all times. If he felt he had to point out undesirable behavior and attendant results (for the clients were woefully impoverished in social experience and skills), he merely would suggest, something like this: "You did this . . . and she got angry with you, right? Say, would it be better if you did it that way? Let us try it out." Then the therapist would play roles himself, with a supporting cast, and conclude with "Well, what do you think?" This way, the therapist pointed out undesirable behavior and its consequence and "taught" new behaviors by offering suggestions. And, at all times, the client was free to accept or reject, or to improve or modify what was suggested. The therapist took extreme care not to give the impression that he was criticizing or "teaching." Of course, and almost invariably, communication by therapist constituted an amalgam of sign language, gestures, pantomime, etc.

It is significant in that, when the members of the group learned to act out their thoughts and feelings, and to generally express themselves better by whatever communication avenues were open to them, they were better able to touch upon thoughts and feelings relative to their early childhood experiences, relationships with parents, family members, and with other people. This in turn opened up valuable diagnostic channels for the therapist, and lent to his greater understanding of each group member.

Further progress was noted in that each client was able to openly talk about their disabilities other than deafness. For example, one client, for the first time in his life, discussed his epileptic condition, and the abject embarrassment of having seizures in public. Because he opened up, the therapist learned that he had not faithfully taken medication to control his seizures. It was soon discovered that he hadn't taken the medication because he did not know what it was for! After a painstaking explanation of the function of the medication, and after supportive admonishment and encouragement from the group, the client went back on medication, took it faithfully. He also learned to secure from the physician prescription renewal and to have it refilled at the pharmacy. His family was pleased to note this new self-responsibility in him, the results of which was a diminution of and milder epileptic attacks.

Group topics included sex, sexual relations between male and female, homosexuality, dating, marriage, and children. The group showed keen interest in drug use and abuse since some of the clients resided in areas infested with drug addicts and pushers. A burning issue with the group was attitudes of society toward the physically disabled, particularly deaf people; all of the clients had at one time or another suffered ridicule, ostracism, and discrimination by the nondisabled. The world of work was broached and encompassed the role of vocational rehabilitation, vocational training, occupations, work attitudes and habits.

To be sure, ventilating sessions abounded, but particular gripe sessions were given over to the clients' complaints about rehabilitation counselors, other rehabilitation personnel, psychologists, psychiatrists, and social workers. Perceived shoddy treatment by those professionals and their inability to communicate with deaf people were predominant themes. Nonetheless, some of the clients waxed retrospective, recounting their "failures" on the job and in DVR-sponsored training and evaluation programs.

RECAPITULATION

The group therapy was an unique experience in more ways than one for those eight severely handicapped deaf individuals. One aspect of the experiential tapestry, however, should be pointed out. The group afforded each member to be themselves, apparently for the first time in their lives. Accustomed to a life style of regimentation, overprotection, rejection, neglect, and having other people do things, speak, and think for them, they found the predominantly *nondirective* atmosphere of the group somewhat unsettling at first, to be sure. The clients never had so much freedom: freedom to talk about what was on their minds without fear of censure. Not to be criticized for their feelings was indeed a strange experience.

As with group therapy in general, this one was not without psychological pain for its members. Nonetheless, each client, in his own fashion, learned to accept such pain as being necessary for improvement and change. Instead of destructive feedback from his fellow group members, he found respect, acceptance, understanding, empathy and support. When criticism was due, it was given in a constructive manner; each client had by then learned that one is more responsive to gentle and supportive criticism . . . they also learned the power of positive reinforcement when due.

During the fifth session, the group members complained that one hour was insufficient and requested an additional half-hour. This was granted. Around the fifteenth session, the group pointed out that they met only once a week and felt that they needed two hours. This, too, was granted. However, all fought and protested against the impending termination of the group. The last three sessions were given over to the phasing-out process; discussion revolved around what had happened within the group, what each member had learned, observable changes in individuals, and what the group generally meant to each client. During this phase, each member became increasingly retrospective and introspective, and compared their former selves with their present selves.

Interestingly, attendance, which was spotty at the beginning, became impeccable from the fifth session on. Only illness precluded attendance. Punctuality became ritual with each group member.

Around the seventeenth session, the clients became more active; the therapist less active. They required less prodding; spontaneity increased by leaps and bounds. They would take the initiative by opening discussion rather than wait for the therapist to do so. They would stage *role-playing*, entirely on their own, assigning roles, switching roles, and directing "scenes." The director-client even would assign to the therapist a specific role for him to play.

A FINAL WORD

This group of eight individuals represents severely handicapped deaf people generally considered by educators, rehabilitation counselors, psychologists, psychiatrists and authorities in deafness to be the most difficult of deaf people to work with. This therapist would concur, but only up to a point. While it is a difficult task, it is *not* impossible. And he is of the opinion that group counseling or therapy can be effective with such a population group. True, it is an enormous challenge, and necessitates the marshaling of every resource within the therapist and resources at his disposal. But the greatest resource is within the client himself, and his innate *desire* for self-improvement and enhancement. It is believed that we are on the threshold of developing practical and workable therapeutic techniques and approaches with what after all may not be so difficult a population group.

Still, the key lies with the therapist himself. This therapist suggests the following basic ingredients: high-level training in group counseling and therapy; ability to communicate with the deaf individual according to his conceptual level and within his perceptual world. Also needed is an inordinate amount of patience, perseverance, and doggedness in the teeth of frustration and setbacks. Further, he should possess characteristics such as willingness to experiment, to be creative—and even daring—at times. On top of these, he should have the ability to learn from failure as well as success. Finally, he should be on the ready to learn from the clients themselves. They have so much to teach us. This therapist has learned so much from the group of eight deaf individuals. He is very grateful to them.

This presentation is based on Dr. Sussman's 1972–73 experience with one certain group of severely handicapped deaf clients at Maimonides Medical Center's Community Mental Health Center, where he formerly served as director of its Psychological and Mental Health Services for the Deaf. Dr. Sussman is currently Assistant Professor of Counseling with the Department of Counseling at Gallaudet College's Graduate School. Dr. Sussman continues to do extensive group counseling on the college campus and, as psychological consultant, group therapy with deaf clients at the Maryland Rehabilitation Center in Baltimore.

11

Psychopathology Associated with Myasthenia Gravis and its Treatment by Psychotherapeutically Oriented Group Counseling —MELVIN L. SCHWARTZ and ROBERT CAHILL

M YASTHENIA gravis is a neuromuscular condition characterized by progressive muscular weakness upon exertion. By nature of this symptomatic presentation it can frequently be confused with syndromes such as chronic fatigue, peripheral myopathy, metabolic deficiency, and brain stem and extrapyramidal disorder. Even when such simulators can be ruled out, there still remains the differential diagnostic task of distinguishing between MG and psychoneurosis, particularly of the hysterical or conversion reaction type. Fullerton and Munsat[1] have described seven cases of pseudo-myasthenia gravis based upon diagnosis by physical and psychiatric history, clinical examination and laboratory work-up. These authors concluded that there is a particular constellation of factors which make the pseudo-myasthenic state unique. They found a clear history of previous conversion reactions in their patients as well as hysterical stigmata such as globus hystericus, fainting, urinary retention, dyspareunia and headaches. One group of investigators[2] reported as a further diagnostic complication the fact that 7 of 25 Ss in their sample had the onset of their illness at a time of distinct psychic stress. Similarly, Schwab and Perlo[3] have detailed several specific sources of error in making a proper diagnosis, including incorrect evaluation of the history and physical findings, incorrect interpretation of the Prostigmin or Tensilon tests, incorrect interpretation of response to oral anticholinesterian medication and false positive Tensilon and Prostigmin tests. Despite these differential diagnostic problems, several factors do exist which enable positive diagnosis of MG. Usually the muscles of the neck, shoulder girdles, upper limbs and flexors of the hips are more frequently involved than those of the lumbar area, abdomen and legs below the knees. Furthermore, the MG patient usually has his abnormalities confined to muscle, without involvement of the central or peripheral nervous system.[4]

From the opposite point of view, when in fact the disease has been correctly diagnosed, a perusal of the case history may often reveal that the patient was initially referred for psychiatric consultation at a rather early stage in the diagnostic work-up. Meyer[5] has reported that 20 per cent of his sample of 99 patients had such consultation prior to final diagnosis. Therefore, it can be seen that patients with confirmed diagnoses are certainly not immune from emotional disorders. Furthermore, upon the establishment of an accurate diagnosis of MG, the patient frequently presents difficulties in psychological management. MacKenzie *et al*[2] found 11 Ss (44 per cent) exhibiting major difficulty in adapting to their illness. These may occur secondarily to learning of the diagnosis, or more importantly, secondarily to adjustment to living with a chronic and partially disabling disorder. Although there are several case reports and subjective observations bearing upon mental difficulties occurring in treatment of patients,[6,7] the present authors were unable to find any detailed empirical evaluations of the psychopathology associated with the condition. The illumination of this associated psychopathology was, therefore, taken as a major purpose of this investigation.

The prevalence of psychopathology in MG patients can only be very inaccurately estimated from a perusal of the literature. These estimates are subject, of course, to several sources of bias among which are the method of report (case history information, etc.), as well as the particular emphasis or deemphasis placed upon personality dysfunction by the diagnostician. Nevertheless, Meyer[5] has reported that in addition to the 20 per cent of patients who had earlier psychiatric consultation, another additional 28 per cent had significant emotional problems as had been judged from notations in their clinical charts. Grob[8] has reported that 20 per cent of his sample had emotional problems. With such sparse literature, it would, therefore, seem that the range of 20–50 per cent would approximate the prevalence of MG patients with emotional difficulties subject, of course, to the aforementioned, as well as some unmentioned source of error.

If appropriate treatment of the patient's total disorder is to ensue, it then becomes essential to study the specific nature of these emotional components of MG. There are no attempts in the literature to specify any personality profile which might be common to MG patients. In fact, the only substantial evidence of a statistical variety pertaining to the interrelationship of MG and personality disorder, other than that already cited, is the report by Meyer[5] of a higher mortality rate (particularly in younger patients) among those patients with significant emotional disorder. Much more often, the literature has provided clues as to the nature of the psychodynamics operating in individual patients. Most authors who have addressed the problem of evaluating the psychodynamics of their patients have concerned themselves with the problem of overall adjustment to the disability and cooperation with medication regimes. For example, Chafetz[9] has noted that increase in dosage seems to be perceived by the patient as a worsening in his condition. On the other hand, Chafetz also noted that a decrease in prescribed dosage levels may be perceived by the patient as a threat to his control over the manifest symptomatology.

In considering the overall psychological adjustment of the patient to his disease, Osserman[10] reported that there are two types of personalities who tend to adjust rather poorly. He has labeled these as the dependent person with marked ambivalence about his dependency and the super-independent person. Similarly, Chafetz[9] in commenting upon dependency problems has noted that patients may frequently wish that they had more observable symptoms so that acquaintances would not think them to be lazy, crazy, or more importantly, faking. He also found that the patients who cooperate best in treatment are those who deny their dependency needs. Still on the issue of dependency, Brolley and Hollender[11] have observed that patients who try to be independent are prone to more serious psychological setbacks in the face of exacerbations in the disease.

The role of the physician in contributing to problems with dependency has not gone unnoticed. Goss[12] has reported that the physician may occasionally join the patient in denying the existence of physical and/or emotional problems. On the other hand, he goes on to say that if the physician feels helpless in treating the disease, he may be too much the nurse to the patient. In summary, then, viewing these reports of dependency problems of MG patients, it seems clear that their psychodynamics are not unlike those of patients with other disabling conditions characterized by necessary limitations of physical activity. Hence, one would not necessarily expect to find a particular configuration of personality traits and/or disturbances which would differentially characterize the patient with MG. Nevertheless, the review of psychodynamics, as well as the data reported on prevalence of emotional disorders in MG, certainly suggest that it would be valuable to conduct an empirical investigation of the emotional components of the disease and to attempt to modify these problems in a therapeutic setting, which was the second major purpose of this investigation.

METHOD

The local Myasthenia Gravis Association chapter contacted the senior author to consider the possibility of instituting a counseling program for its patients. The need for the program arose primarily out of the requests to the organization from many patients who desired to discuss their psychological problems. As a result, a pilot project was developed with two primary aims: (1) to evaluate the nature of the psychopathology manifested by these patients; and (2) to conduct a series of counseling sessions devoted to helping patients attain a more satisfactory adjustment to their disease.

SUBJECTS

The Ss were two groups of MG patients, comprising a total of 17 patients. Group I consisted of 11 Ss who were solicited from the rolls of approximately 150 diagnosed MG patients maintained by the association. Each patient was sent a letter briefly describing the aim of the project and asking his cooperation. Replies were received from 12 patients, 11 of whom (4 male and 7 female) were able to concur on a specific time and place for weekly meetings. Background data was elicited via a questionnaire sent to all patients. Subsequently, a second group of 6 patients, 3 male and 3 female, were selected in the same manner, as an extension of therapeutic services seemed both feasible and realistic, given the success achieved with the first group.

The mean age of all Ss (n=17) was 44.6 yr (range 24–66 yr) and they had a mean educational level of 12.7 yr of school completed (range: 12–16 yr). There were 7 males and 10 females, a sex ratio very close to what has been reported for the disease. The males were all gainfully employed as were the unmarried females. All of the Ss were married with the exception of six (two separated, two single, one divorced and one widowed). All of the patients resided in a large urban center or one of its surrounding suburbs. They were asked to rate the severity of their myasthenia on a three-point scale with the following results: mild=5; moderate=8; severe=2; two patients preferred not to make a self-rating.

It is difficult to assess the representativeness of this sample in that the patients were volunteers for a counseling program, and, hence, may be self-selected for a higher than average degree of psychopathology. On the other hand, it is conceivable that many patients who had considerable overt psychopathology would find such a program too threatening to their psychic integration and thereby refuse participation. Hence, it would appear that these factors could balance each other, perhaps resulting in a relatively accurate reflection of psychopathology in MG.

Procedure.   Patients were informed that there would be a series of eight 1-hr per week counseling sessons aimed at helping them make a more satisfactory psychological adjustment to their disease. Subsequent on-going evaluation of the project demonstrated the need for extension to an additional eight counseling sessions and all patients were agreeable to a continuation. The sessions were conducted by the authors in the MG Association conference room. They were run in an open-ended manner with encouragement for patients to bring to discussion any matter pertaining to themselves or their disease. The therapists had an eclectic orientation, making use of principles from several therapeutic persuasions, including psychoanalytically-oriented therapy, client-centered therapy and behavior therapy. All sessions were tape recorded with the awareness and approval of each patient.

Personality assessment was conducted during the first session and again after the 16th session. The Minnesota Multiphasic Personality Inventory (MMPI) short form, consisting of 366 true-false items, was given to each patients to take home and to return to the therapist at the next meeting. Questions and feelings about the evaluation were discussed during the first hour when the test was handed out, also at the second hour when patients returned their answer sheets. All patients indicated that their responses were solely their own, given without consultation of other family members or friends.

RESULTS

Findings from the intial MMPI assessment have been previously reported[13] in a brief abstract. The essential finding was that these Ss present MMPI protocols with scale elevations (peak disturbances) similar to those found in patients with medical illness of almost any other variety, i.e. with pathological elevations on Hypochondriasis, Depression, and Hysteria scales. What was somewhat remarkable was the relatively elevated score on the Schizophrenia scale, which we interpreted as more likely reflecting embarrassment, physical limitation, and minimization of social contact, rather than overt or covert psychosis.

However, presentation of such quantitative findings, although quite valuable from the point of view of experimentation, makes only a limited contribution to the actual demonstration of the psychopathology in the daily living situation of the patient. Hence, we also wish to draw upon our clinical observations made during specific counseling sessions to demonstrate some psychodynamic patterns and their variations, as well as the changes in such patterns as a result of psychotherapeutically-oriented counseling.

In order to give a preliminary characterization of the therapeutic changes occurring in the group as a whole, the criterion of the number of MMPI T scores at or above 70 (2 standard deviations above the mean) was used as the index of change from before-to-after counseling. According to this index, of the 13 patients (from both groups) who cooperated with follow-up after 16 sessions, 6 were improved, 5 were unchanged and only 2 were worse. It is interesting to note that of the 5 whose 'change' score remained the same, 3 were patients who had, on initial pre-therapy MMPI, no T scores in the pathology range. Hence, one would not expect that much therapeutic change could be hoped for, or even desired, in such persons. Four patients did not cooperate with MMPI follow-up. Actually, with such small n's, which would be reduced even further by inter-sex comparisons, we feel it to be unwise to present conclusions based on comparison of pre- and post-therapy means until larger samples can be evaluated. In fact, in terms of MMPI measurement, it could be misleading to compare patients in this fashion in that score decreases may not necessarily indicate improvement, but rather the opposite.

We would like to provide specific empirical documentation of improvement based on MMPI changes in one case correlating with a clinically observed improvement.

Case Report—S.O.F. 39-yr-old, white, married, female high school graduate, suburban mother and housewife, rating her own MG as of 'moderate' severity.

By inspection of Table 1, a comparison of pre-therapy scores of this patient with scores after 16 hr of treatment reveal an improvement on *every* MMPI pathology scale with the most marked improvements occurring on

TABLE 1.   *S.O.F.: MMPI K-corrected T-scores at Three*
           Stages in Therapy

	L	F	K	Hs	D	Hy	Pd	Mf	Pa	Pt	Sc	Ma	A*
Pre-therapy:	60	68	57	62	73	72	90	49	79	74	86	63	(6)
After 8 sessions	63	60	49	66	78	70	62	41	62	65	87	63	(3)
After 16 sessions	63	62	51	54	65	61	55	34	50	51	60	50	(0)

*Total of pathology scales with *T* scores over 70, i.e. scores of 2 or
more standard deviations above normal, indicating very high degree
of disturbance on that scale.

the Psychopathic Deviate, Paranoia, Psychasthenia and Schizophrenia
scales. In fact, it can be noted that therapeutic change seemed to be occurring throughout the sessions with some improvement noted even after the
initial 8 hr of counseling. The therapists were pleasantly surprised to note
that following 16 sessions, the patient's MMPI did not have even a single
score in the range of values characteristic of serious psychopathology.

Clinically, the woman initially presented to the group as an intense but
withdrawn, superficially feeling person. Her initial problems revolved
around guilt feelings which had been stimulated by the dependent position
in which she found herself as a result of acquiring the disease. Subsequently, she reported that she had been beaten and robbed in the weeks just prior
to the onset of her disease. Her associations in therapy suggested that this
event had also had considerable sexual meaning for her and that it carried a
hostile charge which then manifested itself in decreased sexual interest and
increased hostility toward her spouse. In the course of therapy, and in
response to the patient's own inquiry, it was indicated that it was extremely
unlikely that the incident was of any etiological significance in her disease.
Upon noting this lack of connection very early in therapy (session 3), the
patient became considerably less anxious and more communicative. She
regularly cited instances of increased socialization, both with friends, family
and with other patients; furthermore, she reported briefer and more infrequent bouts of both depression and feelings of passivity.

DISCUSSION

(a) Methodological Considerations.   The results of this investigation are
only preliminary in nature. They, nevertheless, suggest that group counseling seems to be an effective method for helping patients cope more effectively with the psychological difficulties stemming from Myasthenia Gravis.
However, certain reservations must be noted so as not to allow an un-
critical acceptance of these findings.

From an experimental point of view, the present study did not employ
any control groups. Rather than view this as a methodological oversight,
the authors viewed the research as a demonstration or pilot project undertaken with patients having a disease with psychological concomitants about
which little had been understood. Also, the question of the stability of the

findings over time can be raised. At this point, we do not have any follow-up data to report; however, we do intend to follow these patients at yearly intervals. Other limitations of the present study which can be overcome in subsequent investigations are the relatively small number of subjects, the use of only a single measure in personality assessment, the choice of criterion for therapeutic change, and the interaction of neurological deficit, chronicity, and medication levels with the psychopathology. Also, it is very difficult, if not impossible, to get accurate pre-morbid personality assessment of such individuals to use as a baseline for the study of personality changes induced by the myasthenic state. Finally, although not necessarily a limiting methodological factor, but of considerable interest, would be a very cautious comparison of personality function of MG patients with patients having diseases with some similar manifest organic pathology such as multiple sclerosis and various neuromyopathies.

(b) Myasthenia Gravis and Modification by Group Counseling: Psychodynamics. In the course of the therapeutic sessions, the most important psychological configuration observed in the Myasthenia Gravis patient involves his manner of coping with pressing dependency needs. He is directly confronted with a relative loss of autonomy or self-sufficiency, and this situation certainly threatens whatever image he has of himself as being an adequate, healthy person with mastery over his own behavior. To the degree that the MG patient may have already felt threatened in this respect, owing either to particular personality defects or to psychological conflicts of a neurotic or psychotic nature, this confrontation may be seriously disturbing. Yet even those relatively free of emotional symptoms would be expected to have a difficult time adjusting to this illness, and, in fact, this is seen to be the case. Our impressions about dependency dynamics seem, therefore, to concur with those of Osserman.[10]

Though an evaluation of pre-morbid psychological health could be made only in retrospect and only through what was reported by the patients themselves during the group sessions, it was apparent that many of them had attained a relative degree of emotional maturity and stability preceding the onset of the symptoms of myasthenia gravis. One group member, for instance, spoke of his long-time employment at a hospital as having been highly gratifying, and, even more significant, were indications that there had existed an extraordinarily good relationship between himself and his wife. Not only did the symptoms of his illness make it impossible for him to continue at his job, but it precipitated feelings of guilt and depression in his having to depend so heavily on his wife. He found himself unable to provide financial support for her and unable to help with many of the household chores. Though he never openly showed any anger or resentment toward her during the group sessions, it was evident that his exaggerated accolades and frequent allusions to the fact that his wife must 'put up with me' thinly disguised some negative feelings toward her which resulted from the distress he felt over his imposed position of dependency.

The group counseling enabled this man to reassess his own worth, since the communications from others in the group were inconsistent with his self-image. He had remained isolated in his home most of the time since contracting the disease, but with the therapy group he felt socially alive again. Near the end of the counseling program, he reported that he and his wife were planning on adopting a child. This decision seemed to reflect to some extent a significant positive change in his sense of self-esteem.

In dealing with the psychological conflicts attendant to MG, the defense mechanism most frequently used was *denial,* i.e. in their behavior or verbalizations the patients would deny the existence of physical symptoms, the severity of these symptoms, or the emotional stress experienced as a result of the physical symptoms. On the latter issue, a young man who had only recently discovered that he had myasthenia gravis was never able to focus on the very intense feelings he was experiencing, but spent most of his time in the group discussing the varieties and quantity of medication he was using. This particular maneuver occurred very frequently in the groups and was used at one time or another by almost every MG patient seen. The fact that MG patients do require a large and varied medication regimen makes this an especially easy topic to turn to in order to avoid discussing other thoughts or feelings which are fraught with anxiety or depression. At other times, this same patient talked about his hobby, bringing in some of his creations for the group to see. He could not reveal the sources of the anxiety he was overtly exhibiting, even to the extent of initially hiding from the group the fact that he had lost his job. Following a confrontation regarding his feelings about this loss, he stopped coming to the meetings and did not respond to follow-up.

A middle-aged male patient typically denied both physical and psychological aspects of the disease, though he was one of the most verbally active members in the group. When he did discuss the particular problems that a myasthenia gravis patient is faced with, he suggested that much of this had to do with his attitude, as if one could talk himself out of experiencing any physical or emotional disability associated with the disease. Most of the patients revealed that there was a very lengthy adjustment period before they could accept the fact that myasthenia gravis was incurable. An elderly woman who showed a number of religious concerns said that it was 4 or 5 yr before she could admit to herself that there was no cure for the disease. At the other extreme, one member immediately accepted the grave implications of the disease, which represented to her a punishment from God for her sinfulness.

Another serious problem observed in almost all of the MG patients seen in the counseling sessions was a fear of social contact with strangers. Many of the patients indicated that they felt very self-conscious about visible symptoms (such as ptosis and weakness of the facial muscles) which could not be completely controlled by medication, and most of them feared that their symptoms would become more pronounced in social gatherings. From experiences related to the group, it seemed that myasthenic symptoms did in fact become exaggerated for many of them when they were in situations where there were several unfamiliar persons. It was apparent from this and other information provided by group members regarding reactions to stressful experiences that anxiety, either by contributing to muscular fatigue, or through some other mechanism, could lead to a temporary exacerbation of symptoms. Much of the members' fear of socializing can also be attributed to their difficulty, alluded to above, in dealing with dependency needs. Expressions from others of sympathy, pity, or fear were especially upsetting to those patients who did not wish to be perceived as needing help or support from others. On the other hand, many of the counselees would at times also show exaggerated dependent needs, which resulted in their being unable to remove themselves too far from home or spouse for fear that they would have an attack and be left helpless.

An overriding concern for most of the patients who participated in the group counseling program was that a myasthenic crisis could occur at any time and could be severe enough to result in death. The fact that such crises, though infrequent, could occur unpredictably represented a tremendous source of anxiety to the group. Again, in this instance, the defense mechanism of denial was used to help alleviate this anxiety. The patient who had the most difficulty accepting the fact that myasthenia gravis was incurable also reported feeling deeply depressed following the deaths of her parents and brother. These deaths occurred separately during the period she was struggling with her feelings about MG. Other patients also talked about the death of relatives, but their reactions were not as intense. Probably the most anxiety-arousing session was one in which a member mentioned having had a minor crisis the night before. The group was relatively quiet that evening, and it was apparent that this news had depressed them. Such a direct confrontation with the gravity of the disease made it difficult for them to maintain their psychological defenses.

Some interesting comparisons with respect to anticipation of death can be made between MG and other chronic on-going, potentially fatal diseases. MG is frequently accompanied by a lack of pain and hence the patient may not have the constant reminder of illness so common in fatal conditions. Psychologically, therefore, MG would seem to allow for more effective utilization of the protective mechanism of denial. Also, the fact that most patients maintain an ambulatory, non-hospitalized adjustment (excepting those reaching the crisis state) supports this denial. However, although there is less of an immediate life-threatening situation confronting MG patients, they may nevertheless experience massive anxiety due to the ambiguity and lack of predictability of their condition.

Another interesting observation which arose very early in the therapeutic program was the fact that many patients were rarely following their prescribed levels of medication which had been set for them by their physicians. Interestingly, in our patients there was a far greater tendency to increase dosage, rather than to omit the prescribed requirement. One patient who was remarkable in this respect noted that she would uniformly increase her regular dosage whenever she had to leave home to attend a social function, being fearful of an exacerbation of muscle weakness. (In this respect, we would modify Chafetz's[9] finding of correlation between increased dosage and perceived worsening condition to refer to 'potential' worsening and to 'psychological' condition.) This patient, as well as some others, had often noted an increase in symptomatology in situations requiring multiple social interpersonal relationships. We could not clearly determine whether such overdoses were accompanied by disturbing side-effects. Nevertheless, for some patients this behavior obviously had anxiety-reducing properties and hence the anxiety reduction reinforced its continuation. Sufficient warnings about possible toxic reactions by the therapists apparently contained enough noxious value so that most patients discontinued this habit. Of course, without therapeutic intervention, such a habit could generalize to the point where anxiety from any source whatsoever might call forth a dosage increase. The importance of such a possibility is obvious, though most of our patients had *never* discussed their self-imposed dosage changes with anyone, much less their physicians. Having become aware of these factors, some patients began to achieve a much more frank relationship with their physicians

With respect to the literature relating psychopathology to MG as cited earlier, our initial MMPI findings suggested that 8 of our 17 patients (48 per cent) had psychopathology which was of sufficient degree so that either of us, having tested these patients as psychological evaluation referrals, would have recommended psychiatric consultation for them. These estimates are quite close to those reported by Meyer,[5] but somewhat higher than the 20 per cent reported by Grob.[8] Aside from differences in method of assessing psychopathology, self-selection for a group therapy program may be partially responsible for the high figure as compared to the latter investigator's findings. With respect to the number of patients who had previously sought psychiatric consultation, we knew of three cases in our sample, but suspected that the figure was, in reality, somewhat higher.

CONCLUSION

Psychotherapeutically-oriented group counseling can produce empirically verifiable changes in the direction of more positive mental health in selected MG patients. The lack of empirically verifiable positive change in other patients may be due to several factors including the possible inappropriateness of the measuring rod, the MMPI, for those patients, or the limited number of counseling sessions, among other factors. Nevertheless, the authors were encouraged by the continued participation at group meetings of patients who did not improve with respect to the MMPI. It was our subjective impression that these people were beginning to 'warm up' to the counseling and that were the program to be extended beyond 16 hr, the positive changes might have then been measurable. On these bases, it is anticipated that other investigators in MG would consider group counseling as a treatment method for patients with associated psychopathology. Perhaps more importantly, this might serve as an important adjunct to the initial phase of medical management, immediately following as a prescription after diagnosis. Herein lies a potential preventative method for coping with a problem in chronic disease.

SUMMARY

A project was undertaken to: (1) study the psychopathology associated with Myasthenia Gravis; and (2) to treat this psychopathology in a series of psychotherapeutically-oriented group counseling sessions. Seventeen patients with MG were seen, in two separate groups, for 16 counseling sessions. MMPIs administered before, during and following the intervention revealed striking changes in the direction of more positive mental health for 6 patients; 5 patients were unchanged and 2 appeared to be worse, of the 13 who cooperated with follow-up. Some characteristic psychodynamic patterns were revealed in a case report which was supplemented by empirical documentation of change. In particular, self-imposed medication overdoses in response to socially generated anxiety were noted. All findings were integrated with the existing literature. The study was interpreted as implying that a series of group counseling sessions are helpful to many MG patients. Furthermore, such a procedure may produce important psychodynamic changes in selected patients who may then be considered as candidates for more extensive individual or group psychotherapy. The group counseling procedure may also have utility shortly after diagnosis in helping to prevent particular patients from developing psychological disturbances centered around this chronic disease.

REFERENCES

Drs. Schwartz and Cahill are affiliated with the Departments of Psychology and Neurology, respectively, Wayne State University, Detroit, Michigan.

This study was supported in part by a research grant from the Myasthenia Gravis Association, Detroit. The assistance of Dr. John Gilroy and Miss Sandra Rovsek is gratefully acknowledged.

1. Fullerton, D. T., Munsat, T. L.: Pseudo-myasthenia gravis: a conversion reaction. *J. Nerv. Ment. Dis.* 142: 78, 1966.
2. MacKenzie, K. R., Martin, M. J., Howard, F. M.: Myasthenia gravis: psychiatric concomitants. *Canad. Med. Ass. J.* 100: 988, 1969.
3. Schwab, R. S., Perlo, V. P.: Syndromes simulating myasthenia gravis. *Ann. N.Y. Acad. Sci.* 135: 350, 1966.
4. Gilroy, J., Meyer, J. S.: *Medical neurology—a textbook of neurology.* New York, Macmillan, 1969.
5. Meyer, E.: Psychological disturbances in myasthenia gravis—a predictive study. *Ann. N.Y. Acad. Sci.* 135: 417, 1966.
6. Hayman, M.: Myasthenia gravis and psychosis: report of a case with observations on its psychosomatic implications. *Psychosom. Med.* 3: 120, 1941.
7. Marcus, J.: The interrelation of myasthenia gravis and psychic stress: presentation of a case. *Israel Med. J.* 21: 178, 1962.

8. Grob, D.: Myasthenia gravis—current state of psychogenesis, clinical manifestation and management. *J. Chron. Dis.* 8: 536, 1958.
9. Chafetz, M. E.: Psychological disturbances in myasthenia gravis. *Ann. N.Y. Acad. Sci.* 135: 424, 1966.
10. Osserman, K. E.: *Myasthenia gravis.* New York, Grune and Stratton, 1958.
11. Brolley, M., Hollender, M. H.: Psychological problems of patients with myasthenia gravis. *J. Nerv. Ment. Dis.* 122: 178, 1955.
12. Goss, J. D.: The physician's reaction to myasthenia gravis. *Ann. N.Y. Acad. Sci.* 135: 428, 1966.
13. Schwartz, M. L., Cahill, R.: Personality assessment in myasthenia gravis with the MMPI *Percept. Motor Skills* 31: 766, 1970.

12

Social Group Work as a Treatment Modality for Hospitalized People with Rheumatoid Arthritis —CINNIE HENKLE

THE Rheumatic Diseases Unit of The Wellesley Hospital, Toronto, is a 40-bed ward, devoted to the treatment of rheumatic diseases, of which rheumatoid arthritis is the most commonly known. Treatment on this Unit is based on the team concept, which includes not only the medical staff physicians, residents, and interns, but also the allied health professionals, nurses, occupational and physical therapists, the dietitian, and the social worker. In cooperation, each discipline involved in the treatment program carries out its protocol of assessment and appropriate therapy, sharing the results of various interventions in order to provide comprehensive total patient care.

Social work activity on the Rheumatic Diseases Unit involves, for the most part, casework practice, family and marital counseling, an education program for family members, and coordination of a volunteer "Friendly Visiting" program. Group work has recently become an extension of social casework on the Rheumatic Diseases Unit and an integral part of the treatment program for hospitalized rheumatoid arthritis patients.

PERSONALITY VARIABLES AND SYMBOLIC MECHANISMS—MAJOR CONSIDERATIONS IN RHEUMATOID ARTHRITIS

Because the causes and underlying mechanisms are not known, this condition has been the focus of interest for the medical profession and psychiatrists and sociologists alike.

Reprinted by permission from *Rehabilitation Literature* 36 (11): 334–341, 1975.

Whether certain personality factors predispose a person to rheumatoid arthritis, or whether certain personality characteristics result, has been a matter of extensive research. Furthermore, the question is not whether background and emotional factors "cause" the disease but rather how they contribute to its causation. The part then, which personality variables, background, and precipitating emotional factors and mechanisms play in rheumatoid arthritis cannot be underestimated and, for social casework and group work, they are significant considerations.

Some of the commonalities that are reported in the rheumatoid studies done on personality variables of the rheumatoid arthritic, are that arthritic people, "tend to over-react to their illness, are self-sacrificing, masochistic, rigid, moralistic, conforming, self-conscious, shy, inhibited, perfectionistic, and interested in athletics, in sports and games. They tend to describe their parents as strict, rigid, and domineering."[15] Furthermore, emotional trauma, such as death or separation, is attributed by many as the cause of exacerbation of their condition.

There are several reasons, however, why the evidence, which indicates prevalent commonalities across the various studies, is not conclusive but awareness of these commonalities is helpful.

MECHANISMS

"One of the most important aspects of the relationship of psychologic and social factors with rheumatoid arthritis is that of the mechanisms by which emotions or interpretation of environmental events are related to physiologic changes of the disease."[2]

Muscle Tension

Various studies have implied that, in some cases, emotional factors can result in rheumatoid arthritis symptoms. Though many interpretations and generalizations have been presented on this theory, the following statement is of interesting significance for the social worker.

Many persons with or without clinically obvious arthritic deformities habitually exteriorize their psychic tensions through sustained regional or generalized hypertonia of somatic muscle, which may in turn give rise to musculoskeletal symptoms. These psychogenically induced symptoms can be exceedingly severe. Some patients obtain relief from symptoms when they can be taught not to exteriorize mental tensions through sustained hypertonia of somatic muscle, or when their mental tensions are lessened through directed psychotherapy or through changes in the environment.[11]

Symbolic Manifestation

Some authors suggest that symptoms of rheumatoid arthritis may be a symbolic manifestation of conflict. The localization of the disease seemed to one investigator to be in the joint(s) in which conflict was focused. The joint might play an important part in an activity that was disliked or be essential to the assumption of an attitude expressing symbolically the patient's general demeanor (being stiff-necked), or the joint may have been subjected to physical trauma that had psychological significance.[12]

Symbolic Control

Some investigators hve indicated that arthritic symptoms represent means for the control or prevention of expression of hostile aggressive impulses; if the joints are stiff and rigid, motion is limited and the anger will be encapsulated, and the danger to others and self will be averted.[12]

Projective tests on arthritic patients have concluded that the "outer rigidity of the body represents a way of inhibiting something bad within, the bad being unacceptable—hostile, aggressive feelings."[1]

The area of personality variables is no more conclusive than the matter of mechanisms in the etiology of arthritis. However, the evidence on these subjects suggests that these areas should not be ignored in their relevance to social work and in considering their contribution to the disease process of rheumatoid arthritis.

THE ADULT WITH RHEUMATOID ARTHRITIS—
PSYCHOSOCIAL PROBLEMS

The fact that a person becomes ill with a chronic disease and requires hospitalization carries with it the concept of deviation in relation to our society, with many of the implications that accompany deviation and abnormality. The numerous social-emotional consequences of this particular condition have significance for casework and group work.

These consequences include: the often sporadic nature of the condition itself, the necessity for continuous drug therapy (with resultant side effects); the physical effects—pain and deformity; the effects on activities of daily living and the limitations and resultant frustrations with the simplest of tasks; frequent necessity to change jobs with consequent financial loss, humiliation, and nonachievement of ego ideal; the effect on families who might need to alter and adapt roles; the change in social life; the numerous effects of the various mentioned alterations on one's self-image; the financial burden, with the cost of drugs and appliances; the time off work; and the emotional reactions (depression, guilt, fear, shame, etc.) to trying to cope with even one of the above alterations in one's normal life-style. These are, briefly, some of the psycho-social implications that chronic disease has for the person faced with the diagnosis of arthritis. The emotional reactions are especially significant and in need of a medium for ventilation. Verbalizing is the one certain way the person who is physically limited and in pain can express what it is like to have arthritis.

THE METHOD "SOCIAL GROUP WORK" AS A
TREATMENT MODALITY

The concept and term *social group work* is used here in the context of groups with hospitalized arthritis patients. Based on assessment of various group theories, it is most applicable to what the initial general objectives were in the organization of groups for arthritis patients:

"Intrinsic to social group work is *voluntary* participation, and freedom of decision to attend or not. . . . [It] is based on self-satisfaction as the only necessary conscious basis of membership in the group."[7]

"Social Work Practice uses the small group as both the context and means through which its members support and modify their attitudes, interpersonal relationships, and abilities to cope effectively with their environments."[16] The small group is most effective in bringing about positive growth and change in its members if it combines effective psychological support for efforts to change with adequate stimulation from others to act as a motivation toward change."[16]

In S. R. Slavson's interpretation, "group guidance" would for the most part describe the type of social group work applicable. Two essential elements in guidance are support and clarification, which help to reduce the ego load through communication and objectification. Slavson pointed out that the discovery that one is not alone or peculiar in having problems and in seeking help reduces stigma and guilt and raises one's self-esteem. The significance of a group disposes him toward more socially approved reactions and relationships, in addition to the release and help supplied by the group. This homogeneity crystallizes the group into a unit in which each member identifies with the others and all are able to help each other because of emotional empathy and mutual understanding. Such homogeneity also favors universalization, from which results reduction of feelings of guilt and uniqueness.[18]

SUPPORT

Frey states:

> Improved functioning is brought about by environmental changes, by the effects of catharsis, by the influence of an encouraging, anxiety-relieving relationship with a caseworker, and by better perception of external reality. Supportive treatment does not involve, by intent, any uncovering of hidden material.[5]

CLARIFICATION

Hollis has discussed the benefit of clarification:

> The dominant note in clarification is understanding. . . . It is directed toward increasing the ego's ability to see external realities more clearly and to understand the client's own emotions, attitudes, and behavior.[9]

THE HOSPITAL AS A SETTING FOR SOCIAL GROUP WORK

In hospitals, because it is a secondary setting, the proper use of "group psychotherapy on the wards would . . . depend on its being integrated with, and taking full advantage of, the group influences inherent in the social structure of the hospital society."[3]

Structure

Hospitals represent, for many, a bureaucratic and authoritarian setting usually characterized by a great gap between patient and staff system.[6]

The structure of the hospital social system consists of two interacting groups, the patients and the treatment staff. The patient population has no fixed structure and its membership is constantly changing. Patients differ in the nature of their illnesses and in their expectancies from treatment. They are, however, held together by a common dependence on the treatment personnel, and by the bond of suffering. Patients on the same ward, besides being placed together geographically, come under the care of the same personnel and may have similar illnesses with similar symptoms, often leading to similar apprehensions. These common features may cause them to exert considerable influence on each other for better or worse.[3]

I would agree with Frank's statement:

> It would seem highly probable that hospitalized patients are emotionally affected by the pervasive and persistent influences emanating from the treatment staff and other patients. Being sick, they are in a state of heightened emotional dependence on their environment and the hospital environment is full of implications for their welfare.[3]

Furthermore it was stated,

> The proper use of group psychotherapy on the wards would therefore seem to depend on its being integrated with, and taking full advantage of, the group influences inherent in the social structure of the hospital society.[3]

Interdisciplinary Approach

A brief word is warranted on the fact that, before organizing groups for arthritis patients, consideration was given to the fact that cooperation and approval of the group program was required by the other staff team members and physicians. This applied not only to the medical staff, who have always acknowledged the psychosocial factors and approved of the group program, but also to those in the allied health areas, for the purpose of encouraging group participation and to prevent planning treatment with group members for the time designated for group meeting.

The interdisciplinary process can view and use the group as a vehicle for improving patient care. It functions then, "to examine not only the internal group dynamics, but encourage analysis of external factors unique in the medical setting which impinge upon the group process."[20] Obstacles in effective teamwork emerge when the purpose of group is unclear, when administrative leadership is lacking, or when interdisciplinary conflict is not resolved around patient needs.[20]

Individual goals of the group for patients and the method to be utilized were shared with the physicians and allied health members to this end. The outcome of the group's activities and the information of importance to the health team are shared by way of written reports on a regular basis (4 months) and when especially pertinent—in weekly ward conferences. The group has consequently fit into the routine with other services provided by the team.

PURPOSE

General Purpose

Besides "engaging the sick person as a collaborator in his treatment,"[6] the "development of a group climate that is supportive of the members' strengths and permits their participation in a self-satisfying but also socially positive way,"[6] is a purpose of a group in a health setting.

Frank says that the purpose of most group therapy with medical patients is:

> . . . to maintain patients at the optimal level of functioning and feeling of well-being consistent with their disability. This is done primarily through the mutual support that comes from the presence of a common goal and from hearing of the successes of others similarly afflicted. Instruction in the nature of the illness and its management, which such groups also offer, is indirectly a powerful builder of morale because it gives the patient a feeling of being the master of his condition instead of being at the mercy of it.[3]

"Socialization"[7] has been suggested as another goal of social group work and this idea was presented by several theorists, in terms of providing a medium in which people with common concerns (i.e., sickness, hospitalization) can share their feelings.

It is further referred to by Margaret Yeakel, who formulated a theoretical approach that also illustrates other purposes of group work with the following considerations:

— *Social Response.* Need for social response, for acceptance and approval of peers for a place in a group is a common human need. Hunger for satisfaction of this need leads to loneliness and isolation. Therefore, the commonality of the experience for the members of a group is a way of universalizing and discovering they are not so different. The group medium then provides people with an environment within which reality can be geared to the current level of functioning of the ill person, designed to foster identification with others in a variety of social roles other than the sick role.

— *Social Reality.* Reality testing is described as a function of a group, since social reality depends on others. The concept of being able to distinguish reality from unreality is especially important for the hospitalized person so that his or her perspective is not lost by the absence of familiar cues. The boundaries between fantasy and reality of the setting and the illness need to be made clear and this can be a purpose of the group as well.

— *The Sick Role.* This role has been sanctioned only conditionally since illness, with its emphasis on passivity and dependence, flies in the face of expectation in our society that puts particular emphasis upon independent achievement.[4] This means that the deviancy of the role has to be recognized by the patient and others who share it with him, and that the goals of the individual and the group are expressed in steps taken to move back into a healthy role. It is often evident that a role conflict exists for the patient between gratifications from dependency in illness (freedom from social responsibility) and striving to get well. So, "to provide the opportunity for identifications (even partially) with others who can collaborate in eliciting or supporting protest against valuing illness" is an important function for the group and in helping to resolve the role conflict.[6]

This author's summation of this material emphasizes that the focus is on group process in terms of consequence of the "immediacy to create within the group, reciprocal roles that meet individual needs for social response and group's need for survival."[6]

Purpose of the Group for Arthritis Patients

— To provide a supportive milieu for hospitalized patients with rheumatoid arthritis, in which they can share common concerns regarding their illness, hospitalization, and psychosocial problems that result because of their condition (to devalue sickness and strengthen coping mechanisms).

— To enable patients to use the group experience to share and ventilate common problems, experiences, and feelings in the areas of work and social relationships with friends and family. To find ways of solving them (effect possible attitude and behavioral changes).

— To provide the opportunity to recognize that one is not alone, that others emphathize and have similar experiences and emotional reactions (depression, fears, hopes).

— To help patients discuss and share problems and solutions in "activities in daily living" (managing to maintain independence with labor-saving devices) and community resources affecting positive group norms in the rehabilitation program (not valuing illness and dependency).

— If, in fact, there is some evidence of "symbolic manifestation" of disease for some, and if the personality variables regarding contained hostility, anger, etc., might be true for some who attend, to provide them with the opportunity to relieve tension and ventilate—*not* to uncover repressed conflicts or challenge defenses.

— For the worker on the staff team— to have the opportunity to gain further insight into "what it's like to have arthritis" from a group, who, as a group, might offer significant and useful information in this regard.

These points, plus the objectives presented in the previous section on general purposes of groups, are the goals intended to be attained by social group work with arthritis patients.

As, H. Wilson, ACSW, Ranchos Los Amigos Hospital, California, points out in her paper "Method and Process of Working with Groups of Hospitalized Arthritic Patients,"

> The process of group interaction is to help the patient explore and understand their feelings about themselves and others in the group. In this process, the patients will uncover neurotic conflicts, develop understanding and, through an emotional re-educational experience, will be better able to cope on the outside. . . . Our focus is to help him to strengthen his coping defenses and to gain support.

ORGANIZING THE GROUP

Based on the type of group method considered to be most applicable to both the hospital setting and the Rheumatic Diseases Unit per se, and considering the structure of the hospital system and the interdisciplinary approach in treatment, our group work with arthritis patients was organized for the above purpose with the following guidelines.

PREGROUP PRIVATE PHASE

This phase of development has been referred to by various theorists and is basically when there is a "recognition of the mutual value of collective action for the fulfillment of individual interests."[2]

Because the Rheumatic Diseases Unit is a segregated medical unit, with people having a common diagnosis, the same physical protocol, common psychosocial concerns, commonalities in some personality variables as personally evidenced and as indicated in the research, in my estimation, it presents a natural milieu for social group work.

Patient social interaction is generally quite high and patients are already affecting each other and cooperating with the treatment plan in, usually, a dependent and passive manner. As suggested by Weiner, "The goal is to enable these group processes to aid in the treatment plan."[20]

PREGROUP PUBLIC PHASE

This "is the period in which the decision to have a group is made known to others, beyond the originator."[8]

It was at this point that the plan for group activity on the Rheumatic Diseases Unit was shared with the head nurse, with the intention of cooperating with her in the group. The reasons for including the nurse are multifold and based partially on the premise that the complexities of patients' health needs are matched only by the difficulties of any one professional group in meeting them.[17] The reasons for feeling that the collaboration of the skills of both the social work and nursing disciplines would be effective are as follows:

— Good communication and interaction exist regarding appropriate

verbal casework referrals, sharing of information, delineating overlapping services, and sharing of appropriate responsibilities, i.e., discharge planning.
— The nursing division is, in essence, the backbone of the ward structure, and it was hoped that collaboration with this discipline would
aid communications by recognizing the overlapping of some of the
services to patients. Also, the other members of this discipline are
kept informed of the group activity since they meet more regularly
and pertinent concerns of the group can be presented that might not
otherwise be brought out in a weekly ward conference.
— Nurses are often seen by patients more as a part of the medical situation than is the social worker. Relevant anxieties regarding physical
condition, drugs, and so on are often presented to them and the nurse
is well informed as to the effects of drugs on emotions, physical
manifestations, and their repercussions. Furthermore, as Frank
points out, "the nurses occupy the crucial position from the standpoint of the patients' emotional welfare, since they are continuously
present, administer most of the treatments, and look after their comfort."[3] Nurses carry out the execution of the medical plan.
— We share a common conviction regarding the importance of emotional factors in illness and the need for the ill to express their anxieties.
— The head nurse makes daily rounds and gets to know *all* patients on
the Unit to some extent. She is in a good position to encourage
patients to attend group meetings.

With the head nurse's agreement and interest in this plan, the appropriate supervisors were consulted and a memo of the plan was given to the
staff physicians for their approval. No objections were raised. Also, in this
"pregroup public phase," the plan was discussed with potential members
about their possible participation, interest, suggestions, and goals, not only
to get their ideas but also to give them an opportunity in the formation of
the first group. Northen refers to this time as a "phase of origin in which
the focus is mainly on the social worker's actions in the determination of
group purpose and composition, the establishment of a contract with individual members about the service to be provided."[16]

COMPOSITION

Composition depends on reasons for forming the group.[6] The purpose
had been established prior to this phase. Numerous persons with other
arthritic conditions are hospitalized on the Rheumatic Diseases Unit, but it
seemed most feasible to work with the condition that is most common,
about which we had more knowledge (i.e., physical, psychosocial, research
on personality variables), and with which more commonalities seem to exist. This is rheumatoid arthritis.
The main initial consideration in selection was whether to invite all of

the rheumatoid arthritic patients, who are usually approximately 25 in a total of 40 patients. We were aware that the concept wouldn't interest all, that some would have visitors, be tied up in some other area of treatment, or be bedridden, either due to an imposed restriction (i.e., injection), or by nature of their condition. In fact, the average number attending is 8. Though we felt some might benefit more than others and we planned to encourage attendance individually, we were concerned about including the newly arthritic or less disabled people with the long-term, often quite crippled, or incapacitated persons. Forming two separate groups was not considered feasible at this time.

Because the tone in education classes and on the Unit generally is positive and optimistic and emphasis is on the fact that each patient is different and is treated differently (drugs and dosages, therapy, surgery, etc.) with different results, we felt that we would include all patients with rheumatoid arthritis.

Moreover, the group was planned to be open-ended ("constantly in the process of composition"[6]) with attendance contingent upon the ebb and flow of admissions and discharges to the ward and dependent on the patients' interest in attending. It was felt, for these reasons and because the purposes of the group are generally applicable to all rheumatoid arthritis patients, that the integration of varying involvements of the condition would not necessarily be detrimental to the newer people. One of the roles of the group worker in this regard would be to be perceptive and aware of any deleterious effects that might result for individuals from the integration in the group and look into the problem by the process of "individualization."[6] It is important to note, however, that some reactions, while appearing negative, might actually have a reality base and be important for the denying individual.

RECRUITMENT

For recruitment, it is important that patients be made aware of the purpose and proposed goals of the group. It was to this end that we chose to inform each rheumatoid arthritic on the Unit by the way of a "flyer" explaining the what, why, where, and when of the proposed group. This invitation is given to new admissions weekly (the day of the group meeting) and a verbal reminder is given to the members from the previous week. Sometimes one of the members does this. As mentioned, encouragement is given individually to those people who, it is felt, might best benefit or offer more to the group.

The day and time (from 4 to 5 PM) were chosen because the physicians are away at medical rounds, the physiotherapists are in regular meetings, and most lab tests, etc., have been completed. One hour was chosen as the block of time because many cannot sit much longer; also supper arrives at 5:00. Some thought has been given to an evening program, and this will be reconsidered, depending on participation, interest, and suitability.

GROUP FORMATION PHASE

The "Pregroup Convening Phase"[3] was, in essence, combined with the Formation Phase, mainly because patients are on the Unit an average of 3 weeks. Since time is a factor, the elements of a convening phase are continuously incorporated, as the group forms and reforms. It could be said that the group is, in fact, at most times in the beginning stages of group formation and development, based on the above facts of composition, recruitment, nature of setting, attendance, and open-endedness.

THE GROUP MEETING

WHAT HAPPENS

Each group meeting begins with introductions by each member—on a first-name basis. The concept of confidentiality and a "contract" among us based on the purpose of the group is introduced at the beginning of each group. If a member from the previous week or if a patient "leader" has been self-designated, he or she reiterates to the others what has passed in the previous week and some of the concerns presented. If there has been a complete turnover, one of the workers refers to the written invitation and opens it up to the group to share a "common concern." Either introduction inevitably sparks some reaction, and interaction flows quite easily.

When silences become too lengthy or are felt to be not purposeful, normally one of the workers suggests a topic, such as "In what ways do you feel your families and friends might benefit from education about arthritis?" or "Sometimes people feel that upsets exacerbate a flare-up; has this been anyone's experience here?"

Termination of each group is done by one of the workers and might involve a summation, an introduction of a possible subject for next week, a thank you for attending, a reiteration of the confidentiality code, and an invitation to attend next week. Sometimes patients attend only once, depending on interest, length of hospitalization, whether they are available (if no other treatment is being administered). Even if a patient has attended for the number of weeks he is in hospital (usually three), termination does not present a major problem in preparation for separation,[6] since the intensity of relationships, group sentiment, interaction, and so on have not, so far, presented major issues for which alternatives to the group are needed.

GROUP PROCESS

Homans'[10] three mutually dependent elements in group behavior—interaction, sentiment, and activity—do occur.

Interaction, the response of one piece of behavior to another,[10] is normally quite high depending on subject matter presented and personalities present.

Group sentiments develop in what is perceived mainly to be an empathic reaction to others sharing common concerns. People's drives, feelings, and emotions[6] in many areas resemble each other's as a result of experiencing many of the same psychosocial problems. Partly because of this there seems to be no conflict: Agreement is evident. Also this may result because personality variables such as contained hostility or anger and passivity do not find a medium for expression in a group with people who are possibly similarly inhibited. Moreover, affectional ties such as identification, complementarity, cordiality, togetherness, acceptance, and interest are evident in the group.

The group is not task- or activity-oriented but focuses on discussion. Some topics are: what it feels like to have arthritis; to be ill in a healthy family and society; the frustrations experienced by imposed physical restrictions and fatigue; psychosocial problems incurred in trying to function (work, socialize, etc.); exchange of practical ways to cope with tasks (labor-saving devices); can emotional upsets that coincide with flare-ups be prevented; the need to learn to cope with inactivity (alternatives such as hobbies); need to alter values (meticulous nature—if one can no longer scrub the floors on one's knees, to be satisfied with alternate cleaning methods); how to cope with solicitous bystanders. Topics are related and ventilated and solutions considered.

ROLES

Despite the constant change of composition of the group, roles do emerge. One that is basic to each member is being a member of a group and with this come some affectional ties, such as identification, mutual understanding, and empathy. This association, or being part of the group, not only gives support and a feeling of acceptance but denotes a collaborative role in relation to other members and the role of the social worker, i.e., mutual-aid-system interdependence.[6]

Again, because of the constant patient turnover and relatively short hospitalizations, there is not much time to see people develop into the depth of a role. Certain ones take on the leader role and help bridge the gap from the previous meeting. For the most part, time and changing composition do not allow for roles to become well defined. The shy person, the calm talkative one, the bitter one, all appear at some time but are short-lived. A scapegoat has been virtually nonexistent, and role delineation is normally on a fairly superficial level, with a more aggressive, talkative member often leading the group and encouraging everyone's participation. Dyads and subgroups do not seem to form significantly, probably because of the nature of the group and patient turnover.

ROLE OF THE GROUP WORKER(S)

The group worker informs and reminds Unit patients with rheumatoid arthritis that the group is to take place on the designated day. She encourages those for whom the group is considered beneficial or those who have been especially referred by the physician or psychiatrist.

The team of allied health disciplines and staff physicians is kept informed of the group's activity, keeping them similarly aware of the process. This is done verbally whenever especially relevant, as in the ward conference, and by a written evaluation.

Casework relationships are carried on in conjunction with group work. Those seen in casework who also attend the group are advised that confidentiality is assured. I had some concern that relationships in which some dependency or transference had occurred, as a result of the casework relationship, might interfere with my role as a group worker. This has yet to happen, but it is an area that I feel it is necessary to be aware of and that should be worked out individually with the client if it arises.

Individualization[6] and the life space interview[19] are used when the need is presented.

The role of the worker changes as the group develops, but the basic role remains that of being a catalyst for the accomplishment of the purpose of the group. This is achieved in various ways, at different times, in group process. In the initial group and continuously, the worker presents trust and acceptance to the group, with an objective understanding of the meaning of the new experience on members, who are apt to be uncertain and anxious. To develop a working relationship and sustain the members, the worker shows enthusiasm in presenting the purpose and the confidentiality code and in clarifying norms and values of open sharing, while establishing and developing mutuality of expectations.

Supporting each member's entry into the group is also important, as is giving direction, while at the same time setting the tone for freedom of expression and self-direction.[16]

Lang[14] describes three group orders, with "allon-autonomous" best encompassing the roles of the worker meant to be performed in the arthritis patients' group.

The "allon-autonomous" stage is described as an intermediate stage in which the worker is concerned both with individual development and functioning and with the developing entity, the group as a whole. The worker addresses himself to all levels of social process. He is focused on the social functioning of individuals and the achievement of group-defined social goals. The group is both an instrumental socialization medium and an intrinsic social reality. The group, formed with the worker as a significant constituent, is structured for greater autonomous functioning, with the worker moving between a central and a peripheral focus, in keeping with the readiness of the members to deal autonomously. The worker pivots between surrogation in group processes when necessary and facilitation of autonomous functioning when possible. The client has some capacity for autonomous group engagement, not yet fully developed in all areas. The means of service may combine worker-mediated interaction, behavioral conditioning, ego strengthening and developing, socialization, worker facilitation of group processes, worker and member role modeling, and social action. The worker deals with all group processes attempting to create growth-supportive norms but encouraging group-direct processes to the extent possible.[14]

Based on these and various other theories, I saw my role compatible with the head nurse in terms of a collaborator with each member and as a group for the purpose of achieving mutually accepted goals. A tone of positiveness, I feel, was set by an informal, open, objective, positive, and interested attitude. I feel that, as a model for identification, by communicating opening, freely, and in a manner that connotes genuine concern, support, and empathy, I may help others feel comfortable doing the same. Reciprocally their reaction encourages others to do so as well.

Since not all patients who attend group are seen in a casework relationship (a social work assessment is not done on all patients—only those referred), the group presents an opportunity for the life space interview or individualization. This entails the worker's awareness of how the individual copes (verbal and nonverbal cues) in the group.

At times, the workers have had to be directive, as in checking out messages to see if they are correctly perceived. Clarification is sometimes necessary when the nurse has medical questions posed to her. Clarification is also used in checking out reality, attitudes, and reactions.

The worker is often active in explaining environmental resources that might reduce the patients' stress in the community. Acceptance of prosthetic appliances and aids is another matter for discussion in which the worker can facilitate communication.

Since the conscious and preconscious are still the area of a worker's focus, the worker must be aware of "threat areas" and recognize the onset of anxiety beyond permissible levels. "Much of his efforts have to be bent upon *avoidance instead of unrestricted exploration* invclved in uncovering and free catharsis."[18]

Alan Klein says, "The task of the group worker is to help the person select more appropriate and constructive alternatives for action within his behavioral range."[13] I feel this relates to Northen's statement that "support alone is not enough. Stimulation toward different attitudes and behavioral patterns is essential also."[16]

It was based on these two statements that I, as worker, with a directive approach, referred to some of the issues presented, in terms of what can be done. This was done with the hope that, in achieving the purpose of providing a supportive milieu for the sharing of common concerns, members might find alternative ways of coping with their problems—not just talking about them.

EVALUATION

Based on the outline for Diagnosis of the Group[6] as developed by the Boston University School of Social Work, the guidelines for evaluation applied to the arthritis group were adapted. An assessment is done on regular intervals, every 4 months, to evaluate the group in time.

The guidelines adapted include the following areas: the environment; history of the group; group characteristics; group goals and purposes; elements of group behavior-interaction and structures; group sentiment; nature of activity; group norms; worker in relation to the group; and limitations—group, setting, method.

CONCLUSION

In conclusion, I feel that the group for arthritis patients does, in fact, provide a supportive milieu for inpatients and that the group achieves a number of the purposes set down. I feel that, if people are only to find in the group that others understand them and their plight, it accomplishes something important for someone.

The limitations of the open-ended, constantly changing, group are evident in terms of trying to effect behavioral and attitudinal changes, but it is felt that, for some, the group presents a good opportunity to test reality, consider alternatives, realize some insight, and gain understanding and acceptance by others.

The group certainly gives me, as worker, more insight, empathy, and understanding for the ill arthritic person both in the hospital and in our society.

REFERENCES

Mrs. Henkle is a social worker with the Rheumatic Diseases Unit of the Wellesley Hospital, Toronto Canada.

1. Cleveland, Sidney E., and Fisher, Seymour. A comparison of psychological characteristics and psychological reactivity in ulcer and rheumatoid arthritis groups. I. Psychological measures. *Psychosomatic Med.* July-Aug., 1960. 22:4:283–289.
2. Coyle, Grace Longwell. *Social process in organized groups.* New York: Richard R. Smith, 1930.
3. Frank, Jerome D. The effects of interpatient and group influences in a general hospital. *Internatl. J. Group Psychotherapy.* Apr., 1952. 2:2:127–138.
4. Freeman, Howard E.; Levine, Sol; and Reeder, Leo G., *eds. Handbook of medical sociology. (2d ed.)* Englewood Cliffs, N.J.: Prentice-Hall, 1972.
5. Frey, Louise A. Support and the Group: A generic treatment form. *Social Work.* Oct., 1962. 7:4:35–42.
6. Frey, Louise, *ed. Use of groups in the health field, report; com. members, 1959–1966.* New York: National Association of Social Workers, 1966.
7. Gifford, C. G.; Landis, E. E.; and Ackerly, S. Spafford. The use of social group work as a therapeutic factor in the hospital setting. *Am. J. Orthopsychiatry.* Jan., 1953. 23:1:142–157.
8. Hartford, Margaret E. *Groups in social work: Application of small group theory and research to social work practice.* New York: Columbia Univ., 1972.
9. Hollis, Florence. The techniques of casework. *Social Casework.* June, 1949. 30:6:235–244.
10. Homans, George C. *The human group.* New York: Harcourt Brace, 1950.

11. Kaufman, William. The over-all picture of rheumatism and arthritis. *Ann. Allergy.* Jan.-Feb., 1952. 10:1:47–52.
12. King, Stanley H. Psychosocial factors associated with rheumatoid arthritis. *J. Chronic Diseases.* Sept., 1955. 2:3:287–302.
13. Klein, Alan. Role and reference group theory. In: *Social science theory and social work research.* New York: National Association of Social Workers, 1960.
14. Lang, Norma C. A broad-range model of practice in the social work group. *Social Service Review.* Mar., 1972. 46:1:76–89.
15. Moos, Rudolf H. Personality factors associated with rheumatoid arthritis: A review. *J. Chronic Diseases.* Jan., 1964. 17:1:41–55.
16. Northen, Helen. *Social work with groups.* New York: Columbia Univ. Pr., 1969.
17. Robinson, Sally S. Is there a difference? *Nursing Outlook.* Nov., 1967. 15:11:34–36.
18. Slavson, S. R. When is a "therapy group" not a therapy group? *Internatl. J. Group Psychotherapy.* Jan. 1960. 10:1:3–21.
19. Vernick, Joel. The use of the life space interview on a medical ward. *Social Casework.* Oct., 1963. 44:8:465–469.
20. Weiner, Hyman J. The hospital, the ward, and the patient as clients: Use of group method. *Social Work.* Oct., 1959. 4:4:57–64.

13

Group Rehabilitation of Vascular Surgery Patients —MARTIN R. LIPP, M.D., and SANDEE T. MALONE, S.W.A.

THE value of group support for patients with disabling or disfiguring or chronic illnesses has been a part of medical folklore for decades. Joseph Pratt, a Boston internist, began organizing group meetings for tuberculosis patients as long ago as 1900 to 1906, using the meetings both for teaching patients about their disease and to allow them to express feelings about their shared experiences. Since that time, the popularity of group meetings for persons with physical ailments has followed an erratic course. In recent years, reports in professional literature of such activities have been remarkably few.[1]

We have believed for some time that group support approaches to enhance rehabilitation have been vastly underutilized in general hospital settings. This paper concerns the development and functioning of one such group, comprised of vascular surgery patients, either facing amputation or postamputation, in the San Francisco Veterans Administration Hospital (SFVAH). These particular patients were chosen for several reasons. (1)

Reprinted with permission. *Archives of Physical Medicine and Rehabilitation* 57: 180–183, 1976.

The idea of the group was supported enthusiastically by the corrective therapist with whom the patients had daily contact. (2) One of us (S. T. M.) had regular contact with the patients in her capacity as social work associate on the ward on which most vascular surgery patients are bedded. (3) These patients often have prolonged hospitalizations, allowing time for group cohesiveness to develop among them. (4) Most of these patients have unimpaired intellect and are capable of participating in ordinary social intercourse. (5) It seemed to us that many of this number have emotional needs which could be met optimally by their peers, rather than either calling in mental health professionals or allowing these needs to go unmet.

THE PATIENTS

Vascular surgery amputees at the SFVAH are distinguished by several features. Demographically, they are all veterans, almost all men, with a mean age of about 60 years. Over half are diabetic, about four-fifths have had previous direct arterial surgery and one-third have had sympathectomies. Most have multiple health problems which have been disruptive of their personal, occupational, and family lives, with prolonged hospitalizations which dominate their recent personal histories. Though many had obtained medical care privately until they could no longer financially afford to do so, the patients uniformly regard themselves as fortunate to be receiving medical care on the vascular surgery service at SFVAH.

The latter comment deserves elaboration. The SFVAH is one of several medical centers in this country which in the mid-1960s pioneered use of immediate postoperative prosthesis fitting techniques (IPPF) for vascular insufficiency.[2, 3] Though not every patient is an appropriate IPPF candidate, the program and its history in the institution nonetheless lends a certain cachet to the vascular surgery department and to its chief, Wesley Moore, M.D., for whom the patients have an almost reverential respect. Much the same can be said for the corrective therapist, Zane Grimm.

The hospital itself is a 350-bed general medical and surgical hospital affiliated with the University of California School of Medicine, San Francisco. During any given year on the vascular surgery ward, the patients can reasonably expect to be looked after by 24 medical students, 12 interns, 6 or 8 residents, numerous nursing and physical therapy students, a variety of consultants, perhaps several psychology and dietetics trainees, plus the daily rotation of nursing staff and the normal turnover of personnel of a complex general hospital. Since our amputees have spent a major part of their recent lives in the hospital (varying from 3 to 23 out of the past 24 months), they frequently have more tenure in the hospital than many of the people who are caring for them.

THE GROUP

The group first met in April 1973, with two staff (the authors) and four patient members present, and has continued to meet since on almost an uninterrupted weekly basis. During the first several months, the meetings often seemed to be labored affairs, with patient attendance bolstered by the coaxing of the corrective therapist, with patients physically taken from the ward to the meeting room by staff nurses and invitations to participate repeatedly being tendered by both staff member participants. Even so, attendance seldom exceeded two to four patient participants, which represented about one-third of the potential inpatient membership.

After about four months, we began to provide coffee on an intermittent basis, with one of the staff members going to the hospital canteen, buying the coffee, and bringing it back to the meeting room. The group atmosphere became noticeably more relaxed. Sometime after that, the patient members began offering to buy the coffee themselves and coincidentally, attendance began picking up. Involvement in the group may have been bolstered by other factors as well. The personalities, needs, and contributions of the specific patients on the vascular service at the time clearly played a part. The fact that several of these patients were able to take major control of their own health care and their environment also seemed contributory. Examples of the latter include a patient who assumed complete responsibility for dressing his own wounds, another who voiced his own desire for immediate amputation and was able to alter a conservative policy of watchful waiting, and a third who was able to alter janitorial procedures by complaining to the hospital director. Since that time, attendance has ranged from 8 to 12 people, including 1 to 3 staff persons and an occasional outpatient who chooses to continue to participate after discharge. New members are most often brought in by patient members, with staff coercion being absent to minimal. Increasingly, the meeting has come to belong to the patients with staff attending, rather than vice versa.

In style, the group bears little resemblance to a formal psychotherapy group. The atmosphere is primarily social, though rehabilitation issues are very much a part of the interactive fabric. The emphasis has been primarily on shared experiences, with one patient teaching another, and intrapsychic issues are only rarely explicit foci of attention. More recently, the group has taken on educational overtones, with a variety of professionals (vascular surgeon, prosthetist, corrective therapist) attending frequently, both to share their expertise and to learn from the patients.

CONTINUING GROUP THEMES

When this very informal, social group is examined in terms of conventional psychotherapeutic variables, a number of specific themes emerge.

First, the group is supportive in nature, with anxiety-provoking techniques rarely used and anxiety-filled subjects seldom becoming primary foci. The emphasis is on coping, with personal strengths repeatedly reinforced. Patients share personal testaments of "how to do it." Principal topics include techniques of living with amputation, ways of combating wound infection and fostering wound healing, grievances with hospital personnel, phantom limb pains, medications, and coping with bureaucracies in obtaining financial support.

The principal function of the group has been to foster interpersonal support for individual coping skills. For instance, one member will tell another that "You've been spending too much time in bed; you've got to get up and get going." Another will say, "The only way to get the dressings changed the way you want is to learn how to do it yourself. That's what I do." Or, "Worrying won't make it happen—you got to tell the doctors what you want." The continuing enemies are passivity, fatalism and dependency—and the group members attack these relentlessly.

A natural concomitant of this provides the second theme: that there are a number of subjects which are taboo in the group, especially depression, fearfulness, hopelessness, and seemingly insurmountable problems related to family interaction.

On the rare occasion when the group focuses on these issues, it does so only obliquely, briefly, and with scant emotion expressed. Typically, a member will say, "I don't know what is ahead of me, but you can't worry about it." The latter remark will immediately elicit agreement from other members.

Psychiatrically, this constitutes denial, but denial of an enormously adaptive sort. In fact, these men know exactly what is ahead for many or most of them: in this group, progressive vascular impairment, sometimes gradual and sometimes fulminant, is the rule rather than the exception. The relentlessness of their disease process is all around them. All have gone through surgical procedures of increasing seriousness as their disease has progressed. Several who joined the group at the time of their first amputation are now bilateral amputees.

Inevitably, the group members intermittently become weighed down by the gravity of the problems they face. Since depression is not a welcome topic per se, personal distress is expressed in other ways which group members find more tolerable. In particular, anger and somatic complaints are used as depression-equivalents. Though these men frequently have valid reasons for voicing physical complaints (for example, pain and infection) or expressing anger (for example, at the veterans administration or specific health personnel), they in fact rarely do so. In general, if an amputee begins to complain or get angry, it is likely that he is feeling stressed in many respects but is selectively choosing the most acceptable way of expressing this distress.

Another continuing theme is the specialness which the patients feel about themselves. By virtue of their amputation(s), these patients form a population apart: they are identifiable in appearance and they are generally wheelchair bound at least for much of their hospitalizations. They share numerous common experiences, operations and problems which separate them from the mainstream hospital population. And they share a matrix of hospital personnel (surgical team, prosthetist, physiatrist, corrective therapist, special radiodiagnostician, discussion group leaders, etc.), which makes them unique in the hospital.

CONCLUSIONS

During the evolution of the amputee group, we developed a set of goals, both to focus our energies and to set a standard against which our efforts could be judged. Each of these will be discussed separately as follows:

1. Assisting amputees with feelings of helplessness, isolation, and depression. Since these feelings are so frequently denied by amputees, our impact in these areas is very difficult to measure. The group is clearly a socializing experience for those who attend, thereby diminishing actual isolation and fostering "interval therapy" (interaction of group members between sessions).

This camaraderie is evident on the ward, in the hospital canteen, in the physical therapy and wherever the patients come in contact. More mobile individuals run errands for less mobile ones, and profound friendships have developed through such sharing. We presume that sharing of experiences helps to mitigate against feelings of helplessness and depression, but we have not been able to prove this. We believe, given the climate of the group, that the group is not sufficient therapy for patients with genuine clinical depressions.

2. Facilitating staff awareness of psychosocial factors in each patient's rehabilitation. Under ordinary general hospital circumstances, complaints and anger from patients tend to elicit like behavior from staff. The group helps to foster more positive responses by titrating each patient's subjective distress in a formal way on a weekly basis, and by encouraging all patients to help staff understand what would otherwise be regarded as negativistic behavior. Patients thereby become staff-extenders, both as perceivers of potentially useful information and as reinforcers and implementers of rehabilitation policy.

The mere fact that the group meets regularly encourages staff to consider psychosocial factors. The ordinary myopia of all specialists which tends to restrict observations to one's own field of expertise can be overcome when we are reminded to broaden our scope. In fact, when psychosocial issues come up, all staff members have generally been sensitive and sympathetic.

3. Integrating ward management with physiatric treatment. While neither physical therapy nor ward nursing personnel are able to participate in the group on a weekly basis, the group presents a forum where issues common to amputees can be openly expressed. The patient peer group and the staff members who are present then all act as message-bearers of treatment strategies evolved either in physical therapy or on the ward. Where such strategies are mutually inconsistent, over-ambitious, or otherwise inappropriate, the patient group supports the individual amputee in bringing this to the attention of the staff. The important consideration is that skills learned in physical therapy are carried over onto the ward.

4. Mobilizing patients' coping skills. The principal enemies of these men are fatalism, passivity and dependency. Conversely, they strive for a

sense that they can actively control or influence their destiny and look forward to a life of reasonable self-sufficiency. The emphasis on self-help in the group continually pushes the individual towards coping. Dumont[4] believes that such groups are part of a nation-wide phenomenon, which he calls a dramatically growing "movement toward a peer-oriented self-help approach to care giving [which] has profound consequences" for health care delivery in this country.

5. Motivating patients to participate in rehabilitation of other amputees. In many respects, this has been the most useful aspect of the group. By formally focusing on the specific rehabilitation needs of each individual in front of the group of amputees, each amputee has a built-in opportunity to participate. One person can and does assist another by sharing experiences or expertise, by encouraging or goading, by cheering up or acting as an external reinforcer of desired behaviors. In the months since the group has begun, vascular surgery amputees have become a distinctive subgroup in the hospital, referring to themselves as a special sort of fraternity. With members in all stages of the rehabilitation process, they are able to teach one another by example as well as the sharing of information. Each group member can and does choose among a full array of coping techniques displayed by his peers.

In sum, the weekly discussion group for amputees has been primarily a mutual support group, with social, ventilative and educational overtones. It has not been a psychotherapy group in the traditional sense of the word, but it has brought to light psychosocial issues in a way that has facilitated informed surgical and physiatric management.

REFERENCES

Dr. Lipp is from the Psychiatric Service, Veterans Administration Hospital, San Francisco, California. He is now with the Permanente Medical Group at Kaiser Hospital, Hayward, California.

This article was presented at the 51st Annual Session of the American Congress of Rehabilitation Medicine, San Francisco, November 22, 1974.

1. MacLennan, B. W., Levy, N.: Group psychotherapy literature 1970. *Int. J. Group Psychother.* 21:345–380, 1971.
2. Moore, W. S.; Hall, A. D.; Wylie, E. J.: Below knee amputation for vascular insufficiency: Experience with immediate postoperative fitting of prosthesis. *Arch. Surg.* 97:886–893, 1968.
3. Moore, W. S.; Hall, A. D.; Lim, R. C., Jr.: Below knee amputation for ischemic gangrene: Comparative results of conventional operation and immediate postoperative fitting technic. *Am. J. Surg.* 124:127–134, 1972.
4. Dumont, M. P.: Self-help treatment programs. *Am. J. Psychiatry* 131:631–635, 1974.

_____ **14** _____

Group Counseling for Multiple Sclerosis Patients: A Preferred Mode of Treatment for Unique Adaptive Problems
—PAUL W. POWER, Sc.D., and SALLY ROGERS, M.A.

C HRONIC, deteriorative illnesses, such as Parkinson's Disease, Multiple Schlerosis, and Rheumatoid Arthritis, adversely affect the afflicted person, resulting in uncertainty, apprehension, and isolation. As these diseases slowly limit physical functioning there are continued adaptive demands involving the person's family, occupation, and social life. Unfortunately, patients are often left alone to cope with the illness and its impact on their life.

One such disease that causes a distinctive emotional impact is Multiple Sclerosis. A neurologic illness of the central nervous system affecting the person's mobility, vision, sexual capacity, speech, and sphincter control, the disease is variable and uncertain in its course (McAlpine et al, 1955). Some patients become bedridden within a few months and others remain unscathed for many years after an initial attack. Even in those patients whose disease begins to be progressive, the progression can halt and reverse at any time. Uncertainty magnifies the emotional problems in these patients, causing anxiety and confusion over an unknown personal future (McAlpine et al, 1955; Shontz, 1956). Learning how to adjust to the uncertainty of disease progression is a recurrent necessity. One alternative in learning coping skills is group therapy which offers the opportunity for persons to learn how to deal successfully with this chronic illness.

During the past 25 years, several group programs have been established to help Multiple Sclerosis patients cope with a range of problems, such as those related to medical management, clarifying for the person's family the impact of chronic disease on family life, or providing patients with an opportunity to share their experiences and reactions with others similarly afflicted (Barnes, Busse & Dinken, 1954; Bolding, 1960; Day, Day, and Herrmann, 1953; Hartings, Pavlou, and Davis, 1976; Huberty, 1974; Long, 1954; Mally and Strehl, 1963). The reports from the literature concerning group strategies with Multiple Sclerosis patients identify three factors that become strongly evident in group counseling; 1) ambiguity and uncertainty of health status "which can leave the patient apprehensive, distressful, and sometimes fearing the worst" (Hartings, Pavlou, and Davis, 1976, p. 68); 2) great relief expressed by patients in the knowledge that they have a forum to discuss Multiple Sclerosis with other interested people (Hartings, Pavlou, and Davis, 1976); and 3) more experienced group members can provide assurance from their broader perspective on the disability and the adjustment process to the newer members (Huberty, 1974). As group sessions progress, moreover, there are further indications that most of the Multiple Sclerosis patients are able to accept their illness and its implications (Day, Day, and Herrmann, 1953; Hartings, Pavlou, and Davis, 1976; Long, 1954).

The purpose of this paper is to describe a group therapy program for persons having Multiple Sclerosis that was developed by the authors to meet some of the distinctive needs of their patients. The focus of the article is on the particular rationale for starting the group, some of the unique aspects of the group process and specific highlights from the group, and certain problems and implications emanating from the group process.

SETTING, RATIONALE AND PURPOSE OF THE GROUP

The setting from which the members were selected for the group is a VA Outpatient clinic which serves over four hundred Multiple Sclerosis patients each year, representing varied ages and differing degrees of limitations. Three full time and two part time neurologists, two full time and two part time psychiatrists, a nurse, a social worker, an EEG and EMG technician, a rehabilitation psychologist and his clinical associate are available to this population. Though many of the patients' psychological problems had been addressed by psychiatrists and social workers on the staff, a group counseling modality for treatment had not been attempted.

As a group, the outpatients brought unique considerations. All of the prospective members were receiving substantial monetary compensation from the government which, for some, brought added tension to interpersonal relations. When friends became aware that the veteran was receiving a large amount of money without working, their attitude towards him often changed, causing the patient much anxiety and embarrassment. Some persons unwillingly withdrew from many prevous social contacts because of their inability to explain and to justify their benefits. Also, many of the outpatients became very passive regarding their disease-related treatment, relying only on help from the clinic and avoiding taking more responsibility for their own care. Consequently, they had particular needs to become more responsible for the treatment management of their disease, as well as to cope with their aloneness, their depression resulting from disease related limitations, and with their uncertainty, fear, and general inability to plan for vocational and family activities caused by the unpredictable nature of the disease. In identifying the factors present among many of the clinic's Multiple Sclerosis patients, the authors believed that a group counseling treatment modality could alleviate many of these difficulties.

Through the group format the authors expected that the group members could provide factual information and support for emotional expression in relation to the disability. The authors also hoped that early in the group process the patients would learn, through reinforcement, encouragement, and support from the members, how to express their feelings resulting from being disabled, e.g., their fears about further deterioration, anxiety about their ability to cope with the illness, and the embarrassment and anger that comes from being dependent upon others. Through an exploration of these feelings the authors expected to assess each member's unique coping strategies and deficits. They further anticipated that many members would learn a variety of new adaptive skills, including the ability both to communicate feelings more readily and to cope with stigmatizing situations. The auhors hoped that with more adaptive coping strategies, the group members would increase their productive functioning and their ability to make use of residual assets.

STARTING THE GROUP

As the neurologists and nurse serving the clinic were aware of the physical and emotional needs of most of the patients, they were asked for names of persons who might be amenable to group counseling and who could benefit from such an experience. It was decided that the group would consist of 10–12 persons because: 1) A larger group would make it even more difficult for the group members to voice their concerns in the alloted time of the group sessions; 2) Though a smaller number would be more ideal, time available in the clinic permitted only one group and there was a concern to provide this opportunity to as many as could be appropriately accommodated. It was felt that while 10–12 is a large number for a therapeutic group of the chronically ill, learning how to deal more adaptively with a serious illness was possible and growth experiences of intimacy were continually available during the group sessions.

Though the clinic treats a very small number of women with Multiple Sclerosis, these women were asked by the neurologist and nurse whether they were interested in joining the group. Because some of them in need of psychological help were already being seen individually by the staff psychiatrists, they decided not to become involved in group activities. The other women explained that they were not interested at this time.

MEMBERS

From the pool of names suggested by the medical staff, twelve were contacted initially by phone and invited to an introductory/exploratory group meeting. Included in the original list of names was one man who, though not afflicted with Multiple Sclerosis, was experiencing similar physical symptoms and emotional difficulties from another neurological illness (Frederick's Ataxia), he asked to be included in the group. Ten people attended the first group meeting. Table 1 describes the basic demographic data for the group members, and Table 2 explains the stages of Multiple Sclerosis in the group members. In turn, the stages identified varied

TABLE 1

Patient	Age	Marital Status	Occupation	Number of Children	Years since Diagnosis of Illness	How Long Unemployed due to Illness (Years)
1	44	married	unskilled laborer	2	9	5
2	46	married	plumber	4	16	10
3	52	married	bank officer	none	23	13
4	44	divorced	salesman	3	20	15
5	52	married	quality control technician	3	30	4
6	39	married	post office worker	2	17	8
7	44	married	manager-food store	3	16	15
8	23	divorced	none	2	3	n/a
9	30	married	printer	2	7	4
10	37	married	policeman	2	8	still employed

emotional problems, differing needs, and assorted adjustmental concerns. Also, eight of the ten persons had never received formal counseling or therapy.

TIME

The group sessions were to be limited to an hour and a half, once every two weeks. The time, length, and frequency of the meetings were determined by transportation arrangements and the schedules of the members when they were receiving treatment at the clinic. Because many of the patients had to come a great distance by cab, it was financially feasible to hold the meetings while the members were at the clinic, and the group sessions were to be scheduled between doctor's visits and physical and occupational therapy.

LEADERS

In planning the group it was decided that there would be co-leaders, namely, a rehabilitation psychologist, the first author, who worked part-time at the clinic and his clinical associate, the second author. The psychologist had been with the clinic for two years but had been working with the chronically ill for six years. His associate was an unmarried, female doctoral student who previous to returning to school had worked four years with a state agency as a rehabilitation counselor.

TABLE 2. *Group Stages of Multiple Sclerosis in Members as Shown by Neurologic Deficits, Behavior, and Life Effectiveness*

Stage Number	1	2	3	4	5
Patients per Stage	patient #9	patient #5	patient #8 patient #1 patient #10	patient #2 patient #3 patient #4 patient #6 patient #7	no patients

1. Minimal signs and minimal changes in mental status, behavior and life effectiveness. History of neurologic deficit but without significant residuals.

2. Slight but recognizable signs of nervous system dysfunction, such as gait disturbance, weakness, incoordination, and only slight change in behavior and life effectiveness.

3. Moderate and easily recognizable signs of nervous system abnormality, gait disturbance, incoordination, visual difficulty and incontinence. Moderate change in behavior and life effectiveness. (Still able to work, but only able to give marginal performance relevant to physical demands. Can engage in full activity at home.)

4. Moderately severe and easily recognizable abnormality of nervous system; severe change in mental status, behavior, and life effectiveness. At-home activity is confined to the wheelchair.

5. Severe and easily recognizable neurologic deficits, such as gait disturbance, incoordination and visual difficulties and incontinence. Bed and chair existence at home.

The presence of a woman was expected not only to facilitate the discussion, but also to provide different perspectives when dealing with many questions from the group members. For example, sexual issues are often a paramount concern to men with Multiple Sclerosis. When the group members felt comfortable with a female co-leader, it was believed that they could benefit both from her views on sexual issues and from a woman's view point on many family concerns that re-occur during continuing adjustment to disease implications. It was also believed that a male and female co-leadership may have added advantages, since some members of the group may find that they could relate more easily to a man, while others more easily to a woman.

THE GROUP PROCESS

In reviewing the development of the group, two phases were identified which differentiated the time when the group members began to change in their attitude towards each other and started to express their feelings related to their disease. The initial phase included the first six sessions, and the subsequent and continuing sessions can be called the second phase, for the group still meets regularly as originally scheduled.

INITIAL PHASE OF THE GROUP

In the first meeting the group members expressed a desire to help others in their struggle to cope with the illness, to learn from others, to acquire a more positive outlook on life, and to deal both with the depressing aspects of the illness and with the fear and uncertainty of becoming more physically limited and dependent. The organization of the group in and of itself was encouraging for many members because it was an indication that their problems and needs had been recognized by the clinic staff. But during this first session the potential members seemed ambivalent about expressing their feelings and their need to become involved in a therapeutic experience. Much of the discussion in this meeting was of a superficial and non-threatening nature.

The leaders encouraged exploration and expression of feelings during the first several sessions and promoted appropriate areas of discussion for the group. For example, early in the group one person discussed his arrangements about vacationing with friends in another part of the country. This included his apprehensions about informing his friends about the illness and his physical limitations because of a fear of rejection. The leaders elicited further exploration by the young veteran and provided encouragement when other group members joined in the discussion. Yet the members tended to ignore their feelings or often discussed activities that were irrelevant or inappropriate for group sessions. During these meetings they avoided emotionally-laden subjects, either because they were fearful of such exploration or were uncertain about what seemed acceptable to discuss. Many members, in addition, seemed to "view the world through rose-colored glasses" and adopted a complacent acceptance of their physical limitations and resulting dependence on others. Eventually, the leaders found that these attitudes served as a mask for deeper feelings of helplessness, anger, fear, or ambivalence about their dependency.

In these initial sessions it became apparent that many simply wanted to listen to the leaders and were hesitant to empathize with the concerns of others. One exception was the relationship of an older member who had had the disease for many years and a younger member who had a more recent diagnosis. The former perceived himself as a father figure and became concerned that the younger person might make the same disease-related, adjustmental mistakes that he had made many years earlier.

When the members did initiate some discussion, it was on issues related to information or knowledge of the disease. When a feeling was even suggested in a person's verbal expression, he would immediately change the subject. But in each group session the leaders discussed the importance of identifying their own feelings as an initial step toward a better disease adjustment, then asked the members about their feelings and confronted them on the avoidance issue. Gradually they realized that it was acceptable to express their emotions, became more comfortable with each other and also became aware that other members shared the same emotions relevant to the disease. This awareness slowly stimulated an understanding and closeness between the group members, which manifested itself in the form of humour, positive confrontation, and empathy.

SECOND AND PRESENT PHASE OF THE GROUP

After the beginning six sessions the group moved at their own pace and generally chose their own topics. Instead of directing their discussion to the leaders, they began to talk to each other and a communication pattern developed from their mutual understanding and their need to help many of the members through a particular adjustmental difficulty. Also, after the sixth session, the group members confronted the leaders as to "how do you think the group is going and what are your expectations now?" It appeared that not only did they want some validation for the group process, but also encouragement for their increased involvement in the group. Their own attitude toward the leaders changed from a more "authority-figure–you lead us" perspective to a "you are necessary for the group, yet we will call on you when we need you" outlook. Within the group two of the members became more dominant in their verbalization and when this issue was raised by the leaders, the members in turn began to deal with their own reticence.

After the first six group sessions the role of the group leaders shifted from one of providing structure and acting as dominant guides for the discussion to acting more as a source of encouragement and a reinforcer to verbal statements made by the group members in their efforts to participate. The leaders also realized that they were to model "non-judgmental" acceptance, interpersonal honesty, and spontaneity. For example, the age variation in the group indicated differing values and varied beliefs. Some of the statements made by the younger members relevant to sexual adjustment were contrary to some of the moral beliefs of others. There was the temptation by the latter to impose their viewpoints and make a judgment on the younger members' actions. Realizing that such value judgments would be destructive to the group process, the leaders, each of whom represents differing values and viewpoints, did not assert their own opinions, nor on these occasions did they necessarily act as a reinforcer. The impression conveyed was that each group member was to make his own decision and take responsibility for his actions.

Throughout the group meetings, however, the role of the leaders also included facilitating the ventilation of personal feelings of loss associated with the disease. Though the men gradually became more accustomed to expressing some of their feelings associated with the illness, such as, embarrassment over falling or perceived rejection from others because of their limitations, they were still reluctant to reveal personal feelings about having the disease and the restrictions and hardships it brought to their life-styles. Yet the anger, resentment, and grief were often hidden by indirect statements or references to those emotions that others in the group might possess. When it was apparent that the members could handle the expres-

sion of their own feelings and receive support from others, the leaders
would utilize confrontation to break through this defensive device.

FACTORS FACILITATING COPING AND ADJUSTMENT TO THE ILLNESS IN THE GROUP PROCESS

Since one of the main goals for the group was to help the individual
member cope with the physical and emotional implications of the illness,
the leaders were continually determining those factors in the group process
which were conducive to this coping. There were three such factors identified, namely, acceptance, ventilation, and modeling.

Acceptance. Members, especially those with a more recent diagnosis,
began to realize that despite their illness and the previous failures they had
made in adjusting to it, they were accepted by others in the group. From
the group acceptance they began to have more confidence in themselves,
grew to appreciate their residual strengths and productive capabilities, and
gradually learned how to tolerate the negative attitudes of others and to
assert themselves when necessary in public. Much of this acceptance
resulted from a recognition of the similarity of their disease-related situation with that of others in the group and that to help someone else with a
problem meant an acceptance and a tackling of one's own difficulty. It also
resulted from group support and the suggestions about maintaining one's
feelings of personal adequacy and dignity.

Ventilation. Through the ventilation of personal feelings of loss and anger
much unfinished grief business was resolved. The members were then able
to move on to the task of dealing with present adjustmental concerns. One
person, for example, was bitterly angry that his wife had left him because of
her supposed negative attitude toward his disease. He was reluctant to express these feelings for many group sessions until he was finally confronted
by a group member. The member then verbalized them over many group
sessions, but at the same time also began to make new arrangements for his
life, such as social contacts, a new apartment and an exploration of what he
could do occupationally, even with his limitations.

Modeling. Many members learned how to cope by listening to how
someone else's difficulty had been handled. It was not merely the providing
of information, but with the development of group trust, the patients grew
to believe in the value of the information imparted. While men with MS
have many similar experiences resulting from their limitations, for example,
loss of bladder or bowel control and the resulting embarrassment, or loss of
much of sexual function and the often accruing friction with one's spouse;
so they have many different ways of dealing with these problems. Some are
maladaptive, others are adaptive, but a member who has newly experienced
these problems needs someone who has also encountered them and can relate how they were dealt with successfully. The group environment provides

such a setting for learning how to cope, and the leaders discovered that as the members grew to understand and accept each other the information imparted by the patient was highly valued. This trust between the group members strongly encouraged the following of advice for coping with the disease.

GROUP HIGHLIGHTS

Certain factors helped to make this group counseling with the chronically ill a unique treatment experience. This became evident as the group members began to feel more comfortable in expressing their personal thoughts or learned to trust each other. These factors frequently highlighted the group meetings and can be referred to as: a) religion and shared hope as a coping mechanism in chronic illness; b) group accountability as a source of patient motivation; and c) the utilization of the past.

RELIGION AND SHARED HOPE AS A COPING MECHANISM IN CHRONIC ILLNESS

From the information that was provided during the meetings it became evident to the leaders that common coping approaches toward illness-related problems were held by the group. Rather than talk of the future, a "take each day as it comes" approach prevailed. Surprisingly, many of the members discussed the importance of religious faith, and while never attempting to impose their values upon one another, they felt quite comfortable in explaining how religion helped them to cope with many disease-related problems. Most of the group members were not regular churchgoers prior to illness onset, but became members of varied religious organizations upon the prompting of family and friends when they were encountering serious physical and emotional difficulties related to their disease. In the group the members stated that religion became not a source for a miraculous cure, but a resource to deal with the daily difficulties emanating from their disease.

Also, the members were anxious to convey to others a sense of "hope" and the theme of "never give up hope" was often repeated during the sessions. This philosophy became very important to the younger members and this reassuring attitude from others provided the impetus, in many instances, to make an important life decision. For example, one group member had been separated from his young wife for six months because she was unable to accept the disease and its implications for their marriage. She also took their two children and the patient was hesitant to see them or become more assertive in claiming his rights to visit them because of personal feelings of inadequacy, depression, and uncertainty. The group members helped this person focus on his residual strengths and gave him a sense of hope by repeating often the information that the course of the disease is unknown and a remission could last for an indefinite period of time. They encouraged him to express his feelings after they were identified by the group members and then suggested how he could become more assertive in dealing with his wife. The interest and information represented for this member a form of reassurance and support and provided the stimulus to adopt a plan of action that eventually led to regular visits with his children.

GROUP ACCOUNTABILITY AS A SOURCE OF PATIENT MOTIVATION

During the group sessions, various issues were discussed such as the importance of keeping busy during the day, how to become more involved with the raising of one's children, or how to tell others that you have a neurological illness. In addition, feelings were explored, information was given and the impression was conveyed by the group members that they were responsible to provide some feedback to the group on each planned course of action. Consequently, the group environment was not only able to provide a vehicle for conveying information, but also furnished an atmosphere of support and accountability. When the group members would ask "how did our suggestions work," the patients seemed to realize more the importance of attempting to implement the suggested course of action.

UTILIZATION OF THE PAST

When they were acting as facilitators for the expression of feelings, the leaders stimulated a discussion of the group members' occupational, family, and social past. In order to adjust to present physical limitations and achieve some measure of acceptance of their condition, the patients must first review the past events of their lives, talk about them and re-live many of their memories. This has a cathartic effect which releases feelings that contribute to anger and grief. Then when the patients begin to discuss present adjustmental difficulties, they are more readily disposed to express their anger over what they have lost.

For a group of chronically ill patients such a discussion creates a unique experience in group therapy. Instead of focusing only on here and now issues, or only on how group members are relating to one another, "outside of the room" issues are frequently raised. When past, predisease experiences are brought up, first the leaders and then the group members provoke further discussion and provide some insights into present behavior from past experience.

One group member, for example, realizing that re-occuring, deteriorative loss had now prevented him from driving a car, decided to remain at home and withdrew from many previous social contacts. He lived alone, but was not making any alternative arrangements for transportation to social activities. Becoming aware of this behavior, the group members asked the person to talk about the satisfying times he had with the use of the car and to describe now what the driving loss meant to him. The member stated his feelings and through this expression learned the reason for his behavior. The group then suggested alternative ways of getting out of the apartment and conveyed support in these endeavors. Feeling better about himself, the patient adopted some of these suggestions, reported to the group about his progress and gradually restored some of his social pastimes, which are necessary for his coping with the disease.

PROBLEMS AND IMPLICATIONS

There are several aspects of the present group which may be barriers or facilitators to the change process, aspects which warrant attention when starting a group. First, the size, homogeneity of the group, and the frequency of meetings have an impact upon the group process. As mentioned earlier, time restrictions in the clinic impelled the leaders to consider a group of 10–12 members, even though this may not be ideal for facilitating change. Since the group has proven beneficial to the members and has been well received by the staff, consideration may be given in the future for two groups. In organizing an additional group, the authors will consider the advantages and disadvantages of a more homogeneous group in terms of physical stages of the illness and age of the members. Our group is heterogeneous and because of this offers a wide range of emotional reactions to the disability, knowledge of the illness, and experience in coping with it. However, precisely because of this diversity, members who are in the intial stages of coping with the disability may find it difficult to relate to members in which the disease is in advanced stages (and vice versa).

Another important issue is the frequency of the meetings. Less frequent meetings, we believe, would not offer as great an opportunity for the development of group trust, cohesion, and change. While weekly meetings are more costly to the agency and inconvenient for the disabled members, it may provide more continuity and a more concentrated process of therapeutic change.

Two other important issues are the inclusion of females and family members in the group. (see Schwartz, 1974). Both of these alternatives may offer an opportunity to understand the dynamics of familial and/or interpersonal problems from a broader perspective than is afforded with the members alone. Those spouses of Multiple Sclerosis patients who have adjusted well to living with the disease could offer valuable suggestions to the other family members who are having a difficult time adapting to the illness. Including family members could also have specific implications for medical management. In as much as increased understanding of the medical and psychosocial aspects of the illness by the family members could enhance their ability to cope with the illness and in turn help the member cope more constructively, this would be beneficial. However, the inclusion of family members could inhibit the members' expression of feelings or discussion of particularly sensitive topics, such as, incontinence, low self-esteem and sexual problems.

A question entertained by the leaders as the group developed was: "Would the group members have a hard time relating to the leaders because they were not disabled?" Yet with this group it did not seem to become a concern. They related to the leaders as professionals who could provide information and facilitate group interaction. But the leaders realized as the group continued that a disabled group leader who was a professional member of the staff could have enhanced the group process. More than likely the men would have found in such a leader an important model for coping with adjustmental difficulties, and learned to become more open to each other earlier in the group meetings.

Initially the members experienced difficulty in identifying and revealing their feelings. Some of the reticence to discuss feelings may have been overcome by the use of structured interventions or "exercises" designed to encourage discussion and group trust (Pfeiffer and Jones, 1977). More direct interpretation of avoidance may have been helpful when the members became tangential in their discussion. This interpretation may have been useful in establishing the norm of self-disclosure earlier in the process. In addition, it is helpful to be aware of significant underlying issues that some members may have difficulty discussing, such as incontinence or sexual problems. If these issues are masked, dealt with superficially, or completely avoided, gentle confrontation should be used at appropriate times to facilitate exploration in these areas.

CONCLUSION

The group continues to meet regularly, as initially planned, for there are continued adjustmental issues and the men themselves have found an environment in which they are comfortable to talk about personal feelings. The focus of treatment, however, in a chronic deteriorative illness, such as Multiple Sclerosis, is often upon the physical aspects of the disease. This group has provided a balance to that treatment by recognizing and attending to the psychological component of the illness and, in general, appears to have had a rather significant impact upon many individual members. Because of the shared experiences within the group the veterans gained a sense of commitment and responsibility to each other. In turn, this encouraged some patients to function as "helpers" to members who needed to learn new coping strategies or ways to function more productively within their limitations. The group has also provoked in many members a willingness to share their feelings and expressions with others and recognize that there is validity and importance in this sharing. There seems to be an increased awareness by some members of the necessity for change in their coping strategies and that they have control over and responsibility for these behavioral changes. Specifically, the group has encouraged a more active response in some members as opposed to passive acceptance of their limitations. As a result most of the group members are dealing more constructively with their illness.

The group has also had a significant impact on the leaders in terms of understanding the medical, psychological, and social impact of a chronic deteriorative illness upon the patient and patient's family. The leaders have become aware both of the varieties of reactions to the illness and the unique coping mechanisms of some patients. The process of constructive change in the group has demonstrated the potential of group therapy for the chronically ill in dealing with the effects of their illness.

REFERENCES

Dr. Power is an associate professor and Director of the Rehabilitation Counseling Program, School of Education, University of Maryland, College Park, Maryland. Ms. Rogers is a doctoral candidate, Department of Rehabilitation Counseling, Boston University.

Barnes, R. H.; Busse, E. W.; and Dinken, H. The alleviation of emotional problems in multiple sclerosis by group psychotherapy. *Group Psychotherapy,* 1954, 6: 193–201.

Bolding, H. Psychotherapeutic aspects in the management of patients with multiple sclerosis. *Diseases of the Nervous System,* 1960, 21: 24–26.

Day, M.; Day, E.; and Hermann, R. Group therapy of patients with multiple sclerosis. *Archives of Neurology and Psychiatry,* 1953, 69: 193–196.

Hartings, M. F.; Pavlou, M. M.; and Davis, F. A. Group counseling of MS patients in a program of comprehensive care. *Journal of Chronic Disease,* 1976, 29: 65–73.

Huberty, D. J. Adapting to illness through family groups. *International Journal of Psychiatry in Medicine,* 1974, 5: 231–242.

Jaques, M. E., and Patterson, K. M. The self-help group model: A review. *Rehabilitation Counseling Bulletin,* 1974, 48–58.

Long, R. T. Insights gained through group therapy with multiple sclerosis patients. *Journal of Nervous and Mental Disorders,* 119, 1954.

Mally, M., and Strehl, C. B. Evaluation of a three-year group therapy program for multiple sclerosis patients. *International Journal of Group Psychotherapy,* 1963, 13: 328–334.

McAlpine, D.; Compston, N. D.; and Lumsden, C. *Multiple sclerosis.* Edinburgh: E & S Livingstone Lts, 1955.

Pfeiffer and Jones. *Handbook of structured experiences,* Vol. 1–6. La Jolla, California: *University Associates,* 1977.

Shontz, F. Some psychological problems of patients with multiple sclerosis. *Archives of Physical Medicine and Rehabilitation,* 1955, 37: 633–640.

Schwartz, M. Group psychotherapy with multiple sclerosis patients and their spouses. *Proceedings American Psychological Association,* New Orleans, 1974.

15

Group Therapy with The Terminally Ill
—IRVIN D. YALOM, M.D., and CARLOS GREAVES, M.D.

A spate of recent publications has reflected a renewed commitment by the medical and paramedical professions to the care of the dying patient.[1-8] Workers in this field have identified the special psychological needs of patients facing imminent death, studied and outlined "stages" of dying, and sketched rough guidelines for the psychotherapy of the terminally ill. During the past four years we have employed a group therapy format in the care of dying patients. Initially we assumed that the group members would profit from continued close contact with others facing the same tragic experience. We thought that sharing, open communication, and the opportunity to be helpful to others would be an antidote to the bitter isolation so many dying patients experience.

A second reason for organizing a therapy group for terminally ill patients was the conviction that such a group could teach us much about everyday psychotherapy with the living. Although it is common knowledge that a serious confrontation with death often triggers a profound reappraisal of one's basic relationship with oneself, others, and the world, it is uncommon for a concentrated contemplation of death to enter the psychotherapeutic dialogue. One important reason for this is that the psychotherapist's basic theories of anxiety (and hence his/her chief consideration in psychotherapy) rest not on the bedrock of the dread of nonbeing but on such derivative phenomena as separation, castration, and loss of ego boundaries. Another reason issues from the magnitude of the threat. Most psychotherapy patients and most therapists will not stare at death very long before they lower the blinds of denial. Psychotherapy groups occasionally deal with death when prodded by such stimuli as the death of someone close to one of the members or the departure of one of the members from the group. However, the focus is rarely sustained for more than a single session; depression, avoidance, and denial soon obstruct the work.

Both of these considerations prodded us to organize a group of patients with terminal illnesses—patients who are so close to death that continual denial is not possible. We hoped to help them if we could, to learn from them, and to apply what we learned to the everyday therapy of the living.

Reprinted from the *American Journal of Psychiatry*, vol. 134, pp. 396–400, 1977. Copyright 1977, the American Psychiatric Association. Reprinted by permission.

DESCRIPTION OF THE GROUP

Four years ago, with the aid of a patient with metastatic cancer, we began a group for patients with metastatic carcinoma (breast carcinoma in most cases). Since then the group has met once weekly for 90 minutes. (Occasionally there have been special 1-hour sessions before the meeting wherein training is offered in meditation and in autohypnosis for pain control.) The patients are all fully aware of the nature and prognosis of their illness. Our experience is that it is best to exclude patients who exhibit massive denial of their illness and its implications. We also exclude patients whose cancer has been contained and who have excellent prognoses. It is an open group; members come as often as their physical condition permits and as long as they continue to profit from the experience. Almost all are outpatients, but a few have attended while hospitalized. The number attending meetings ranges from 3 to 12, averaging 6–7 members. We have found 7 members to be the approximate maximal effective size; when more than 7 members attend, we divide the group into 2 small groups for an hour and reconvene as a large group for the final 30 minutes.

Patients generally enter the group by self-referral or by referral from cancer organizations such as the American Cancer Society's Reach to Recovery program. At first, physicians rarely referred patients to the group; they feared that a group in which dying was discussed would severely unsettle their patients. However, after physicians observe the group, speak to members, and learn that the group's major focus is not dying but living, their fears are alleviated, and many physicians have referred patients to the group. During the course of 4 years more than 40 patients have attended at least one meeting; the group maintains an active roster of approximately 20 members, some of whom attend regularly and some only periodically when in deep despair. Twelve members have died. There have been several therapists during the course of the group—2 faculty members of the department of psychiatry, 3 psychiatric residents, a psychiatric social worker, and 2 guidance counselors. Usually there are as many as 3–4 therapists present at every meeting—not because of the needs of the group but because its unusual nature has aroused much student interest.

COURSE OF THE GROUP: MODES OF HELP

A number of mechanisms of change (i.e., curative factors[9]) have operated in the group. Members were helped by such factors as altruism (being able to be helpful to others), catharsis, group cohesiveness, universality, and existential factors.[10]

The group began in a significant and memorable way. Five desperately anxious women filed into the room and sat down. One of them, a 50-year-old woman with metastatic breast cancer who had been a prime force in organizing the group, began the meeting by passing out copies of the following Hassidic tale:

A rabbi had a conversation with the Lord about Heaven and Hell. "I will show you Hell," said the Lord and led the rabbi into a room in the middle of which was a very big round table. The people sitting at it were famished and desperate. In the middle of the table there was a large pot of stew, enough and more for everyone. The smell of the stew was delicious and made the rabbi's mouth water. The people round the table were holding spoons with very long handles. Each one found that it was just possible to reach the pot to take a spoonful of the stew, but because the handle of his spoon was longer than a man's arm, he could not get the food back into his mouth. The rabbi saw that their suffering was terrible. "Now I will show you Heaven," said the Lord, and they went into another room exactly the same as the first. There was the same big round table and the same pot of stew. The people, as before, were equipped with the same long-handled spoons—but here they were well nourished and plump, laughing and talking. At first the rabbi could not understand. "It is simple, but it requires a certain skill," said the Lord. "You see, they have learned to feed each other."

The parable was prophetic—much help was destined to flow between the members of the group. In fact, the group was unusual in that there was such a wide range of support. Not only did the patients help one another in *quid pro quo* (giving-receiving) fashion, but altruism, the act of giving, was intrinsically valuable to the members. As in any therapy group, the members themselves were the prime agents of help. In this group that fact took on an added dimension since terminally ill patients are so imbued with a sense of powerlessness and uselessness. They dread nothing so much as helpless immobility, being not only personally burdensome but without value to another. Consequently, learning that they had much to offer others imbued many of the members with a renewed sense of worth.

Furthermore, being helpful to others brings patients out of a morbid self-absorption which, for many, had stripped life of its meaning. The more they are able to move out of themselves, to extend themselves to others, the more they experience a sense of fulfillment. Nietszche once wrote, "He who has a *why* to live can bear with almost any *how*."

Members are able to be helpful in a number of ways. They telephone and visit members who are in despair. They share books and coping techniques that have been useful to them. For example, one of the members taught other members in the group the meditation techniques that had been useful to her in dealing with pain.

Another mode of offering help (and thus helping oneself) is to teach by sharing one's experiences with others. (The patients often felt before joining the group that "We are teachers but the students will not listen.") The patients are very willing to speak to medical students and to permit observation of the meetings through a one-way mirror. There is rarely a meeting without observers (e.g., nurses, physical therapists, medical students, psychologists, oncologists, radio-therapists).

These patients are especially desirous of reaching and influencing the medical profession because, almost without exception, they have a complex and ambivalent set of feelings toward their doctors. At first, much anger was evident; in fact, the group's initial cohesiveness resulted at least in part from a common bond of enmity toward the medical profession. Some of this enmity was justified, some was irrational. Both types of anger were dealt with: the irrational by understanding and working through, the realistic by ventilation and development of adaptive coping strategies.

The irrational anger stems from the doctors' failure to meet extremely unrealistic demands. At deep, unconscious levels the members expected the doctors to be all-knowing and all-protecting. They put their faith in the doctor to the same degree that their ancestors had placed their faith in the hands of the priest. And, of course, the doctor could not be the ultimate rescuer. Patients are forced to confront limits and finiteness, and the ensuing anger and dread is often displaced to the physician.

However, much anger is justified. The surgeons and oncologists either lack the time or arrange their schedules in such a way that they cannot provide the time for the kinds of support and information the patients crave. The patients felt their physicians were too impersonal and too authoritarian. They resented not being kept fully informed and being excluded from important decisions regarding their own treatment. Many patients reported that physicians withdrew emotionally from them when metastasis occurred. They felt abandoned just at the time when they needed the most support.

Patients learn from one another what they can and cannot expect from their doctors. They compare notes and role-play methods of asking doctors questions. They come to grips with how much they really want to know—were the physicians concealing information, or were the patients asking questions in such a way that the physicians were merely complying with their wishes to avoid gaining the information they ostensibly wanted?

Over time it became abundantly clear in the group that the patients had a strong need for a sustaining relationship when their illness was no longer deemed curable and that many had physicians who were so threatened or discouraged that they could not provide the sheer presence the patients required. Presence was the overriding need and the chief commodity provided by the group. Almost without exception, patients facing death feel cut off and shunned by the living. We agree with Kübler-Ross that the question is not *whether* to tell the patient that his/her disease is one that has no cure, but *how* to tell the patient. The living, by a multitude of signals, always let the patient know that the illness is terminal. Nurses, paramedical personnel, and physicians cue the patient, often in the most subtle ways—a hushed shrinking away, a tendency to be less intimate, a slightly greater physical distance. One member commented that her doctor always ended his meetings with her by giving her a gentle pat on her fanny. When he became more solemn and, instead of patting her, shook her hand, she recognized the seriousness of her illness for the first time.

Not only are patients isolated because they are shunned by the living, but they increase their isolation by their reluctance to discuss their most central concerns with others. They fear that friends will be frightened and avoid them; they are reluctant to burden and depress their families further.

It became apparent that the most basic anxiety of many group members was not so much a fear of dying, of finiteness and nonbeing, but of the absolute utter loneliness that accompanies death. Obviously, basic existential loneliness cannot be allayed or taken away; it can only be appreciated and, in a curious way, shared through the sharing of it. The other kind of loneliness, secondary interpersonal loneliness that is a function both of the shunning of the dying person and his/her self-imposed isolation, can be dealt with effectively in the group. First and most important, the group offers an arena in which all concerns can be aired and thoroughly discussed. There are no issues too deep or morbid to be discussed openly in the group. These issues include physical concerns (e.g., loss of hair from chemotherapy, disfigurement from mutilating surgery), fear of the actual act of dying, fear of pain, the possibility of afterlife, the fear of becoming a "vegetable," the desire to have decision-making power concerning the time of death, euthanasia, the "living will," funeral arrangements, etc. These concerns are foremost in the minds of many patients, but they are unable to discuss them with any living person. The group affords considerable relief by simply allowing patients to share these thoughts.

In this group, as in all therapy groups, one becomes ever more cognizant of the overarching need that people have for other people. The group spends much time and does much effective work with the patients who, because of characterological style or particular methods of coping with recent stress, have cut themselves off from others. For example, one patient never asked for any personal help from the group. For months she tended to speak in extremely concrete terms. When she was asked about herself, she responded by giving a long summary of her physicial condition, her examinations by doctors, and her recent chemotherapeutic regimen. The therapist helped this patient by repeatedly asking her, when she had finished talking about her physical self, to respond again to the question, "How are *you*? How is the person feeling to whom all of these things are happening?" Gradually, she became more able to relate to others and to discuss her own needs. Although she could not easily discuss her feelings, she once reported to the group a dream of a poor injured kitten for whom she had wept. She was able to accept the interpretation offered by group members that she was the kitten and that she wept for herself. Later in the group she became more open to discussion of all affect; she even reported, after attending one member's funeral, the anger and fear that the sterility and impersonality of the service had aroused in her.

Another member had planned a large dinner party and learned from her physician that morning that her cancer had metastasized. Her chief concern at that point was less a fear of death than of isolation and abandonment. She feared that her illness would cause her so much pain that she would respond to it in a primitive, animalistic fashion and therefore be shunned by others. She held her party and kept her illness secret from friends. It was with much relief that she was able to discuss these concerns in the group and to hear how other members with more advanced disease had experienced and dealt with pain.

Another member began the group in bitter isolation. She was a widow who felt she had been isolated by all of her former friends and abandoned by her only child. The group at first empathized with her, and many members felt extremely angry toward her son, who had apparently behaved in an extremely ungrateful manner. Gradually some members became aware of the fact that neither the patient nor her son acted independently but were instead locked together in dynamic interaction. The patient had for years (long before her cancer) been an embittered and angry woman who had in effect driven her son away from her. With the help of the group she became softer, more open and responsive to others. Her son reciprocated and she became even more generous; eventually, before her death, she became a source of considerable strength for other members of the group.

A woman who was desperately ill with advanced leukemia came to the group for only one session. She spent the entire meeting discussing the fecklessness and coldness of her only child, a daughter, who was a psychologist and "should have known better." One of the other patients helped this woman appreciate the triviality of her charges against the daughter and suggested that she make the most of her remaining time by saying to her daughter, "You are the most important thing in the world to me, and I want us to be close before I die." The patient died only a few days after this meeting, but we learned from the nursing staff that she had followed the group's advice and had a final, deeply fulfilling meeting with her daughter.

THE THERAPIST IN THE GROUP

The presence offered by the therapy group must, of course, include the therapist. One cannot effectively lead such a group by making a dichotomy between "us," the living therapists, and "them," the dying patients. Therapists lead effectively when they appreciate that it is "we" who face death; the leaders are members who must share in the group's anxiety. The anxiety that the leader must tolerate is considerable, and it has been our experience that a period of several months' apprenticeship is necessary for therapists to deal with their own dread of death so that they can work effectively. We found, for example, that when the group interaction was superficial, the therapists were often responsible. The considered certain topics too threatening for the patients to discuss, but ultimately they were protecting themselves. Given the opportunity, the group was willing to plunge deeply and meaningfully into any area.

Sometimes the therapist proceeded with extreme caution because he regarded the patient as too anguished to tolerate any additional anxiety. Not infrequently this spawned an overly conservative approach that merely enhanced the patient's sense of isolation. Victor Frankl once suggested that Boyle's law of gaseous expansion in a physical space could be applied to anxiety, in that anxiety expands to fill any space offered to it. Many people who are relatively unburdened find that trivial anxiety fills their life space completely. Thus, the absolute amount of anxiety in the dying patient is often no greater than that of patients facing a number of other life concerns. It seems that we get used to anything, even to dying. At times the group provided a type of desensitization experience, as patients repeatedly approached and palpated the most frightening issues. Laughter that was neither diversionary nor tension-spawned often occurred spontaneously. For example, during one meeting a member spoke about a seemingly healthy neighbor who had died suddenly during the night. One member stated that that was most regrettable since the woman had had no time to prepare either herself or her family for her death. Others disagreed, and one member said that that was precisely the way she would like to die, quipping, "I've always loved surprises."

At the same time, however, the therapist must learn to respect denial and to allow each patient to proceed at his/her own pace. Even though all of the group members are aware of their diagnosis and prognosis, they often shift their level of awareness, and the therapist renders the most help by respecting the patient's decision regarding what he/she chooses to know at that moment.

It is important to conceptualize the group as a group for living, not for dying. For one thing, physicians are more inclined to refer patients when the group's purpose is to improve the quality of life rather than to focus on dying. Even more important is the fact that an open confrontation with death allows many patients to move into a mode of existence that is richer than the one they experienced prior to their illness. Many patients report dramatic shifts in life perspective. They are able to trivialize the trivial, to assume a sense of control, to stop doing things they do not wish to do, to communicate more openly with families and close friends, and to live entirely in the present rather than in the future or the past. Many report that facing and mastering some of their fear of death dissolves many other fears, particularly fears of awkward interpersonal situations, rejection, or humiliation. We are not being ironic when we suggest that, in a grim fashion, cancer cures psychoneuroses. As one's focus turns from the trivial diversions of life, a fuller appreciation of the elemental factors in existence may emerge: the changing seasons, the falling leaves, the last spring, and, especially, the loving of others. Over and over we hear our patients say (and this is a most compelling message for the psychotherapist) "Why did we have to wait till *now,* till we are riddled with cancer, to learn how to value and appreciate life?"

CONCLUSIONS

Our impressions to date are that the group therapy format for the treatment of terminally ill patients is an exceptionally effective therapeutic mode. The therapy group has become a key support system for many patients and has enabled them to cope more effectively with the enormous stress that invariably accompanies metastatic carcinoma. We are currently in the midst of a three-year project sponsored by the National Cancer Institute that will permit a more systematic evaluation of such groups.

REFERENCES

Dr. Yalom is Professor of Psychiatry, Stanford University Medical Center, Stanford California, and Dr. Greaves is Psychiatrist, Mental Health Service, Maui, Hawaii.

The authors would like to express their gratitude to Mrs. Katie Weers for her inspired guidance in all stages of this work.

This article represents a revised version of a paper presented at the 129th annual meeting of the American Psychiatric Association, Miami Beach, Florida, May 10–14, 1976.

1. Kübler-Ross, K.: *On death and dying.* New York, Macmillan Publishing Co., 1969.
2. Weisman, A.: *On dying and denying.* New York, Behavioral Publications, 1972.
3. Shneidman, E.: *Deaths of man.* Quadrangle/New York Times Book Co., 1973.
4. Lifton, R. J.: *Living and dying.* New York, Bantam Books, 1975.
5. Feifel, H. (ed): *The meaning of death.* New York, McGraw-Hill Book Co., 1959.
6. Abrams, R. D.: Denial and depression in the terminal cancer patient— a clue for management. *Psychiatr. Q.* 45:394–404, 1971.
7. Easson, W. M.: Care of the young patient who is dying. *JAMA* 205:203–207. 1968.
8. Hoffman, E.: Don't give up on me! *Am. J. Nurs.* 71:60–62. 1971.
9. Yalom, I.: *Theory and practice of group psychotherapy,* 2nd ed. New York, Basic Books, 1975.
10. Yalom, I. D.: Existential factors in group therapy. Strecker Monograph Award Series II. Philadelphia, Institute of the Pennsylvania Hospital, 1974.

Personal Awareness: Individual Exercises

1. As a staff member of a rehabilitation hospital, you are leading a group composed of members having any one of the disabilities described in the readings. The group unanimously agrees that being nondisabled, you are incapable of understanding and/or helping them. How do you respond?

2. Earth has been captured by the martians. Interestingly, the martians are just like human beings, physically, emotionally, and intellectually; the primary difference is that they can't hear. Further they despise earthlings who can hear, just because they're different. Therefore privileges usually afforded hearing earthlings have been discontinued (e.g., electric power, jobs, sexual relationships). Only deaf earthlings may continue having these privileges. How do you feel? What might you do?

3. You've just been told you have only one month to live. How would this information affect you? Would you benefit from a group experience with other people with terminal illness?

4. Suppose you had a disability which incapacitated you to a degree, then didn't affect you further for a year; severely incapacitated you for a month and then didn't affect you for three months. There is no continuity in your condition behaviorally or emotionally; you face each situation new, without reference to past experience. Discuss the impact on your social, family, and work relationships.

5. Determine where to get more information regarding a disability group in which you are *most* interested. Volunteer any services you have to offer for at least one week.

6. Determine where to get more information regarding a disability group in which you are *least* interested. Become involved in some form of volunteer work for one week.

7. For the next two weeks, treat your family members as though you only have two weeks to live. Note the behavioral and attitudinal changes you make and how these are experienced by your family.

Structured Group Experience in Disability
—Rollercoaster*

While it is difficult to predict how one would respond if afflicted with a disabling condition, it is important to consider how one might respond to a person who demonstrated an impairment. Would you be sensitive toward the person, could you predict what the person's difficulties were, and how would you feel in the presence of a person who was noticeably different? These and similar questions are examined in this structured group experience.

GOALS

1. To sensitize participants to implications of various physical disabilities.

2. To promote greater awareness of self and others.

3. To examine defenses different people use as they experience various handicaps.

4. To experience the importance of hope even as physical impairment becomes pronounced.

PRELIMINARY CONSIDERATIONS

1. *Level of Intensity:* Medium to high

2. *Group Size:* Groups of four to seven participants
   May also "fishbowl" a group from a larger group

3. *Time Required:* 3 hours

4. *Materials:* (a.) Deck of playing cards for each group (b.) Disability List (one for each participant)

5. *Physical Setting:* Comfortable room with moveable chairs

---

*See Appendices A and B for detailed information on use of the structured group experiences in disability.

PROCEDURE

1. The leader presents a brief introduction on physical disability.

2. The goals of "Rollercoaster" are presented and groups are formed.

3. Participants are told that they will be involved in a game of cards to enable them to experience the impact of various disabilities. The following guidelines are used:

   a. Each player is given the "Disability List" and dealt six cards by a group member. Players are asked to determine if the cards they hold match a disability on the "Disability List." If yes, they are to simulate the disability immediately. If there is no match, the player continues as nondisabled. The player to the left of the dealer picks a card from the deck and discards one card, face up, next to the deck. The first player continues to role-play the disability indicated by his or her hand. Other players take turns trying to determine what cards are held by the role player. The person who is correct becomes the next role player with play continuing in this manner for approximately fifteen minutes.

   b. After fifteen minutes, participants are told to stop and exchange hands with another person in the group and to assume the disability indicated.

4. Following the disability simulation, the experience is discussed from the following perspectives:
   a. How was the loss experienced?
   b. What were some deleterious interpersonal aspects of physical loss? How were these experienced by the person with the loss?
   c. Who was least disabled in the group?
   d. Was hope ever lost for any participant?
   e. What defenses were manifested? For what reason(s)?

LEADERSHIP SUGGESTIONS

1. Encourage observers and participants to share their perceptions of this experience.

2. Be sure to bridge the gap between this experience and losses shared by people having progressive diseases.

3. Explore how hope was affected by loss and gain from the disability.

4. Explore how members felt when they were instructed to exchange hands.

VARIATIONS

1. Group members may be given "ID cards" to display emotional reactions to their loss (e.g., anger, happiness, sadness, no change).

2. Participants may or may not be instructed to exchange hands.

3. Participants may be instructed to pass three cards to their left or right.

DISABILITY LIST*

Card Combinations	*Disability*
All Red Cards	Myasthenia Gravis
(Diamonds/Hearts)	Rheumatoid Arthritis
All Black Cards	Neurological Impairment
(Spades/Clubs)	Nondisabled
Three Black and Three Red	Quadriplegia
Four Face Cards	Total Hearing Loss
(Jack, Queen, King)	Terminal Illness
No Face Cards	Select Any Disability
Deuce of Any Suit	
Ace of Clubs	
None of the Above Combinations	

*Players are encouraged to simulate the disability in whatever way they interpret the loss of the function as described by the various articles in chapter 2 or other sources.

CHAPTER THREE

Group Approaches with Persons Having Kidney Disorders

_____ Overview

Medical breakthroughs in hemodialysis have given new hope for persons suffering from kidney failure. While many are aware of the benefits of these technical advances, the emotional strain of being dependent on a machine for continued living is frequently over-looked. Both hemodialysis patients and those close to them may experience intense adverse emotional reactions to the life changes imposed by complete dependency on a life support system. In an effort to overcome emotional difficulties related to hemodialysis, several group approaches have been used. Articles in this chapter reveal results of these efforts.

The value of group therapy for patients and their families is the central theme of Buchanan's article "Group Therapy for Kidney Transplant Patients." Kidney transplant patients are in a state of crisis that places a significant strain upon the family system. Group meetings designed to meet the needs of both the patient and family provided a forum where a wide variety of concerns were explored, ventilated, and potentially resolved. As a result of this group experience, support systems were established, role modeling took place, and an emphasis on skill development occurred.

"Group Treatment in a Hemodialysis Center" by Wijsenbeek and Munitz outlines the prevailing concerns of hemodialysis patients that emerged in the group process. Such concerns were found to be related to specific stages in the group. As the group developed, increasingly personal topics were disclosed including family problems, fear of death, and life with the kidney machine.

Family members frequently have difficulty adjusting to the impact of hemodialysis on their lives. The intense emotional stress experienced by spouses of hemodialysis patients prompted Shambaugh and Kanter to initiate group meetings for spouses of patients on hemodialysis, some of whom were dialyzing their spouses at home. "Spouses Under Stress: Group Meetings with Spouses of Patients on Hemodialysis" gives the reader greater understanding of spouses' emotional reactions that can greatly influence the course of treatment of the hemodialysis patient.

While many forms of group intervention may be regarded as traditional, occasional divergent approaches have been used in consideration of the unique concerns of hemodialysis patients. In an article entitled "Modified Group Therapy in the Treatment of Patients on Chronic Hemodialysis," Hollon emphasizes a systems approach for hemodialysis patients. This approach uses the treatment team as participants in the group. The advantages of a modified group therapy approach are discussed with a focus on the implications of therapeutic aspects for hemodialysis patients, their families, and treatment staff.

16

Group Therapy for Kidney Transplant Patients —DENTON C. BUCHANAN, Ph.D.

ALTHOUGH group therapy for chronic physically ill patients dates back to the turn of the century, its popularity has burgeoned only recently.[1] Therapists have reported the benefit of group treatment for epileptics,[2] diabetics,[3] postmyocardial patients,[4] myasthenia gravis patients,[5] and dialysands.[6,7] The paper has two basic purposes. The first is to describe some emotional reactions of recipients and their family in the

Reprinted by permission from the *International Journal of Psychiatry in Medicine*, 6 (4): 523–531, 1975. © 1976, Baywood Publishing Co., Inc.

early post surgical period and to present some observations on a group therapy program for them. The second is to relate the content and process of a short-term therapy group for the physically ill to a theoretical framework of groups for psychiatric patients.

Transplantation is a psychological stress for both the recipient and his family. Preoperatively the patient experiences the anxiety of being an obligation to his family. He is aware of the subtle family pressures to produce a donor[8] or perhaps to exclude some donor candidates.[9] The recipient who hopes for a cadaver organ is placed in the uncomfortable situation of having to wait and hope for someone to die a sudden tragic death.

At the time of surgery, patients report feeling a mixture of elation and fear. The return to normalcy is appealing. However the patient raises doubts of his competency and capacity to again establish himself. The fear of rejecting the kidney becomes acute. Such rejection often is viewed as a sign of personal failure and loss, a quality that plagues the renal failure patient throughout his treatment. The risk of the surgery itself, the issue of life and death, adds to the transplant patient's anxiety. Anxiety and depression have been described by a number of writers as the prominent postoperative psychiatric complications.[10-12] In essence, transplantation represents an acute traumatic experience superimposed upon the problem of adapting to a chronic illness.

METHOD

The members were eight kidney transplant patients and their families. The patients, six men and two women, ranged in age from twenty to fifty-five years. Two male patients had their new kidneys for several months when they entered this study. The rest were within their first month post surgery. The family members included five wives, four mothers (two of which were donors), one sister and one daughter. The therapist did not know any of these subjects preoperatively.

All patients and immediate family members were invited to attend the meetings. Attendance was not compulsory but no one declined the invitation. The potential members were told that the meetings had three primary purposes, social, educational, and emotional relief. It was suggested that the members would be interested in meeting one another to discuss common problems and exchange ideas. From the therapist's standpoint this was an attempt to reduce any tendency to withdraw or "tune-out" to other patients as is sometimes seen in dialysands.[13] It also set an expectation for identification and group cohesion. The meetings were to provide a vehicle for the patients to learn techniques in coping and adapting to the routine problems in surgical recovery such as physical therapy, diet, daily laboratory studies, home care of wounds etc. The members were told that they could both gain from the experience of others and contribute their own solutions to help someone else. This purpose was of most interest to the potential members and clearly represented the primary incentive to attend.

The third purpose was an opportunity for emotional relief. Renal failure was frightening and frustrating for the whole family and transplantation also had emotional tension associated with it. The members were told that such problems are common and they were given reason to believe that there would be support within the group and from the group leader for such discussion. The intent was merely to set the stage and give an air of permission for such topics.

The group meetings were held once a week for one hour just prior to the regular weekly renal outpatient clinic. Those patients who were still hospitalized in the postoperative period were brought to the clinic for the meeting.

RESULTS AND DISCUSSION

At the end of three months (10 meetings) the transplant recipients were asked to evaluate their experience. All agreed it had been beneficial for a variety of reasons to be described below. They felt that similar meetings would have been useful prior to their transplant surgery in order to relieve preoperative anxieties and provide a more realistic expectation of postoperative progress.

The attendance at the group meetings was as expected. The members were invited to attend whenever it was convenient and not necessarily every week. All eight patients attended every meeting held on a day when they had a clinic appointment or occurred while they were still in the hospital. Five family members (3 wives and 2 mothers of unmarried patients) attended with equal regularity. The remainder of the family participants attended only once or twice. Group size ranged from six to twelve over the ten meetings.

Yalom has described ten curative factors involved in group psychotherapy with psychiatric patients.[14] These will be used as a heuristic framework for assessing the content and value to this style of open group meetings for transplant patients and their families. As Yalom points out, these factors are conceptual in nature and overlap.

GROUP COHESIVENESS

The meetings produced an attitude of solidarity amongst the membership. A sense of comfort developed which allowed the members to offer their feelings for public scrutiny. This environment of acceptance and respect from others helped in the development of a positive self-image for the members.

The overt communications of acceptance and caring were less in intensity than is seen in psychiatric groups. Indeed, there was very little cathartic interaction between the members. A quiet, respectful discussion would be more descriptive of the meetings.

Undoubtedly, the patients in particular felt a conflict between an affiliation developing from common medical conditions and an attitude of denial and avoidance of all things related to renal failure.

Outside of the groups a social cohesion was evident.The wives seemed particularly active in this aspect of group therapy. They formed a "telephone community" by calling one another to share common problems and thoughts as well as to seek advice and support. They also arranged car pools to commute to the clinic. Two male patients became good friends through these meetings and met regularly in each other's homes for chess matches.

IMITATIVE BEHAVIOR

All too often renal failure patients are afraid to leave their dependent position in the sick role. The opportunity to observe other members gain their independence served as an encouragement. Some participants were motivated to take risks when they saw others with similar problems make attempts at solutions without harm befalling them. After a young transplant started a new educational course to gain employment, a fifty-five year old small business owner returned to manage his company although previously he had doubted his stamina and ability to do so. His son, who had had to quit his studies to operate the business, then returned to school and much of the family tension dissipated.

DEVELOPMENT OF SOCIALIZATION TECHNIQUES

Group discussions provide a means to acquire the social skills that enable a departure from the sick role and a reentrance into society. Hospitalized psychiatric patients gain from discussion of how to explain their illness to friends and how to approach prospective employers. In a similar manner the transplant patients became comfortable about discussing their illness and their concerns in the social setting of the group. A prominent topic was their previous occupation and how they might reenter it. Their ambivalence about reentering employment was demonstrated through their discussion about disability payments and the advisability of working part time. However, when one transplant patient announced that he was undertaking a program in radio repair in order to seek a new occupation he received much support and encouragement from the group. Merely being in the group meetings forced several patients to socialize and converse about topics that ordinarily were avoided.

GROUP AS A DEMONSTRATION OF FAMILY DYNAMICS

The action of a member within the group mimics his activities within his family. Maladaptive behaviors and attitudes become apparent and the group members can serve as a source of corrective feedback. Unfortunately, the group did not serve this function very well. The excessive overprotectiveness of one mother toward her recipient son and the dependence of a recipient upon his wife were obvious in the group setting. Both women were the unwitting accomplices to a process of regression and entrenchment into a sick role. However, the group members never commented upon the behavior and it went unchecked.

VENTILATION

Ventilation represents the benefits obtained by expressing strong emotional feelings and the consequent relief of pent up frustration. Abram has pointed out that renal patients often meet resistance to overt negative statements.[15] "The patient picks up messages, both overtly and covertly, that it is safer to keep submerged any feelings of disillusionment with or hostility toward the treatment. Otherwise he will get the reputation of being a 'bad patient' or a complainer and eventually be labeled as uncooperative."

A group of peers can provide a receptive medium for the expression of anger. Two male patients ventilated their intense frustration with their ailment and projected the entire blame upon the medical personnel. One of these patients recounted his frightening story of misdiagnosis until he was rescued from death through peritoneal dialysis. Although the other members were quiet, they appeared to gain some vicarious relief through the experience. The inhibition of anger in the presence of medical personnel was more dramatically demonstrated in one meeting when the transplant surgeon entered the meeting midway through the session. His presence totally ended the conversation revolving around the frustrations of various side effects of immunosuppressant drugs. Eventually the conversation changed to some technical aspects of wound care and record keeping in the home.

INTERPERSONAL LEARNING

This aspect of groups refers to the changing attitudes and altered goals of the participants as they progress through the therapy. Group members initially entered the group to be spectators. Their intent was to be entertained, to be passive and to learn from the therapist what steps could be taken to relieve their suffering. Their experience with illness has been to have external forces, i.e., doctors, nurses, medicines, and machines impinge their demands upon the patient. Although unrealistic this became the expected means to have their problems solved. A function of group therapy was to alter their attitude gradually over the sessions and develop a more active role in their own welfare and responsibility for their well-being.

Some critical incidents within the meetings allowed the members to experience emotional situations which previously they doubted they could handle. The angry outbursts of a patient toward his doctor stimulated him to take an active role in controlling his treatment while in the hospital. He insisted upon recording his own body chemistry readings, measuring his own urine output and taking his body weight daily. On another occasion, two wives expressed a fear of their husbands' death. This had a profound effect upon one of the husbands. He told the group that he too lived with an awesome dread of dying but had never mentioned it. His affect seemed to brighten after this admission and he eventually made plans for a more normal life.

INSTILLING OF HOPE

In entering the post surgical period, the threats and fears of the future become more apparent. Patients and family fear rejection of the kidney, death and even the possibility of normality is viewed with trepidation. Hope is an essential ingredient in the motivation and rehabilitation of the patient. It was offered to the members through the testimonials of recipients and their families who experienced similar stress yet survived and were in the process of reestablishing their lives. The expression of doubt of the future was expressed in almost every meeting, yet someone always pointed out their achievements to date.

ALTRUISM

Altruism represents the benefit derived by the group member from offering his experience, suggestions, reassurance, and insights to others. In some respects it is the opposite of the Instilling of Hope, as it represents the benefit to the contributor.

Patients seemed to gain more than family members from altruism. The meetings offered a means of contributing to the welfare of others by sharing experiences. It was an opportunity to feel needed instead of a burden to others. Although the family members often described their situation first, it was the suggestions offered by the patients that seemed to have the greatest impact upon both the contributor and the receiver. The group leader had to make a particular effort to encourage the patients to contribute opinions and solutions to the problems of others. They were too willing to let their families be the spokesmen or assume they had nothing to offer. One exception was a patient and his wife who were particularly anxious during a period of organ rejection. They attempted to dominate the meetings for two weeks by offering advice and suggestions. Unfortunately, their behavior really only served to dampen the enthusiasm of other members.

INFORMATION DISPERSAL

A benefit was derived from the factual information about renal failure and transplantation that was dispersed. It provided a realistic expectation of postoperative recovery and reduced the anxiety of the unpredictable and unknown future. Braatz reported that dialysands have an "almost insatiable desire for information about their condition and about dialysis."[16] It may be that the hidden message in such a desire is "How am I doing in comparison to others?" This group offered a means of answering this question.

Information came from three primary sources: the leader, the transplant surgeon, and the members themselves. The leader primarily tried to remove himself from the position of a guest lecturer and play the role of a facilitator, re-directing questions to other members and supporting those that offered opinions or experiences. A more didactic presentation was offered in one meeting by the transplant surgeon. He explained the process of rejection and the function of immunosuppressant drugs. Several members expressed a fear that their new kidney was fragile and easily damaged. One spouse even feared that the abdominal strain of defecation might damage the kidney. The surgeon's reassurance and information on their concerns was a source of relief. The group members offered advice on how to obtain discounts on drug purchases and to apply for welfare support. The most potent topic was a discussion of the organ rejection process that two recipients had gone through. Several members had not understood that rejection could be reversed and could recur. The topic had been raised by an acutely depressed recipient who was rejecting his kidney. His spirits raised dramatically upon hearing the experience of others. It demonstrated the impact of information from a peer. Although he had been informed about rejection by hospital personnel, it was not until he heard of similar experiences, including the depression and anxiety, that he was able to alter his attitude. Eventually his rejection was reversed as well.

UNIVERSALITY

Dialysands tend to be seclusive and avoid contact with other patients.[13] Their colleagues serve as stimuli for anxiety as they graphically represent their fears. However, this social isolation also promotes the belief that they are alone in experiencing physical and emotional difficulties of renal failure. A feeling of uniqueness can develop and be perpetuated. The family also has a limited opportunity for contact with their peers. The group, however, provided a means by which the members could experience a commonality of their experiences.

Within the first four meetings several members expressed a sense of relief that they were not alone in their misery. Merely hearing that others had similar problems and anxieties was therapeutic. The topics were on more neutral issues at first, i.e., the care of open wounds and the cost of parking at the Medical Center, but quickly more emotionally laden topics such as financial burdens, sexual desire and anger toward health professionals were expressed. They discovered that their own reactions were more universal and that the sense of uniqueness was inaccurate.

CONCLUSION

A primary deficiency in these group meetings concerns the degree of interaction between a patient and his family. The communication between spouses or parent and child was generally superficial. Supportive, constructive suggestions were expressed to other group members but seldom to one another. It is assumed that this breakdown in communication was the result of a chronic tension state in the family and a fear of disrupting whatever mechanisms were operative. In general, the whole tone of the meetings was somewhat reserved in comparison to psychiatric patient groups.

Several features of the group should be considered. The limited number of meetings may have prevented the members from perceiving some situations and offering feedback. Also the lack of a consistent weekly membership undoubtedly detracted from group cohesion. Despite these features the group was successful in most areas.

The group appeared to be an effective means of dealing with the average dialysand's low motivation to talk with a psychiatrist.[17] Meetings with one's peers did not seem to present a threat of social stigma and the opportunity to learn more about their condition seemed to compensate, at least in part, with the problems of denial and avoidance. The meetings also provide an economical and effective means of providing long term emotional support and follow-up. The lack of such follow-up is a frequent complaint of psychiatric consultation.[10]

REFERENCES

Dr. Buchanan is a psychologist in the Department of Psychiatry at the Vanderbilt University Medical School in Nashville, Tennessee.

1. J. H. Pratt, The home sanitorium treatment of consumptives, *Boston Med. Surg. J., 1954,* p. 210, 1906.
2. L. H. Brulleman, Group-therapy with epileptic patients at the "Instituut voor Epilepsiebestrijding," *Epilepsia, 13,* pp. 225–231, 1972.
3. C. P. Leeman, Dependency, anger and denial in pregnant women: A group approach, *Psych. Quart., 44,* pp. 1–12, 1970.
4. P. Hahn and R. Leisner, The influence of biographical anamnesis and group psychotherapy on postmyocardial patients, *Psychother. Psychosom., 18,* pp. 299–306, 1970.
5. M. L. Schwartz and R. Cahill, Psychopathology associated with myasthenia gravis and its treatment by psychotherapeutically oriented group counseling, *J. Chron. Dis., 24,* pp. 543–552, 1971.
6. E. R. Sorenson, Group therapy in a community hospital dialysis unit, *JAMA, 221,* pp. 899–901, 1972.
7. T. H. Hollon, Modified group therapy in the treatment of patients on chronic hemodialysis, *Am. J. Psychother., 26,* pp. 501–510, 1972.
8. J. P. Kemph; E. A. Bermann; and E. P. Coppolillo, Kidney transplant and shifts in family dynamics, *Amer. J. Psychiatry, 125,* pp. 1485–1490, 1969.
9. C. H. Fellner, Selection of living kidney donors and the problem of informed consent, in P. Castelnuovo-Tedesco, (ed.), *Psychiatric Aspects of Organ Transplantation,* Grune and Stratton, New York, 1971.
10. J. P. Kemph, Psychotherapy with donors and recipients of kidney transplants, in P. Castelnuovo-Tedesco, (ed.), *Psychiatric Aspects of Organ Transplantation,* Grune and Stratton, New York, 1971.
11. I. Penn; D. Bunch; D. Olenk, et al., Psychiatric experiences with patients receiving renal and hepatic transplants, in P. Castelnuovo-Tedesco, (ed.), *Psychiatric Aspects of Organ Transplanation,* Grune and Stratton, New York, 1971.
12. W. A. Crammond, Renal transplanation—experiences with recipients and donors, in P. Castelnuovo-Tedesco, (ed.), *Psychiatric Aspects of Organ Transplantation,* Grune and Stratton, New York, 1971.

13. F. G. Foster; G. L. Cohn; and F. P. McKegney, Psychobiologic factors and individual survival on chronic renal hemodialysis: A two year follow-up, *Psychosom. Med., 35,* pp. 64–82, 1973.
14. I. D. Yalom, *The Theory and Practice of Group Psychotherapy,* Basic Books, New York, 1970.
15. H. S. Abram, The "uncooperative" hemodialysis patient: A psychiatrist's viewpoint and a patient's commentary, in N. B. Levy, (ed.), *Living or Dying: Adaptation to Hemodialysis,* Chas. Thomas, Springfield, 1974.
16. G. A. Braatz, the psychological climate of the dialysis unit, paper presented at the American Psychological Association, Montreal, 1973.
17. H. S. Abram, Psychiatric reflections on adaptation to repetitive dialysis, *Kidney International, 6,* pp. 67–72, 1974.

17

Group Treatment in a Hemodialysis Center
—H. WIJSENBEEK and H. MUNITZ

INTRODUCTION

ALTHOUGH recommended, group therapy is seldom discussed *per se* in the pertinent literature on the treatment of chronic renal failure in an intermittent hemodialysis program.

The authors treated a small group of such patients during one year in weekly sessions. Frequent topics, discussed in the groups were family problems, death problems, aggression and submission, the shunt as a visible reminder of the disease, and changes in the body image.

The task of the psychiatrist in the unit towards the patients and the medical staff was discussed. It seemed that his task was more to add to modern technology a human understanding than assisting the medical staff in the selection of patients, although the authors do not exclude a scientific way of finding the right patients for such a program.

Patients will receive and work with a psychiatrist in their group in a better understanding, knowing that he is not a member of a selection committee. This knowledge will improve the doctor-patient relationship.

It is too early to evaluate the results of this form of treatment. The account which follows deals with psychiatric group treatment under exceptional circumstances, with a group of patients who are undergoing intermittent hemodialysis.

This is a group of people who live under continuous, extraordinary stress. Their lives are wholly dependent upon recent technological advances in medicine. This very progress, however, raises new problems for the patient as well as the physician; the mechanization of medicine.

From Wijsenbeek & Munitz, *Psychiatria, Neurologia, Neurochirurgia, 73* (1970), 213–220, with permission from the publishers.

The patient is required to cooperate not only with medical personnel, but with a machine as well. This is a natural outgrowth of increased sophistication in laboratory techniques, and it is also in tune with our computerized technology. The introduction of the computer in medicine, however, is not only a means to precision in data processing. Many physicians tend to use the machine as a defense against human contact with the patient.

The physician, educated to exert all his powers toward the saving of human lives, is now faced by a contradiction: economic considerations force him to limit the number of patients who may benefit from this therapy. In effect, then, the physician must choose: not who will live, but who will die. His position is made still more difficult since the definition of death is changing. We have reached an era when technology permits us to prolong an individual life by providing him with the healthy organs of another individual. Some of these organs, however, have been the focus of human emotion and imagination as the kidneys in the Old Testament and the heart as the site of love and courage, and not merely a specialized muscle to be transplanted. It is to be expected that these factors as well as others will lead us to revise our approach to death.

It is not surprising then that in some centers group therapy is being carried out not with the patients but with the medical staff itself.[3]

We divided the problems of the patients in a renal unit as follows: (i) problems of the chronically ill; (ii) specific problems of hemodialysis; (iii) the problems of the person permanently threatened by death. We concentrated in this paper on points (ii) and (iii).

The psychological reactions of these patients vary both in form and in intensity.

In the last years interest has grown in the psychiatric aspects of chronic renal failure. The psychiatrist may be called upon to aid in the selection of patients, or to treat them. Sometimes he fulfils both functions. It seems to us that anyone dealing with the selection of patients must ask himself: "Am I able to foretell accurately how a person will withstand hemodialysis and/or renal transplantation?"

An extensive review of the literature on the psychological aspects of chronic hemodialysis was published recently by MacAfee Husek.[2] Most of the papers reviewed here were studied by us but we feel that her review relieves us from again discussing several separate papers. From her review it becomes clear that the criteria for selecting patients for a dialysis program is still wide open for further deliberation. We want to point out that the patients forming our group were not selected per se and we started our work only after the patients were received in the unit. This relieved us, perhaps, from the severe guilt feelings between members of the staff, as described by Kaplan DeNour and Czaczkes.[3] Nowhere in the literature we found the observation about the difficulties connected with selecting patients in a small country. In Israel these difficulties are obvious because everyone knows everyone and this leads to personal relations building up unscientific pressures on members of the staff. This again is connected to socio-economic factors and possible changes in familial patterns and interaction between the patient, the doctor, the family of the patient, and his role in society. These interactions were examined by Harari from our Department.[1] Most authors feel that group therapy is the most beneficial therapeutic approach to help counteracting the stress experienced by these patients.[2] But we did not find a more detailed report of working in a group of patients in the literature.

Group therapy is well suited to a group of patients faced by a genuine threat, as opposed to a neurotic fear. This was well understood by the medical non-psychiatric members of the unit and led to the request put to us for psychiatric group work in the unit. Our impression was that the medical staff felt that giving care to the patients will help the staff to cope better with their own problems. We understood that they, and later on we ourselves, feel that the death of one patient under its care means also the death of another, the patient who had not been chosen for care—but if he had, might then have lived. We accepted their invitation with mixed feelings and only after prolonged consideration.

The presence of the group diminishes the threat of a psychiatrist. The group's dynamics reflected their position in society and the ability to interact successfully within the group enhanced the individual's adjustment outside the group.

Within the group patients were able to express their anxieties freely. The group atmosphere also accepted their aggression and encouraged them to verbalize it. They were treated as people and not as patients. Within the group they learned from one another how to cope with certain of their difficulties. They also had direct communication with the nephrologist attending the sessions, and a simple clarification from him could reduce anxiety and resolve many daily problems.

Some of the patients felt the need for psychiatric assistance. However, others perceived the psychiatrist as a compounded threat: *i.e.* expressing danger to sanity as well as life. This fear, however, disappeared very quickly, and they initiated contact. On the other hand, the nursing staff felt that their patients were being taken from them and that the going-on in the group seemed mysterious. These feelings led to a certain measure of resistance in the nurses.

COMPOSITION OF THE GROUP

The group under treatment is comprised of the patients, the psychiatrist, the nephrologist and a secretary, writing protocol. There were 8 patients, in age ranging from 17 to 57, 7 males and 1 married female. They met once a week for one year in the unit. After the meeting in the late afternoon hours, they were connected to the machine. Many times we went then to the treatment room and talked with the patients separately. An interesting aspect was the psychiatric atmosphere in real "clinical surroundings," something like a psychiatrist in an operation theatre. A second group of patients who were not participating in the therapeutic meetings became aware of the therapy group. The mere existence of the therapy group influenced this second group. A closer examination of such a secondary group seems indicated.

MATERIAL

The material brought up in group meetings may be divided into 3 parts, distinguished by the time and the topics of conversation. In the first stage patients confined their discussion to very superficial problems, such as those concerned with employment. Any attempt to touch upon their personal problems was warded off.

In the second stage the central topic was the medical regime and its effects upon the patient's life. Matters such as the diet, the shunt and the machine were discussed. At this stage patients were helped to overcome their difficulties in self-expression. They also used this opportunity to verbalize a large measure of aggression against the medical staff.

In the third stage the patients discussed the place of the patient within his family, his feelings as a sick individual, and the reactions of the family to the patient's illness. They described the problem of overprotective attitudes within their families. Others, on the contrary, voiced fears that their families would neglect them. One patient remarked that families could be divided into ". . . those who don't want to hear about the patient, and those who protect him too much . . . ." He added ". . . actually all families do some of one and some of the other . . . ." Some patients used denial as a defence against their feelings of illness: these patients expressed a feeling of illness only when connected to the machine. Most patients, however, acknowledged a constant feeling of illness.

The patients describe stages in their feelings. When they first learn of the severity of their illness they often develop a condition similar to a reactive depression. They withdraw from social activities, remain at home, and welcome the family's protectiveness.

One of our patients told us that since he became ill he feels he has lost social status, and that his worth as a human being has diminished.

The next stage is a conpensatory one. The patients attempt activities outside the home. They try to learn to live with the illness. Their efforts meet varying degrees of success. Often the family refuses to accept the possibility that a "sick" person can maintain activity. It seems to us that this conflict is the problem preventing the establishment of family equilibrium. The third stage is one of acceptance and leading to integration: "we learn that we are ill, we must live and accept our fate."

We should now like to discuss specific problems raised during group meetings. The following points were raised.

FAMILY PROBLEMS

These are complex; not only is the patient chronically ill, but there is the compounded threat that another family member will be asked to donate a kidney. The patients requested that their families be interviewed and be provided with psychiatric support as well. All described their own families as overprotective, but declared that "other" families would be rejecting. One patient stated: "my parents wrap me in cotton until I cannot move." Another described his elderly father of 70 snatching a heavy hoe away from him every time he began to work.

All the patients felt considerable resistance to the familial attitude of overprotection. At the same time, some added that they did indeed need some measure of protection since they were, in fact, sick. Some individuals tried to overcome their families' protective attitudes by initiating a deconditioning-like process. They would increase their activities gradually, and in turn the family would become accustomed to the new level of activity and cease objecting. Occasionally the patients would rebel. This could take the form of a sudden disappearance from home or neglect of their diet. One patient married when he learned the nature of his illness. He explained that he was seeking someone who would protect him.

DEATH PROBLEMS

A major problem, of course, is the fact that these persons are living in the shadow of death. All of them are aware of this. There is an unofficial organization of renal patients: they know one another, and even know patients in other medical centers. Some patients regularly read the obituary notices in the newspapers. They respond to the death of another renal patient with increased anxiety, feelings of aggression and sometimes with attempts at suicide. Their awareness of the closeness of death dominates their thinking: a member of the group expressed it by saying: "whenever I go for a walk, I take my little daughter with me in case something should happen to me." It is well known that patients with chronic, life-threatening diseases such as diabetes may use their illness as a means to suicide. Our group shows similar tendencies. We have seen patients attempt suicide by violating their diet requirements. Alternatively, they may neglect the shunt, hoping for infection and complication. They may suddenly cease taking medication. When these acts are discussed with the patients, it becomes clear to them that some are instances of suicide attempts. One patient explained that he takes revenge on the doctor by suicidal acts which involve disobeying medical orders. We believe that some sudden deaths in this group may have resulted from such suicidal acts.

AGGRESSIVE FEELINGS

All our patients expressed aggressive feelings towards the medical profession. They felt improper care had led to their illness. They reason further that since the medical profession failed them it is now obliged to save them. They feel, accordingly, a large measure of aggression toward the medical personnel. This leads to a psychological dilemma, since they are dependent upon medical aid and therefore inhibited from expressing their anger and rage. As a result, they face a threat that if they manifest their hostility they will be rejected. Their aggression is displaced into petty quarrels between patient and fellow-patient, and patient and nurse. In turn, the staff finds it difficult to tolerate their "ingratitude," and there are occasionally outbursts of hostility.

After the death of 2 members of the group, the remaining patients were aggressive against the doctor and also against the whole group. There was no mention of the deceased patients, but the group atmosphere became tense.

An important place in therapy was the formation of normal outlets and working through the material.

SHUNT

In the beginning of treatment, most of our patients had an external shunt. Lately, however, there has been a shift to the use of an internal shunt and most of the patients in the group now have an internal shunt.

The patients regard the shunt as the symbol of their illness, the tangible evidence that they require constant and highly specialized care. Many try to conceal it with appropriate garments or in some other way. A difficult thing to do in our subtropic climate. They fear an accident to the shunt, resulting in blood loss; or they imagine the shunt will be caught up by some object and be torn out of their body. The patients are aware that change of colour in the shunt is an indication of blood clots, and yet they are reluctant to wash it out, fearing the pain. They repeatedly inspect the shunt to reassure themselves that it is in good condition. Fears concerning the shunt are experienced not only by the patients but by their families as well. This is still another source of family problems. The shunt becomes part of the patient's body, and at the same time symbolizes his illness and his pain. It is a weak point as well, a possible focus for infections. It is understandable, then, that psychological problems associated with the shunt are numerous, and that much of the patient's anger is directed at it.

It is interesting to compare above problems with similar problems encountered after amputation of limbs. The shunt having become a part of the patient's body, becomes in addition a part of his body image. The extent to which it is integrated into his body image can be seen in an example: Jewish ritual law dictates that a body be buried with all its organs in place; and one of our patients asked a rabbi whether his shunt should be buried with him too.

An internal shunt is a source of tension prior to the puncture by needles, particularly if this procedure has caused difficulty on preceding occasions.

LIFE WITH THE ARTIFICIAL KIDNEY

Patients have to live with the machine for 28 hours each week. Initially, the process of connection to the machine rouses tension and fear. Patients have fantasies of mechanical breakdowns, bursting pipes through which all their blood will drain away, or less specific but equally catastrophic fears of accidents to the machine and thus to them. Many are disgusted by the sight of their blood flowing out of their bodies.

We noticed that simple technical explanations by the nephrologist in the group helped the patients to understand what is going on and to relieve their fears.

The patients at first lie motionless, fearing that the needle will be disturbed in the blood vessel by the slightest motion. In the course of time they learn that they do have some freedom of movement, though limited. The connection to the machine renders the patient completely dependent on the medical staff, and increases his anxiety. Some patients prefer not to undergo hemodialysis at night because the number of nurses is smaller on the night shift. This dependency on the machine can be seen in one of our patients who felt increased anxiety as he walked away from the machine and the hospital. Moreover, most patients are unable to sleep while undergoing dialysis spending all their time anxiously observing the machine to be certain that nothing has gone wrong with it. The same we observed during night flights in a plane, where anxious people don't sleep, fearing that sleeping they will loose control.

In the course of time these reactions decrease in intensity, and eventually some may disappear.

Diet

Keeping the prescribed diet poses difficulties. They learn to know the exact composition of their food. After some time in the group they will discuss food in technical and nutritional terms. In addition, the fact of keeping a diet stresses their exceptional status. Social occasions become problematical. At home they must weigh all food and drink consumed. It is not surprising that rebellion against the illness, the staff or the family may take the form of overeating. Patients observed that in periods of stress they reacted with a tendency to bulimia, sometimes leading to serious consequences. In the group it became clear that some of these episodes were frank suicidal attempts; others arose from aggression directed against the staff. Nearly all the patients remarked that they experienced food fads. Some ate prohibited foods before coming to the unit.

Food restrictions make the patient increasingly dependent. He strives naturally to free himself of this dependency and as inevitably, he fails. Coping mechanisms were frequently discussed in the group.

Body Image

We suggest that the attachment to the machine and the concomitant flowing of blood outside the natural boundaries of the body are potent causes of disturbances of the integrity of the body image. In addition, the failure of kidney function is sometimes accompanied by fantasies in which patients imagine empty space in the place of the kidneys. Unlike healthy individuals, the patients are highly conscious of the renal area. The absence of urine leads to sexual fears and fantasies which may be very disturbing. Some patients fear that sexual intercourse may harm their kidneys. The prospect of transplanting a healthy kidney is always in the mind of the patient and in cases when the donor is a family member can add to disturbances in the body image. We know of a case in which a kidney was transplanted from mother to son, and subsequently a pathological relationship developed between them. This case will be reported separately.

DEPRESSIVE AND PSYCHOTIC REACTIONS

We saw reactive depressions after failure of transplantation, frustrations at work and at home, or in times of exacerbation of the renal state. Antidepressive drugs were effective. Some patients experienced psychotic states at the time of dialysis. These were exogenous psychoses.

All the patients showed signs of lethargy, poor attention span, and disturbances in the ability to concentrate, to work, and to maintain consciousness. These were most marked on the day of dialysis and the day following. This was still more conspicuous if there was a drastic fall of blood urea. These conditions may develop to the point of exogenous psychosis. Symptomatology may include disturbances in the level of consciousness, visual and auditory hallucinations and paranoid thinking.

These clinical manifestations are probable evidence of a chronic brain syndrome as described by Menzies and Stewart.[4] More renal insufficiency may also cause disturbances in the sleep cycle, suffering insomnia at night and sleeping by day. We have already mentioned the patient who dares not fall asleep while connected to the machine. Some patients suffer insomnia under normal circumstances as well. We presume that biochemical and psychological factors are responsible.

RESULTS

As in any group treatment it is difficult to evaluate the results. It seems to us that this form of treatment helps the patient to work through his problems together with fellow-sufferers. We noticed that group therapy improved to a great deal the atmosphere in the unit until it became a real therapeutic community. This does not exclude the possibility or advisability of separate encounters between doctor and patient.

After one year of work in the unit we found that every patient and his family are in need of psychiatric assistance and that group therapy was appreciated by the patients and the medical staff as the best form of treating the manifold coping mechanisms of the patient and his therapist.

SUMMARY

Group treatment in a hemodialysis center is discussed in this paper. Eight patients were under treatment and they met with the psychiatrist and the nephrologist once a week during one year, some hours before they were connected to the machine. Special attention was paid to the specific problems of hemodialysis and the problems of a person, permanently threatened by death. The material brought up and worked through was centered around complex family problems, death problems, coping with aggression, the shunt as the externalized symbol of illness, life with the artificial kidney, body image, and psychiatric reactions.

After one year of work we found, after we studied the reactions of patients, their families and staff members, that this form of therapy is highly recommended in treating the coping mechanisms of the patient, his family and his therapist.

REFERENCES

H. Wijsenbeek and H. Munitz are affiliated with the Gehah Psychiatric Hospital, Beilinson Medical Center at the Tel Aviv University Medical School in Petah Tikwah (Israel).

Authors' acknowledgements: We wish to express our thanks to the physician-in-chief Dr. J. Rosenfeld and Dr. J. Robson, nurses and technicians of the Dialysing Unit of the Beilinson Hospital for their kind cooperation and help in this study.

1. Harari, A., Psychosocial examination of patients and families during hemodialysis, Doctoral thesis, Medical School of Tel Aviv University, 1969.
2. Husek, J. A., *Psychological aspects of chronic hemodialysis; a summary and review of the literature; Suggestions for further research,* School of Public Health, University of California, Los Angeles, Calif., 1966.
3. Kaplan DeNour, A. and Czaczkes, J. W., Emotional problems and reactions of the medical team in a chronic hemodialysis unit, *Lancet, ii* (1968) 987–991.
4. Menzies, I. C. and Stewart, W. K., Psychiatric observations on patients with regular dialysis treatment, *Brit. med. J.,* i (1968) 544–547.

18

Spouses Under Stress: Group Meetings with Spouses of Patients on Hemodialysis
—PHILIP W. SHAMBAUGH, M.D., and
STANLEY S. KANTER, M.D.

O VER the past 25 years a number of investigators have described the emotional reactions of individuals subjected to severe external stress.[12,21] A prominent feature is the clear emergence of primitive fantasies and defenses which are usually obscured in the well functioning personality by mature complexities of character structure. Small groups under stress similarly reveal the deeper forces underlying individual and group behavior. However, we have been able to find only two studies of the psychodynamics of groups under stress.[4,6] Both deal with groups of servicemen under combat conditions, but neither traces such a group from beginning to end or correlates the regressive defenses of the members with the dynamics of the group itself.

We have studied a group under extreme stress which has topical interest. It was composed of spouses of patients whose lives depended on long-term hemodialysis. Some of the spouses had their stress compounded by actually being the operators of the artificial kidney machine.

BACKGROUND

Long-term, maintenance hemodialysis is a recent development. Only since 1960 has it been possible to prolong the lives of patients who formerly died of chronic renal failure. However, dialysis and its related treatment, renal transplantation, are currently available to only a small minority of those patients who are medically suitable.[14] In an effort to reduce the tremendous outlay of money, hospital space, and professional time required for dialysis, the artificial kidney machine has been moved out of the hospital and into the patient's home.[5] Training the patient's spouse to operate the kidney machine has seemed a way to reduce the expense further but has proved to be such a severe stress that some spouses have not been able to continue dialyzing.[18] In order to explore the supportive value of regular group meetings, a psychiatrist met with a group of spouses.

Our study was undertaken at a center where hemodialysis was preliminary to eventual renal transplantation. The nephrologists selected the spouses who were to operate the kidney machines at home; their period of

Reprinted from the *American Journal of Psychiatry,* vol. 125, pp. 928–936, 1969. Copyright 1969, the American Psychiatric Association. Reprinted by permission.

training averaged ten weeks. Nurses dialyzed the other patients, either at home or in the hospital. The spouse used the twin-coil artificial kidney, which has the advantage of requiring a relatively short time for dialysis: five or six hours two or three times a week. The spouse was trained to connect his marital partner's bloodstream to the machine via in-dwelling cannulae in a superficial artery and adjacent vein which were connected between dialyses (the "shunt"). Serious malfunctions of the dialyzing appartus were rare, but when they occurred they could be fatal within minutes.[5]

THE GROUP, THE GOAL, AND THE TECHNIQUE

The group met for eight months and included six spouses, three of whom operated the kidney machine (table 1). Six other spouses, in addition to the parents of an adolescent boy on dialysis (M-5 and F-9), attended the meetings for short periods of time (table 2). Most were from the middle socioeconomic class. Only one spouse, M-4, had ever consulted a psychiatrist. The meetings lasted an hour and a quarter and were held weekly. All sessions were tape-recorded and later transcribed; for several months there was a human recorder as well. We interviewed all spouses except M-4 from six months to a year and a half after their group experience.

At the beginning the nephrologists and the leader approached the spouses, explained that the meetings were intended to be investigative and

TABLE 1.   *Characteristics of Members of the Group*

Case (sex)	Age (years)	Personality Type	Months Attended	Operated Machine
M-1	27	Compulsive	13	Yes
M-2	44	"Depressive"	8	Yes
M-3	63	Passive dependent	6	No
F-1	31	"Hysteric"	4	Yes
F-2	37	"Hysteric"	2	No
F-3	41	Passive dependent	1	No

TABLE 2.   *Characteristics of Others Who Attended Meetings*

Case (sex)	Age (years)	Personality Type	Months Attended	Operated Machine
F-4	32	Compulsive	2	Before meetings
M-4	40	Passive dependent	1	No
F-5	29	"Borderline"	1	After meetings
F-6	30	"Borderline"	1	Discontinued before meetings
F-7	38	Compulsive	2	After meetings
F-8	35	"Hysteric"	2	After meetings
M-5	53	Compulsive	1	No
F-9	54	Compulsive	1	No

supportive of their operation of the machine and adjustment to the disease but not psychotherapeutic, and encouraged them to attend. In accordance with this goal, the leader allowed the members to discuss whatever they wished and took a sympathetic, interested, and realistic role. He always commented on their defensive reactions in terms of general human responses to stress and never interpreted their manifestations of dependence or hostility. His major effort was to help the members find a mutually endurable common ground between denial and despair.

GENERAL FORMULATION

Underlying the behavior we observed in the group were certain dynamic struggles which all the spouses shared.[18] They had to cope with many stresses including their marital partners' severe medical complications, possible death, and regressive behavior. In response to these unhappy changes they reacted with intense feelings of deprivation and primitive urges toward psychological closeness to their partners and with enormous hostility, often giving rise to intense guilt. Those who operated the artificial kidney machine had their infantile fantasies confirmed in reality, for now their partners were linked to their machines and could be destroyed. In response to their anxiety, depression, and guilt, both the spouses who operated the machine and those who did not might resort to primitive defenses—particularly massive denial, which was often supported by blind faith in renal transplantation. This defense was particularly difficult for the operators to maintain, for they were most directly exposed to their partners' precarious state.

In the course of the group experience each member developed enough psychological separation from his partner to recognize the changed relationships and to begin to grieve. Yet he was continually impeded by regressive urges toward infantile closeness and by guilt related to his rage at being deprived and restricted by the burdens of his partner's illness. At the same time, denial and guilt comprised an important part of his motivation to operate the machine.

The members unconsciously perceived the leader as a parental authority, either idealized and supportive (a common ego ideal) or prohibiting and sadistic (a superego figure). On the basis of their shared conception of the leader they became identified with one another and coalesced as a group.[3,13] As the group progressed, the members' views of the leader changed from the primitive ones of ego ideal and superego toward that of a peer as they shared the internalization of mature ideals and norms. Thus our group depicted a complex maturational process common to small groups.[19] We have analyzed the reactions of the individual members and the forces underlying the structure of the group at each stage, cognizant of the limitations of our data.[17]

INITIAL EXPERIENCE

The group started with five members, three of whom were just beginning to operate the kidney machine. Although he was compulsive, M–1 had a limited tolerance for anxiety and depression. For example, when his wife had first fallen ill he had projected his anxious fears of loss of control onto the hospital. M–2 was guilty, pessimistic, and chronically depressed. M–3 had been deeply depressed by his wife's illness and had retreated to a lonely life of heavy drinking. F–1 had endeavored to learn as much as she could about dialysis and had welcomed the opportunity to help her husband by operating the machine. F–4 had warded off depression for a long time by hard-driving activity and works of charity. Although her husband had successfully undergone transplantation a year before, she had joined the group to help the others.

At first the spouses were terrified that their machines would break down and bring about their partners' deaths. These fears receded after a few weeks when they discovered that serious malfunctions were rare and that they could master the technique of dialysis. The discussion then ranged widely and impersonally over the lore of dialysis and transplantation. F–4 had much to add, and the other members often complimented her in idealized terms. Initially the spouses likened the patients to infants, but later most seldom mentioned them or acknowledged the illness. Rather, they demonstrated their extreme emotional closeness to their partners; for example, they spoke of them as "we" rather than calling them by name.

Each member supported his denial and maintained his superiority to the others in the group by imagining that he had a special method of mastery. One member had a particular technique in operating the machine; another, a unique insurance policy; and a third, extensive medical knowledge. In contrast to the others, one husband was able to speak intellectually about his wife's illness; he made the other members extremely anxious and angry by his pessimistic comparisons of renal disease to cancer and his vivid, macabre imagery, such as his references to a new dialysis machine housed in a wooden box with brass handles on the sides.

Instead of airing their concerns about the illness, the members expressed their feelings that various authorities were ill-using them either out of indifference or malice; for example, they thought the doctors were not interested in their plight and were using them as guinea pigs or experimental dogs. They decided that their problem was their tremendous financial drain and that only massive government subsidization could come to the rescue.

Clearly the members' initial anxiety was enormous and their regression severe. At first they projected their fears of loss of control of their hostility onto the machine. Subsequently, most denied all feelings about their marital partners. This denial screened from full consciousness fearful sadistic fantasies; for example, much later M–5, the father of the adolescent boy on dialysis, gave as an example of what people want to deny the case of a mother who used a razor on some teen-age boys who were trying to steal her purse. One spouse, however, admitted these fantasies to full consciousness but denied their emotional relevance. At the same time the members were unconsciously identifying with their partners and were projecting their own depriving urges toward them onto various figures who became objects for displacement of their rage.

At this stage the members' displacement of their primitive perceptions of the leader to other group members and to outside authorities was a frequent mechanism. One member would be focused on as an ideal and a good provider for children, and another as the sadistic bearer of ill tidings about their partners' illness. Authority figures were reviled both for failing to fulfill the members' primitive wishes for support and for persecuting them. Meanwhile, the members were only superficially identified with one another, for each maintained his private denial, his individualized, magical method of coping, and his isolating psychological closeness to his marital partner. In fact, the spouses' most powerful resistances to joining the meetings were their reluctance to face the horrible facts and their idea that the group meetings physically took them away from the patients.

FORMATION OF THE GROUP

As their panic abated the members began to speak more openly about their partners' illness. They questioned whether the patients realized how sick they were, and every week they discussed the latest medical complications. All accused the physician of not telling them how ill their partners were. The discussion took an ominous turn when the members felt that the nephrologists made arbitrary decisions about whom to save, although they eventually concluded that everyone who was medically suitable was dialyzed.

Gradually they realized that they would be able to meet their expenses without outside help and that, in fact, money was only one aspect of their problem. However, F–4 felt she had to do something to help the others and held a large barbecue as a charitable benefit. At the same time she was angrily proclaiming that with her husband's transplantation she no longer shared the problems of the others. The other members, however, were becoming increasingly open both in their criticisms of one another and in their manifestations of devotion.

After two months the group faced its first crisis when F–4 announced her withdrawal. At once the other members also considered leaving. The leader responded by urging them to vent their hostility in the meetings rather than have it erupt at home and to press onward toward the goal of successful operation. Thereupon they furiously attacked various rulers as legalizing murder. One member suddenly asked the leader if the recorder were his slave. Yet they concluded the harangue by praising the governments of states threatened by famine that had arranged for everyone to go hungry but for no one to starve.

This stage was marked by the members reducing their denial, interacting more openly with one another, and reaching a tolerable accommodation with the leader. Despite their increased openness about the disease, the members ascribed their denial to the patients and maintained that the physicians had withheld the facts, thus avoiding a full confrontation with their own denial. Nonetheless, they could increasingly give up their reliance on individualized magic as the communication and support made it possible for them to identify with one another. As one member put it, they acquired "a sense of adversity against the group rather than adversity against the individual."

As the spouses began to realize they were managing both emotionally and financially, they progressively replaced their unrealistic demands for massive financial support and their sense of having been mistreated with less extravagant complaints about the physicians. They reached an endurable though beggarly accommodation with the leader and coalesced about him. But only after the group had concluded could the members admit that earlier they had been terrified that the leader would retaliate by removing their partners from the program and condemning them to death.

In retrospect, F–4's withdrawal was partly the result of erroneous selection for, in fact, with her husband having undergone transplantation, she no longer had dialysis in common with the other members. Yet she could no more modify her compulsive need to give to others than she could adjust to the group. In respect to the other members, she played the role of a primitive nurturer (regressive ego ideal).

OPTIMISM AND PARTIAL SEPARATION

The members of the group then became optimistic and certain that they could save their partners' lives. One member announced: "It's a big problem, but you can beat it. All that's needed is a relative who'll put out the effort." Indeed, they fantastically imagined that the group discussions were resolving all the problems of the world. They were strong in their optimism and could empathize with their partners' medical complications and try to understand what they assumed to be their emotional conflicts.

They described the shunts as the patients' umbilical cords and found it understandable that the patients might rip them out and commit suicide to escape their dependence on the machine or on their spouses. Yet at the same time one husband admitted that he felt as though he were tied to his wife's artificial kidney machine by a rope. The members conceptualized the patients' not facing the facts of their illness as denial and criticized magazine articles and television programs for what they considered to be their unrealistic and rosy portrayal of dialysis. Often they sympathized with the pain of the patients' shunt revisions; one member was terrified that he himself would dislodge it.

During this stage the members spoke of authority figures in less ambivalent terms than before. For example, they felt that the local cardinal was no longer completely dictatorial; yet they sometimes called physicians their idols or "miracle men." They also began to refer to the leader directly—sometimes critically, other times warmly—as "their psychiatrist."

Inevitably their solicitude about the patients' complications led the members back again and again to the prognosis. Reality took its toll, optimism vanished, and the group panicked. Again, the leader urged them on toward the goal with freedom to scapegoat him. This phase was shortly concluded when F–1's husband died and she withdrew from the group.

This stage of the group was marked by the members' omnipotent optimism and partial emotional separation from their partners. Now active in their efforts at mastery, they defended their illusion of omnipotent success by denying their own dependence, suicidal impulses, denial, and hostility, and by using as repositories for these reactions[20] the patients themselves and the physicians who operated upon the shunts. Sometimes the defensive nature of their projections became obvious, as when one spouse felt tied to his wife's machine and another was fearful that he himself would pull out the shunt. At the same time the spouses were developing perspective about their partners for, in fact, the patients were dependent on them and the physicians did have to revise the shunts. Although there was increasing maturity in their conception of the leader, with ability to praise or attack him directly, he was still viewed as omnipotent, though now beneficent and an object for identification.

FINAL STAGE

After the death of F–1's husband, the remaining members of the group recalled their similarities to her and partially regressed to the sadistic fantasies and primitive defenses characteristic of the earlier stages of the group. Yet they admitted for the first time that they were preparing for their own partners' deaths and formulated a person's motivation for having a relative dialyzed as a means of assuaging his guilt about letting him die or of trying to arrange continuation together eternally. Shortly afterward, one member announced that his wife was losing hope and had requested transplantation, another suddenly went on vacation, and the third began to drink heavily. Although the members recalled cases of people killing the physicians who had saved them from suicide, they were able to reunite behind the leader, whom they compared to George Washington commanding his beleaguered troops.

F–2 and F–3 then joined the group. The husband of one of them had always shielded her from concerns beyond her housework and care of their children. He was due to undergo his second transplantation shortly, and she was certain that his "strong, rugged body" would carry him through safely again. The other's initial depression had lifted as she had become unshakably convinced that her husband would successfully undergo transplantation and as their relationship had deteriorated to arguing about his overeating.

The introduction of the new members evoked from the other members of the group frequent expressions of hostility toward one another and the leader. When one of the new members became angry about her husband's berating her about his diet, the two operators averred that their wives could not do the same or they would kill them by shutting off the machine; they even speculated that a person might unconsciously make a lethal mistake in operation if he wanted to stop the expenses of his wife's illness badly enough. After the meeting one husband apparently pulled out his wife's shunt while cleaning it.

GROUP INTERACTION

A month after the new members joined, the group coalesced again by discussing the decision it felt the patients had to make—whether or not to keep on living—and by genially criticizing the leader for his lack of omnipotent, curative powers. Talk then turned for the first time to the prerequisites for a happy family. One member explained that it was necessary that parents instill in their children the need for helping one another. A new member added that the older children could teach the younger ones.

Subsequently the members endeavored to face their changed marital relationships. All agreed that their partners had become short-tempered, self-centered, unreasonable, and demanding—quite different from the people they had married. Sometimes they sadly hoped that their partners would change back to their original personalities after renal transplantation. Some spouses thought of leaving their partners, and one admitted that he was home as little as possible. Several found themselves continually angered by the burden of operating the machine and caring for the patients, which intensified their guilt. One operator was too guilty to let anyone else dialyze his wife, and the other could trust no one but himself to do it safely. Yet they were thankful that the patients had not simply died and felt that a spouse should stay close to his partner during dialysis and should operate the machine if there was no alternative.

During the period of this discussion the two operators' dialyzing apparatus catastrophically broke down, though both patients survived. One operator became furious at soldiers who supposedly murder defenseless women and children. When he regained his composure, he told the group how concerned he was to have been relieved when his wife had seemed to be dying. The other operator sympathized with him; his wife's death would have made him independent again, and he could have pursued his career unfettered.

During this stage the members rarely referred to authorities but instead agreed on the necessity for maintaining law and order in society and for helping others involved in dialysis.

The two new members left the group when their husbands successfully underwent transplantation; at the beginning of the seventh month M-3's wife died, and he then left the group. Only M-1 and M-2 remained.

They dissected in enormous detail the methods their relatives used to deny the probability of their partners' deaths. Though one commented that a physician can tell a person increasingly bad news about a relative's fatal illness and "develop him right down to his death," they concluded that even if their wives had little chance of surviving, they were doing their best, might yet succeed, and could never be criticized later. Now they genuinely called the leader their friend, and when two new members passed through the group they worked in partnership with him to support the newcomers in their anxiety. One of them explained to a new member, "Every person who performs dialysis helps the next one, who can stand on your shoulders and progress."

After the 32nd meeting M-2's wife suddenly died, terminating the group.

COMMENT

The beginning of the final stage of the group was devoted to adjusting to the loss of F–1 and then to assimilating F–2 and F–3 into the group. Although there was a partial regression after the death of F–1's husband, the members bore the loss together and emerged strengthened. They admitted for the first time that they were beginning to grieve for their partners and no longer consciously assigned omnipotence to the leader. The group's discussion of the dreadful prognosis was the milestone that had to be passed to assimilate the new members, just as before it had initiated the coalescence of the group. Then, for the first time, the members compared the group to a family.

Subsequently the spouses perceived more clearly than ever the change in their relationships to their partners as they tried to work on the mourning involved. On the other hand, they partially avoided the pain by removing themselves from home and by turning their loving ties into rebellious hostility, which in turn gave rise to intense guilt. Also, their hostility tended to separate them from their partners and to rekindle their urges toward primitive closeness, which for the operators were realized by their performance of dialysis.

The members' relationship to authorities had changed. They were concerned with their own ideals and guilt and not, as earlier, with regressive projections; by comparing their guilt fantasies they gained some relief.

With the death of M–3's wife there was again a partial regression. Yet, although they expected the worst, neither of the remaining members gave up trying to affect the future. Now they were identified with the leader on a relatively equal basis and had internalized the group's ideals and norms. M–2 and M–3 were not overwhelmed by depression, guilt, and hostility after their wives died, and all three men offered to help other spouses of dialysis patients. Later, one tried to will his body to help humanity.

LATER MEETINGS

We continued to meet with the spouses for an additional five months, and five new members sporadically joined. During the span of the meetings only M-1 was operating the machine. As had happened early in the first group, the discussions were relatively impersonal. The members all relied on individualized denial and magical styles of coping and never firmly identified with one another. M–1 continued to attend although he had retreated to a sardonic, intellectual acceptance of his wife's probable death. Although he had little faith in the leader's powers and felt that emotional involvement with the new members would only lead to further loss and pain, he was willing to support them in a factual way.

All of the new members shared the unverbalized fantasy that nonattendance would lead to their partners' removal from the program. Just at the point when they were beginning to vent their hostility and to discuss the patients' prognosis, one woman's husband underwent transplantation, and two other members began operating the kidney machine alone. All three withdrew and the group disbanded.

DISCUSSION

Our study has practical as well as theoretical implications. Hemodialysis in the home has given rise to much hope.[14] However, both this report and our earlier one[18] point out the serious psychological implications of training the spouse to dialyze his marital partner. The stress is enormous. There is a clear potential for serious regression and disastrous loss of control. Therefore, we feel that the spouse should operate the artificial kidney machine only if he has passed careful psychiatric screening and is provided with appropriate emotional support. Group discussions are one possibility; our supportive, noninterpretive technique proved effective, although it was very demanding on the leader and difficult to sustain. If psychiatric screening and support are not feasible, we feel the spouse should not undertake the responsibility for the dialysis procedure. Scribner[16] has advocated training the patient first, using the spouse merely as an assistant when needed; he felt this virtually eliminated many of the emotional problems we have described.

A review of the literature indicates that this group is a paradigm of the unconscious forces inherent in group structure and process which are obscured in therapy and training groups by the members' more sophisticated defenses. The over-all developmental sequence was that of the usual small group. This sequence was recently examined by Tuckman,[19] who divided it into four stages resembling ours. A number of authors[1,2,3,8,15] have pointed to the regression inherent in joining a group. The dynamics of the first two stages of the group are similar to those Mann[9,10] has described as involving the resolution of intra-group hostilities, while the third stage corresponds to Bion's[2] pairing group in which the relationships tend to be dyadic and optimism reigns. Alexander[1] has explained that an individual on becoming a member of a group reverses the childhood process of superego formation. Scheidlinger[15] has referred to the members' peer identification with the leader en route to internalization of group ideals and norms. Kaplan and Roman[7] have described the development of a therapy group in which the changing role of the leader is similar to that in ours. The individual's early denial of the painful relevance of the other members by means of private fantasies has been described by Semrad and associates.[17]

The most striking accomplishment of the group was the members' progressively increasing sense of emotional separateness from their partners as they lessened their reliance on denial. This sequence clearly illustrates Modell's thesis[11] that the extent of denial is quantitatively linked to the degree of lack of separateness from objects. Yet to the end, denial and guilt remained powerful motives for continued performance.

REFERENCES

At the time this study was done, Dr. Shambaugh was junior associate in medicine (psychiatry) at Peter Bent Brigham Hospital in Boston, Ma.; he is now Assistant in Psychiatry at the Children's Hospital Medical School in Boston, Ma. Dr. Kanter is senior psychiatrist at the Massachusetts Mental Health Center and clinical associate in psychiatry at the Harvard Medical School in Boston, Ma.

The authors wish to thank Barbara J. Fulton, R.N., Henry M. Fox, M.D., Constantine L. Hampers, M.D., Donald Snyder, M.D., and John P. Merrill, M.D. for their assistance with this study.

This research was supported by a grant from the Massachusetts Kidney Foundation and by Public Health Service grant HE–08260 from the National Heart Institute.

1. Alexander, F.: "Introduction," in Freud, S.: *Group psychology and the analysis of the ego* (1921). New York: Bantam Books, 1965.
2. Bion, W. R.: *Experiences in groups.* New York: Basic Books, 1961.
3. Freud, S.: *Group psychology and the analysis of the ego* (1921). New York: Bantam Books, 1965.
4. Grinker, R. R., and Spiegel, J. P.: *Men under stress,* New York: McGraw-Hill, 1963.
5. Hampers, C. L., and Schupak, E.: *Long-term hemodialysis,* New York: Grune & Stratton, 1967.
6. Janis, I. L.: Group identification under conditions of external danger, *Brit. J. Med. Psychol.* 36:227–238, 1963.
7. Kaplan, S. R., and Roman, M.: Phases in development in an adult therapy group, *Int. J. Group Psychother.* 13:10–26, 1963.
8. Klaf, F. S.: The power of the group leader: A contribution to the understanding of group psychology, *Psychoanalysis* 48:41–51, 1961.
9. Mann, J.: Some theoretic concepts of the group process, *Int. J. Group Psychother.* 5:235–241, 1955.
10. Mann, J.: Psychoanalytic observations regarding conformity in groups, *Int. J. Group Psychother.* 12:2–13, 1962.
11. Modell, A. H.: Denial and the sense of separateness, *J. Amer. Psychoanal. Ass.* 9:533–547, 1961.
12. Natterson, J. M., and Knudson, A.G.: Observations concerning fear of death in fatally ill children and their mothers, *Psychosom. Med.* 22:456–465, 1960.
13. Redl, F.: Group emotion and leadership, *Psychiatry* 5:573–596, 1942.
14. Report of the Committee on Chronic Kidney Disease, Bureau of the Budget, 1967.
15. Scheidlinger, S.: *Psychoanalysis and group behavior.* New York: W. W. Norton & Co., 1952.

16. Scribner, B. H.: Discussion of Shambaugh, P.W., Hampers, C. L. Bailey, G. L., Snyder, D., and Merrill, J. P.: Hemodialysis in the home—emotional impact on the spouse. *Trans. Amer. Soc. Artif. Intern. Organs* 13:49, 1967.
17. Semrad, E. V., Kanter, S., Shapiro, D., and Arsenian, J.: The field of group psychotherapy, *Int. J. Group Psychother.* 13:452–475, 1963.
18. Shambaugh, P. W., Hampers, C. L., Bailey, G. L., Snyder, D., and Merrill, J. P.: Hemodialysis in the home—emotional impact on the spouse. *Trans. Amer. Soc. Artif. Intern. Organs* 13:41–45, 1967.
19. Tuckman, B. W.: Developmental sequence in small groups. *Psychol. Bull.* 63:384–399, 1965.
20. Wangh, M.: The "Evocation of a proxy," a psychological maneuver, its use as defense, its purposes and genesis. *Psychoanal. Stud. Child* 17:451–469, 1962.
21. Wright, R. G., Sand, P., and Livingston, G., Psychological stress during hemodialysis for chronic renal failure, *Ann. Intern. Med.* 64:611–621, 1966.

19

Modified Group Therapy in the Treatment of Patients on Chronic Hemodialysis
—THOMAS H. HOLLON, Ph.D.

INTRODUCTION

THE patient with end-stage renal disease who, unless he receives a kidney transplant, can survive only on long-term hemodialysis must learn to cope with disability, the constant threat of death, and the added stress of being attached to a machine six to twelve hours two or three times a week. The emotional distress engendered by these hardships may reduce his tolerance for treatment and present a major obstacle to his rehabilitation. The past decade has seen chronic hemodialysis evolve from a relatively experimental technique for patients with end-stage renal disease to a definite treatment. This has been paralleled by the growing utilization of home dialysis to replace center dialysis.

Currently, long-term hemodialysis is keeping patients alive for considerable periods of time where in the past death would have intervened. Nevertheless, to quote DeNour and Czaczkes[1] "the progress of chronic hemodialysis from an experimental to a therapeutic stage has brought new and intriguing psychologic problems. What are the emotional reactions to a machine-dependent continuation of life? How do patients cope with the continuous threat of death? What happens to their body image?"

Reprinted from the *American Journal of Psychotherapy,* vol. XXXVI, no. 4, October, 1972, 501–510.

REVIEW OF THE LITERATURE

The importance of emotional factors in determining the patient's adaptation to treatment and his capacities for rehabilitation has become increasingly evident. Shea *et al.*[2] find adverse emotional reactions to hemodialysis to be a serious impediment to rehabilitation. Wright *et al.*[3] report that emotional stress experienced by the patient on hemodialysis pervades every level of the patient's life and includes such problems as actual or threatened loss of physical functions, frustration of drives resulting from dietary restrictions, loss of sexual vigor, and damage to body image.

Forced changes in patterns of living create strain for the spouse and other family members as well as the patient. Inability to keep social commitments because the patient may not be feeling well enough, the necessity of cancelling a vacation or putting off the planned building of a house all create guilt in the patient and suppressed resentment in other family members. Disappointment, especially in the spouse, when the patient's improvement does not measure up to expectation, is an added stress. Loss of membership in social groups, possible loss of job with threatened loss of home and possessions creates severe stress of financial hardship and insecurity. Attention has been called by Crammond *et al.*[4] and Medrum *et al.*[5] to the socioeconomic stress caused by cost of hospitalization, reduction in income, and impending financial disaster facing the patient on chronic hemodialysis.

DeNour *et al.*[6] consider the loss or threatened loss of urination as a particular form of stressful loss of bodily function suffered by the patient on hemodialysis. They point also to the persistent threat of death with the concomitant inability to plan for the future. However, they consider the greatest source of stress to be the patient's dependency on the machine and the medical team. This dependency evokes reactive aggression in the patient which in turn must be suppressed.

RESISTANCE TO NEEDED PSYCHOTHERAPY

The obvious emotional stress confronting the dialysis patient, and his family, at all levels of living points to a need for some form of psychotherapeutic intervention.[7] Wright *et al.*[3] call for some form of psychologic support based on a sound doctor-patient relationship and focusing on the patient's feelings about hemodialysis, home life, and work. They consider group therapy useful in supporting the patient's coping devices. Patients exert themselves to conform to the higher level of group functioning with constructive results. This correlates with the observation that chronic hemodialysis patients seek one another out and compare progress in a mutually supportive fashion.[2]

Although chronic hemodialysis patients experience emotional stress calling for psychotherapeutic intervention, emotional reactions within these patients, and their families, make it very difficult for them to recognize this need and accept help with their problems. This is well exemplified in DeNour's report[6] that during the first six months the services of a psychiatrist were available to dialysis patients, merely by having the patient stop in the office and arrange an appointment, not one patient took advantage of this help. In fact, the dialysis patients seemed actually surprised and offended by the implication that they might have emotional problems.

This great resistance of these patients to recognizing emotional problems stems, apparently, from a strong need to deny the full impact of their illness. Denial of the severity of illness and degree of impairment was found to be the most prevalent defense utilized by chronic patients on hemodialysis.[2,8] In addition to denial, patients employ defenses of isolation of affect, displacement, projection, and reaction formation. These defenses, especially denial, may help the patient live with his condition, but they tend to narrow and impoverish the patient's personality. They absorb too much of the patient's emotional energy causing his relationship to others to be shallow and superficial; and due to the rigidity of these defenses, they are apt to collapse under stress leaving the patient vulnerable to even greater emotional distress.[6]

Crammond and his colleagues[4] draw attention to the mourning reaction characteristic of all chronically ill patients which may be anticipated for the hemodialysis patient. They point out that a part of the fatigue, insomnia, itching, and anorexia the patients complain of during early adjustment to the program is due to depression related to this mourning reaction. A study of suicide among hemodialysis patients reveals the incident to be much higher than for the general population.[9]

This study indicated that where withdrawal from programs and deaths caused by not following treatment (actions with obvious suicidal implications) were added to the overt suicides, the incidence of self-induced death rose to 400 times the normal rate. These studies make it evident that either overt or masked depression may be present in the dialysis patient, and, as depression reduces a patient's motivation to seek help for emotional problems this makes him more inaccessible to psychotherapeutic intervention.

ADVERSE EMOTIONAL REACTIONS IN THE TREATMENT TEAM

The presence of marked defensive behavior, especially denial, as well as the possible presence of depressive features including self-destructive impulses, renders the dialysis patient difficult to reach with psychotherapeutic services, even though this type of help may be needed. Adverse emotional reactions which complicate the rehabilitation of the hemodialysis patient, however, are not found exclusively in the patient and his family. Intensive contact over a long period of time and awareness of grave responsibility for the patient's life place great emotional stress on the medical team.

In a two-year study of emotional problems of the medical team on a hemodialysis service, DeNour and Czaczkes[1] found feelings of guilt, possessiveness, overprotectiveness, and withdrawal from patients to be the major adverse reactions observed. All team members expressed the demand that patients do better on hemodialysis than they had done before becoming ill. There were expressed feelings of doubt as to whether the patients were being helped by hemodialysis or whether they and their families would really be better off if they were allowed to die quietly.

A tendency to possessiveness and overprotectiveness was found especially in the nurses, who worked most closely with the patients. This appeared related to the nurse's own precarious role on hemodialysis where she is required to do things not called for by nurses on other services such as make the decision to give a blood transfusion or actually give a transfusion. At a deeper level these attitudes of possessiveness and overprotectiveness are a reaction formation to unconscious hostility and aggression toward the patient.

These emotional reactions in the nurse may well be elicited by the attitudes of the patient and his family. The nurses often are the ones who work very hard and are dedicated to the dialysis program while the patients get all the attention. The patients and their family may give no expression of gratitude and may even be complaining and demanding of more attention, in spite of the great efforts expended by the nurse in the dialysis unit.

These findings indicate that the rigors of hemodialysis engender emotional stress not only for the patient and his family, but for the treatment team as well, and this creates an additional complicating factor in the psychosocial problems of the dialysis patient.

CURRENT STUDY

The chronic hemodialysis center at Rockford Memorial Hospital, a community hospital of 410 beds, is equipped with four Travenol twin cannister hemodializers. These four artificial kidney machines permit four patients to be dialyzed concurrently in the center. Medical supervision, however, is provided to a considerably larger number of patients, as emphasis in the center is on home dialysis. All patients, with rare exception, are in training for home dialysis. In addition, medical supervision is provided to postrenal transplant patients and to patients with end-stage renal disease who will be destined for dialysis.

We have found a modified form of group therapy based upon the systems approach to be the most acceptable to the dialysis patients and their families. As the term implies, this concerns bringing together all members of the system responsible for the patient's treatment. Regular group sessions are held in which all patients receiving medical supervision and their significant family members are invited to meet with the treatment team and—whenever possible—representatives of strategic agencies such as the kidney foundation or the Department of Public Aid to discuss problems encountered by the patients and to participate in joint problem solving. The group meets one Saturday morning a month for an hour and a half.

The significant family members generally consist of the patient's spouse, but currently include a patient's fiancee, parents, and an adult daughter, and, on occasion have included elementary school age and teen-age children, adult brothers and sisters, and even a patient's parents-in-law The treatment team participating in the group is comprised of the physician-director, two dialysis nurses, a dietician, a social worker, a chaplain, and a clinical psychologist. Where members of strategic agencies have attended the group, these have included members of the local kidney foundation, caseworkers from the Department of Public Aid, and hospital administrators from our own hospital. Thus the group is comprised of a relatively large number of members and, when attendance is good, may consist of over 30 persons.

ORGANIZATION OF THE GROUP

The physician, psychologist, chaplain, and social worker assume the role taken by co-therapists in conventional group therapy, encouraging expression of feelings by group members, reflecting questions and problems back to the group, pressing for more information on topics introduced for discussion, and making tentative interpretations for the group's consideration. A unique feature of our group therapy concerns the role assumed by the physician-director. Where in most centers group psychotherapy would be delegated to the psychologist or social worker, here the physician actively participates in an essentially psychotherapeutic endeavor. We have been impressed with the extent to which this reduces anxiety and improves the confidence of patients and families.

As the leader of the treatment team and as the one to whom the patients and families turn for final decisions concerning treatment, the physician's involvement in group therapy bears evidence that the patients are perceived as total persons and not merely as patients on a machine. This is a strong component in establishing the sound doctor-patient relationship cited by Wright *et al.*[3] as essential for helping the dialysis patient cope with the stresses of his condition.

Prior to beginning the modified group psychotherapy, we encountered difficulties and resistance in helping patients cope with emotional problems similar to those described by DeNour *et al.*[6] As an example, we were aware from her actions that one of our female patients was determined on self-destruction, but efforts to help her through individual and conjoint therapy met only with bland denial. She willingly explored and ventilated feelings about her earlier life, and certain of her current relationships, but where questions of her emotional reactions to dialysis or her cooperation with the treatment program came up she consistently denied that there were any problems.

Other attempts at individual psychotherapy with patients or spouses or conjoint psychotherapy with both often elicited a discussion of emotional problems, but it was soon found that the seeming benefit from this was not generalizing to situations of actual stress and the patients and families themselves were aware of this, saying "talking about problems doesn't change anything."

The response to the modified group therapy has been quite different.

The patients and family members seem to derive true benefit for sharing experiences with others, ventilating to one another pent-up feelings, and actually "teaching" one another how to cope with pragmatic problems of dialysis and how to develop more effective emotional responses. This is especially true for those on home dialysis. We have observed that families who are training for home dialysis or have just recently begun home dialysis listen intently as more experienced families describe their experiences. The novices put many questions to the experienced families and it is apparent that their anxieties are greatly reduced and their confidence enhanced by these discussions. The experienced families, for their part, gain much self-confidence and composure as they hear themselves relating to the others how they have coped with alarming and unanticipated problems.

CASE REPORTS

The response to group therapy is well illustrated by the following examples:

Mr. L. N., a male patient in his mid-thirties, had been one of the most difficult patients while being dialyzed in the center preliminary to transfer to home dialysis. He was an immature, explosive man and the treatment team viewed his going on home dialysis with considerable misgiving. He was demanding and critical of his wife, he cooperated poorly with the dialysis nurses, and he maintained denial of the true gravity of his illness by projecting his anxieties in the form of grievances against the hospital, social agencies, employers, and others.

His wife complained bitterly to the nurses of his attitude toward her, but when an attempt was made to discuss this with her in an individual interview, she became quite upset, feeling it implied she had emotional problems and was not doing her part. Both the patient and his wife vigorously resisted psychotherapeutic exploration through individual or conjoint sessions. After an initial reluctance, they agreed to attend the group sessions where they appeared to be much less threatened and were able to share their feelings and experiences with the others. Particularly after Mr. L. N. went on home dialysis, he and his wife seemed to gain emotional support from comparing problems and feelings with other group members.

On one occasion Mr. and Mrs. L. N. related a situation in which Mrs. L. N. was required to give her husband a blood transfusion at home. She did this while maintaining a telephone conference with the dialysis nurse at Rockford Memorial Hospital who instructed her at points where she was uncertain. Some members of the group questioned the response of the N.'s children to this emergency procedure and this led to a group discussion of the fact that where proper attitudes prevail, home dialysis can bring a family together.

Mr. L. N. injected a note of humor, saying, his children stood around like young vampires, saying "when is daddy going to get some more blood," but then he went on to say he had heard one of his children explaining the procedure of dialysis to his playmates. Sharing experiences and ventilating feeling with the group has reduced much of the emotional distress and defensive hostility in Mr. and Mrs. L. N. They, in turn, have contributed a great deal to reducing anxiety and engendering confidence in other group members, especially new families.

The manner in which eagerness to measure up to group expectations serves as emotional support in situations of stress is reflected by the reaction of another male patient who had recently gone on home dialysis:

Mr. H. R. and his wife had been considered the family in the center most reluctant to undertake home dialysis and for this reason training in home dialysis had been delayed. They did not seem to communicate well with each other and the wife felt she was incapable of learning the procedure and could not tolerate the thought of carrying it out at home. Nevertheless, a point was reached where they seemed prepared to dialyze at home.

They returned to the group soon after the first week on home dialysis and the patient reported, with great pride, their success. During the initial home dialysis there had been a storm in their community. The wife confessed she had been "jittery" and unwilling to get out of bed to begin the procedure. The patient, however, was an "eager beaver" who got the machine going and carried out most of the operation by himself. His opportunity to relate this to the group did much to solidify his own confidence and, again, had a very beneficial effect on other group members.

There have been numerous examples in the group where members reported they had been able to cope with stress after hearing of the experiences of others. The patients and families also utilized the group to share their feelings of being helpless victims of their predicament and to express the resulting anger:

During one session, Mrs. D. T., a representative of the local Kidney Foundation, who was herself the widow of a kidney patient, reported that when her husband was being dialyzed, they both feared complaining or expressing their own views as this might lead to the husband being taken off the machine. This allowed Mrs. C. G., a depressed, resentful wife of a critically ill patient, to give vent to intense pent-up feelings.

Mrs. C. G. stated that while her husband was being dialyzed in a large metropolitan center, she had attempted to discuss the expense and other hardships they endured. In response to this, she had been told that if she and her husband could not follow orders, other patients were lined up who would be glad to take his place. This led to a discussion of the fact that emotional needs of the dialysis patient and the spouse do not receive sufficient consideration and that groups such as ours provide an opportunity to deal with these feelings.

Mrs. C. G.'s situation revealed the value of group therapy in helping a family member cope with problems in living even where efforts to prolong the life of the patient were unsuccessful. The patient, Mr. C. G., continued to deteriorate physically in spite of treatment efforts and he eventually died. His illness had been a long, exhausting ordeal for Mrs. C. G., she had been quite ambivalent about hemodialysis, and very guilty over her feelings of resentment. Her husband's death provided all of the ingredients for a reactive depression on her part. She continued in the group, however, for a number of months after his death, and utilized the group discussions to aid her through her mourning and the reorientation of her life.

HANDLING THE DISCUSSION OF DEATH

Mr. C. G.'s death drew attention to the persistent threat of death confronting the dialysis patient and his family. Dialysis does improve the patient's health and the prospect of an eventual kidney transplant engenders hope. Nevertheless, the occasional death of a fellow patient serves as a constant reminder to the others that theirs is, at best, a precarious existence.

When the death of a fellow patient does occur, the other patients, family members, and the treatment team are curiously reluctant to talk about it. This appears to be a function of the taboo concerning any but the most superficial discussion of death described so well by Elizabeth Kubler-Ross.[10]

It was felt, however, again based on the work of Dr. Kubler-Ross, that were the opportunity afforded, patients and family members might welcome a discussion of the death of a fellow patient and that group therapy provides such an opportunity. Following the death of a dialysis patient in our center, it was decided that if this were not spontaneously brought up in the next group session, the chaplain would introduce the topic.

The death was not mentioned by group members in the next session, so the chaplain introduced the subject, saying, "Whenever a member of a family dies, it is important for the family to talk about it; we are like a family in some respects and I imagine a number of you have questions about Mrs. K. L.'s recent death." The group responded in a very active fashion. They put many questions to the physician-director and the dialysis nurses which revealed that they harbored many misconceptions concerning the cause of the fellow patient's death.

This question period afforded the opportunity to clarify these misconceptions and for the physician-director to discuss the fact that patients differed greatly in their ability to tolerate hemodialysis. The discussion then focused on the shared opinion that certain patients do not have the will to live or the desire to exert the effort required to survive on dialysis. Finally, the point was made that though death is an ever-present possibility, the patients are not helpless victims but can do much through their own efforts to safeguard their lives and improve their physical conditions.

ADDITIONAL ADVANTAGES OF MODIFIED GROUP THERAPY

The modified group therapy, in addition to providing an opportunity for group members to share feelings, has provided the impetus for pragmatic problem solving. Group members, especially the wives, collaborated with the dietician in composing a cookbook made of varied recipes adapted to the dietary restrictions of the dialysis patient. The group, in conjunction with the local kidney foundation and the hospital administration, established a procedure for purchasing drugs at cost through the hospital pharmacy.

Discussion in the group also led to the organization of a seminar for case workers, counselors, and others in the community on the problems in living encountered by the patient with kidney disease. The person-to-person talks between dialysis patients, family members, and social agency workers led to beneficial clarification of procedures and actual modification in certain agency policies in dealing with kidney failure patients.

The modified group therapy, as a final advantage, has made patients and family members more accessible to individual and conjoint psychotherapy where this has proved necessary. It has also provided a basis for ongoing psychosocial consultation to the treatment team, especially to the dialysis nurses who bear the heaviest burden of patient care.

SUMMARY

The problems of end-stage renal disease and the rigors of hemodialysis create emotional stress for the patient and his family which require psychotherapeutic intervention. Due to the denial of illness, however, dialysis patients and family members are resistant to conventional forms of psychotherapy and may even resent the implication that they have emotional problems.

A form of modified group psychotherapy based on a systems approach has been found to be most acceptable to dialysis patients and their families. This involves bringing together the dialysis patients, family members, the treatment team, and representatives of strategic agencies for discussion of patient problems and joint problem solving.

The major benefit offered by the group therapy results from the sharing of feelings and experiences among group members, but added advantages consist in making patients and family members more accessible to psychotherapy when this is required, and providing a basis for ongoing psychosocial consultation to the treatment team.

REFERENCES

Dr. Hollon is a Consulting Psychologist at the Rockford Memorial Hospital in Rockford, Ill.

1. DeNour, K. A. and Czaczkes, J. W. Emotional problems and reactions of the medical team in a chronic hemodialysis unit. *Lancet,* II:987, 1968.
2. Shea, E. J., Bogzen, E. F., and Freeman, R. B. Hemodialysis for chronic renal failure. *Ann. Intern. Med.,* 62:588, 1965.
3. Wright, R. G., Sands, P., Livingston, G. Stress during hemodialysis for chronic renal failure. *Ann. Intern. Med.,* 64:611, 1966.

4. Crammond, W. A., Knight, R., and Lawrence, J. R. The psychiatric contribution to a renal unit undertaking chronic hemodialysis and renal homotransplantation. *Brit. J. Psychiat.,* 113:1201, 1967.
5. Medrum, M. W., Wolfram, J. G., and Rubini, M. The impact of chronic hemodialysis upon the socio-economics of a veteran patient group. *J. Chron. Dis.,* 21:37, 1968.
6. DeNour, K. A., Sholtiel, J., and Czaczkes, J. W. Emotional reactions of patients on chronic hemodialysis. *Psychosomat. Med.,* 30:521, 1968.
7. DeNour, K. A. Psychotherapy with patients on chronic hemodialysis. *Brit. J. Psychiat.,* 116:207, 1970.
8. Short, M. J. and Wilson, W. P. Role of denial in chronic hemodialysis. *Arch. Gen. Psychiat.,* 20:433, 1969.
9. Abram, J. S. and Moore, G. L., Westervelt, F. B. Suicidal behavior in chronic dialysis patients. Presented at the 123rd Annual Meeting of the American Psychiatric Association, May, 1970.
10. Kubler-Ross, E. *On death and dying.* Macmillan, New York, 1970.

Personal Awareness: Individual Exercises

1. In recent years, hemodialysis patients have been given new hope that they might someday be free from dependence on a machine and benefit from a kidney transplant. Have you thought about donating your kidney for transplant purposes after your death? Present a rationale for your decision.

2. After carefully reading this chapter, visit a hemodialysis center. Determine if there are any specific difficulties related to the care and treatment of hemodialysis patients. Write an action-oriented program which emphasizes overcoming such difficulties. Present this to the class.

3. How would dialysis affect your life? To help you acquire a better perspective make arrangements to simulate hemodialysis for one month. You may choose to go to a hospital and visit with hemodialysis patients or simulate using a home dialysis unit. For example, sit in a comfortable chair for a prescribed period of time structuring your environment as if you were experiencing dialysis. Keep a detailed log of your experiences and feelings.

4. A close friend of yours has kidney failure and offers you $25,000 for one of your kidneys. Any response? Discuss how much money (*you would want to have*) or how close the person would have to be before you would consider donating your kidney.

Structured Group Experience in Disability
—Donor or Recipient?*

This experience focuses upon complex issues arising for donors of organs for transplant. An intense situation may be created since the person requiring a kidney is someone who is emotionally close to you.

GOALS

1. To explore reactions when a person has the opportunity to consider the donation of his or her kidney.
2. To present a situation which is complicated by the needs of a loved one.
3. To examine differing perspectives when the role of a person in need is reversed.

PRELIMINARY CONSIDERATIONS

1. *Level of Intensity:* High

2. *Group Size:* 6–8 participants

3. *Time:* 2 hours

4. *Materials Needed:* Paper and pencils

5. *Physical Setting:* Comfortable room, moveable chairs

PROCEDURE

1. The leader opens the discussion by asking if there were any questions raised by the readings or Personal Awareness exercises in chapter three.

2. If there are questions they are responded to and discussed in the group.

*See Appendices A and B for detailed information on use of the structured group experiences in disability.

3. Having completed the discussion, the leader states that it is easy to read about and discuss a topical area, but the perspective can change when it relates directly to us.

4. Leader reads the following statement: "You have just received a phone call from the person you are closest to and love dearly. Stop and reflect on who this person would be in your life *now*. This person has just received word of having renal failure and is very distressed about his or her health. Due to medical complications the doctors feel that a kidney transplant is critical; without it, the person is in grave danger of dying."

5. Participants write a one-page statement of their reactions to this information.

6. Group members are selected at random to read their responses.

7. After all members have read their statements an open group discussion takes place.

8. During this discussion particular attention should be paid to the quality of the relationship.

9. The leader introduces the concept of significant others (e.g., if you would be hesitant to donate a kidney to this person, is there anyone whom you might consider?).

10. Having processed this, the leader moves to the role reversal stage, in which the group members become the person in need.

11. The leader reads the following statement: "You have just been informed by your physician that you have renal failure, unless you receive a kidney transplant within three months you are risking death."

12. The leader asks participants to write a paragraph on the initial reaction to this news.

13. Next the group leader asks the group to write down the name of a person they would ask to donate a kidney to them and to list five reasons why they might ask this particular person.

14. Two group members are selected to role play the situation of asking the named person for his or her kidney.

LEADERSHIP SUGGESTIONS

1. Closely consider the shift of reasoning when group members are asked to give up a kidney as compared to when they need a kidney.

2. Focus on the similarities or dissimilarities of the potential donors named by the group.

3. Explore the potential danger to the donor.

4. Be aware that a participant may use denial, anger, intellectualization, rationalization, and similar defense mechanisms when reacting to this structured group experience in disability.

VARIATIONS

1. Have the person who needs a kidney be a/their child.

2. Explore the differential reaction if the person who needed the kidney was younger, older, or racially different.

CHAPTER FOUR

Group Approaches with Persons Having Visual Disabilities

Overview

An ongoing challenge for persons who are blind or visually impaired is to live a satisfying life in a "seeing world" that may be well aware of their limitation, but blind to their potential. The articles in this chapter present group approaches that have been used with blind and/or visually impaired persons.

In "Psychotherapy with the Least Expected," Ross and Anderson describe their work with a group of blind persons who also faced extreme economic hardships. They found the use of male and female co-leaders especially useful in dealing with this group. The authors stress the importance of confronting issues and showing genuine concern for group members.

In "The Use of Encounter Microlabs with a Group of Visually Handicapped Rehabilitation Clients," Goldman discusses the use of action-related "encounter" techniques designed to stimulate participation in a group setting. The use of these physical activities, he believes, allows the clients to overcome initial apprehensions and reveal their concerns more freely.

In "Some Observations on Group Therapy with the Blind" Herman reports that visually handicapped persons often employ denial, depression, self-devaluation, and related dynamics in attempting to cope with blindness. The group addressed these issues and sought to come to terms with them. Because the visual cues used by sighted persons are not available in conducting group therapy with visually impaired persons, the leader found his own intervention had to take the form of more active verbal communication.

In "The Theragnostic Group in a Rehabilitation Center for Visually Handicapped Persons," Manaster discusses how the group process was beneficial to clients undergoing testing at a rehabilitation center. Manaster identifies two aspects of the group process— "gnostic" or understanding and therapeutic. He views the group as a vehicle to reinforce a group member's assets while helping to overcome limitations. The integration of gnostic and therapeutic group processes afford the rehabilitant the opportunity to become an active participant in his or her rehabilitation planning.

In her article, "Para-analytic Group Therapy with Adolescent Multi-Handicapped Blind," Avery discusses the impact of group therapy on each group member, focusing on individual adjustment problems of adolescent girls in relation to their visual impairments. A primary theme in Avery's group is the need for flexible group leadership with adolescents who are disabled. Avery points out that more generic problems can take priority even over blindness. This is a concrete example of the importance of dealing with the person, not the disability per se.

In "Adaption to Visual Handicap: Short-Term Group Approach," Keegan describes the goals and dynamics of group meetings in his work with blind persons undergoing treatment at a rehabilitation center. He stresses that a practical, active, and didactic group format is to be preferred to a more silent, passive process. Keegan also discusses several advantages of a group approach to facilitate the personal growth of visually handicapped persons and suggests that other disability groups could also benefit from a similar short-term therapy model. Highlighted in Keegan's article are a variety of issues to which the group leader must attend, such as hostility toward sighted persons and nonvoluntary group participation.

In Roessler's article "An Evaluation of Personal Achievement Skills Training with the Visually Handicapped" the value and power of a structured group format is presented. By stressing a goal orientation, group members had the opportunity to both define and attain goals as well as increase self-esteem.

Taken as a whole, the articles in this chapter offer the reader a variety of theoretical and practical alternatives to facilitate the use of group practices with persons who are visually impaired. All contributors to this chapter share a common belief that group procedures enhance the rehabilitation potential of such persons. The several viewpoints discussed by these authors provide the reader with a well-rounded perspective for maximizing the personal growth of visually impaired persons through a therapeutic group format.

20

Psychotherapy with the Least Expected: Modified Group Therapy with Blind Clients
—ELISABETH KUBLER ROSS, M.D., and JAMES ROY ANDERSON

PSYCHOTHERAPY has long been regarded as a form of treatment for a special kind of patient. Such a person has a certain degree of sophistication and education; he is capable of thinking objectively and of taking a critical look at himself. He is curious, motivated to gain some insight into his behavior.

Group therapy, in contrast to individual therapy, may be less demanding for many people, as it allows time, observation of other patients, and contemplation before one enters more actively into the group discussion. It allows the person to lose his shyness, reluctance, or inhibition gradually and in the process to participate in the dialogue. For others, group therapy is more difficult to enter, as it lacks the privacy and intimacy of individual therapy, and it may be more difficult for some to speak up in front of other people. For those with more serious disturbances, it may be too stimulating and confusing, thus contributing to their withdrawal and isolation. From an economic point of view, group therapy has the distinct advantage, in that many more people can be helped by the same therapist in the same time span.

In such an agency as The Lighthouse for the Blind, in Chicago, where a psychiatric consultant is available once a week and the number of troubled people exceeds her availability, group therapy is an ideal means of reaching as many as possible. The blind and seriously handicapped at The Lighthouse for the Blind impressed us with their multitude of problems, which ordinarily were not dealt with in an agency. Many of these people came from the low socioeconomic class and lived in deprived neighbor-

Reprinted by permission from *Rehabilitation Literature* 29 (3): 73–76, 1968.

hoods with all their shortcomings, overcrowded living quarters, and environmental dangers. Many who were able to travel independently were afraid to do so because of the dangerous area in which they lived. They were unable to move out and practically remained prisoners in their dark apartments without the energy to do something about it.

Many of these people had convulsive disorders and other afflictions, often continuing to take medication that had been prescribed some time before, without adequate medical follow-up or regular checkups. A great majority were burdened with extreme poverty and had feelings of hopelessness and inadequacy because of their blindness, their inability to earn a minimal living, and, in some instances, because of their being Negro. Only a few had had sufficient education and even fewer had ever had an opportunity to seek guidance, counseling, or psychiatric help for emotional problems.

We were convinced that we had enough "clients" to form a group suitable for exploring the possibility of meaningful group therapy. We hoped to be able to share their daily conflicts and to facilitate their verbal expression. We had little expectation of ever making "good psychotherapy candidates" of them. We did not anticipate high gains, except, perhaps, that they might learn to express verbally what they had suppressed for so many years. They seemed to look at the world in a gloomy fashion, as if there were nothing that could change their "fate."

H AVING two therapists for this group was decided upon for several reasons. First, this assures continuance when one is missing; second, it offers a parental setup for people who come from one-parent homes; and, last but not least, it facilitates the starting of therapy, for the two therapists can have dialogue together until the members of the group feel free to join in.

The male therapist was an experienced rehabilitation and placement counselor who had worked with the blind for many years, knew the staff and the environment of the workshop, and, most important perhaps of all, knew all the facilities and job opportunities for the blind in the state of Illinois. He thus represented the "all-knowing father" who was aware of the realities and set them straight when they were misrepresented.

The female therapist was a psychiatrist who supplied warm, caring support, looked after their emotional needs, and offered them some insight. She turned to the male partner when final job placements or future dispositions were discussed. The two therapists often discussed interpretations openly to show the group how they came to certain conclusions—and to prove that there was nothing magical about their findings. This also created an opportunity for members of the group to disagree with the therapists or to add strength to their statements.

The meeting time chosen for the group was at the end of a working day to facilitate participation without loss of income and to avoid the cost of additional travel, which our clients could ill afford.

The choice of candidates was not easy, as most of our blind clients seemed to be in need of some counseling and guidance, none of them could afford private therapy, and those who could attend a clinic had never even considered such therapy. We hoped to keep the group at between 8 and 10 participants and planned one weekly session of an hour and a half.

Once these technical problems were solved, the therapist approached those considered as candidates, inviting them to join the group on a trial basis. Since few really understood what was asked of them, we felt that trial attendance would be the fairest way of conveying to them the meaning of group therapy. They were given a brief, simple description of the purpose of such a group and they were expected to give a final answer within a few days. The majority of the clients accepted the offer. Rather soon it became evident that they had not joined the group out of interest or curiosity: Fear inhibited their freedom to refuse to join.

D URING the first session it was apparent that few had actually volunteered. Everyone sat in the room stiff and rather stilted, expecting someone else to talk, answering in monosyllables when approached. Each member was asked to introduce himself so that the group might be familiar with everyone's voice. The therapists did the same, adding some personal data that would normally not be offered before other groups. We would say, for example, how many children we had, how long we had lived in Chicago, and what motivated us to work at The Lighthouse.

The new participants mentioned little more than their names and their reasons for being in the agency (either working in the workshop or pursuing some training there), often terminating their statements with "That's all I can say about myself." There was a mixture of passive resistance, paranoid thinking, and great fear and concern that they might "say too much or the wrong thing." This was the ideal opportunity for the two therapists to recapitulate the meaning and task of the group and to share with each other opinions about the reluctance of the participants.

This provoked enough feeling for them to open up and to admit their concern about losing their positions at The Lighthouse if they refused to join. Others were afraid they would be laid off at the next opportunity if they did not cooperate or that they would not be placed in a job after termination of their training period. Naturally, all of these fears were without basis in fact, but, for these guarded, often rather paranoid, people, they constituted a reality that could not be ignored. Some were able to admit that they planned on attending the minimum number of sessions, "to see what it's like," and to disappear at the first opportunity. Two admitted to deciding to sit in the group passively "but not to open my mouth"—an admission that was followed by uneasy laughter. In general, there was a mood of enforced compliance, fear of retaliation if they would not submit, and a guarded, suspicious, "wait-and-see" attitude that made the start a difficult one, to say the least.

Since blind people depend on nonvisual cues, the therapists cannot just sit and look from one to another, hopeful of stimulating one to contribute something. Silence is least tolerated in such a guarded group, whose members are not yet familiar with the people and the process. It would only increase their anxiety and paranoid thinking, thus making it impossible to get meaningful interaction. This can create a valuable opportunity for the therapist-couple; they ask each other what is going on and try to define over and over the purpose and goals of such meetings and their own reactions to the hostility, rejection, or just waste of precious time.

A s we started to talk about our children, one of the participants mentioned proudly that he had seven little ones. Suddenly we found some common ground, some familiar problems and questions that interested all of us, and we started a very significant discussion. When this father, a Negro, realized that he was in the midst of a dialogue that he had planned to boycott, he stopped, finally bursting out with the question, "How can a white, rich, educated, sighted person understand the multitude of problems of our miserable existence?"

Rather than to become defensive, adding to the group's doubts, we threw this question open to all the members, an equal number of white and of Negro participants. Half were male and half, female; the age range was 18 to 55 years. All except the psychiatrist were legally blind or severely visually handicapped, most since birth.

One participant described with anecdotal material the misery in which he lived. He shared an overcrowded apartment with his in-laws, his young wife, and seven small children. He described his struggles as a totally blind man to earn a minimum salary to feed his family. He told of the long hours he worked to make ends meet, his wife's dependency on her mother, his need for more privacy, and his frustration and inability to secure it. He went on describing how he waited at night for his in-laws to go to bed so he could open up the couch and transform it into a bed for himself, his wife, and some of the children. He described the tensions, the arguments, and finally the breaking point, when he could no longer tolerate the situation and left his family.

The reaction from the group was a genuinely human one: They pitied the children for having lost a father, they reprimanded him for seeking solace with another woman, and finally they attempted to seek other solutions. They shared their own experiences and, with him, his isolation, his inner and outer darkness, and his despair. Before we realized it, the group took over and left the therapists as mere catalysts, occasional interpreters or advisors.

This outburst of human emotions, the verbal expressions of years of misery and agony, seemed to open the door for the most reluctant and inhibited. One by one, they started to share their own problems, which they had carried in silence and sometimes in sadness and anger. Since the same reality issues confronted many others in the group, they received little sympathy but faced a rather harsh jury and were questioned as to what they had done to change their "fate." The others offered rather concrete suggestions as to how to get out of debt, where and how to get the long-needed medical attention, and whom to approach for possible training in a much-desired field. We dealt with specifics rather than generalities, we expressed our feelings rather bluntly, and—most important of all, perhaps—we used the same language. The often vulgar slang expressions of their neighborhoods had to be translated occasionally to insure communication. As soon as the group realized that we accepted them the way they were—without any value judgment attached—they used less extreme expressions and often were quite shocked when one of the therapists or a new member used the same idioms.

S OON after the initial introductory sessions, we decided to serve coffee during the meeting. On special occasions, we surprised them with cake, with candles on birthdays. Some of them had a birthday cake for the first time! What seemed at first to be a rather hostile or passive-indifferent group of people impressed us soon by their mutual consideration, their ability to laugh and cry together, and an almost total disappearance of the guarded suspiciousness and paranoid thinking.

The "being blind" was dealt with first and also dismissed first. The "being poor" remained an issue during the whole year but it was no longer a matter of an unchangeable fate, but rather something of a challenge that could and had to be tackled in a planned and constructive fashion. On-the-job training, rather than continued employment in the workshop for the handicapped, became more of a possibility. Two of the members attempted and completed such training. They are now self-supporting, in much more stable and permanent positions in the city.

The race problem was an issue occasionally but was handled in a meaningful fashion that was helpful to both sides. A good example of this was the problem of a young white girl who joined the group late. She shared with us some of her frustrations with boyfriends and the reasons for dropping them. On discovering that a young man was of a different race, she dismissed him as ineligible. An extremely frank discussion ensued, during which each person tried to understand the reasons and motivations behind her actions, rather than just to condemn them.

The group soon elicited the girl's hostility toward her mother, who did not allow her to grow up or to achieve any independence, using the girl's blindness as an excuse. The mother was an extremely limited woman who approved only of people with her own narrow cultural background. The daughter "happened to fall in love" only with boys of a different race, then "happened" to discover their race, and "dropped" the boys instantly. When the group pointed these patterns out, the girl began to realize that this behavior might be a way of acting out against the mother and in actuality really had very little to do with a race problem on her part.

When the mother attempted to discourage her from regular work and attendance at The Lighthouse, as well as from receiving additional training to become self-supporting, the members of the group supported the girl's wish for emancipation and added several examples from their own existence. This girl has completed a training course and has been offered a good position that makes her financially independent. She has become a real pal to her group partners, Negroes and whites. She has traveled an hour and a half on her own from her home to reach The Lighthouse, where she has kept a job while awaiting another opportunity.

ANOTHER member of the group used highly intellectual language as a defense against his feelings of inferiority. After almost a year of mutual confrontations, he has finally had the courage to leave the sheltered workshop and has found employment in private industry, where his sociable, friendly manner is appreciated by his coworkers. He earns a more regular income, which helps him support his wife and newborn baby—both "newcomers" since he entered the group.

Our "favorite son" is perhaps T. X., who presented himself as an extremely shy man, hard-working, but somehow unlucky all along. No matter what he attempted to achieve, something always seemed to happen at the last minute to ruin his plans. He seemed to be very talented in car mechanics and tried desperately to get an agency's approval for such training. He was unlucky in having an extremely passive, unperceptive, and often hostile counselor, who had a talent for delaying decisions for months. Each time our friend had an appointment, additional tests or requirements were asked of him, thus adding to his feeling of hopelessness and despair. We strongly believe that it was the group that kept this man—if not from suicide—at least from giving up all efforts to change his miserable, lonely existence. It was our placement specialist and another member of the group who practically talked him into accepting an opportunity to learn the skills of a darkroom technician, for which he successfully completed training a short time ago. He, too, is currently employed, and his behavior shows no trace of his past chronic depression.

WE are trying to conclude what we have learned after one year of weekly sessions with this unusual group of underprivileged, blind people sharing a multitude of problems in a modified form of group therapy.

Since few of them had ever heard of or had contemplated having such treatment and all shared every sort of fantasy about psychiatry, it was necessary to communicate on their level and to facilitate the expression of their concerns about therapy. They needed a few "trial sessions" in order to understand the meaning of such meetings. Their initial lack of motivation, their fears of retaliation, their unrealistic concerns about retribution or the consequences for failing to attend, their hostility, could all be overcome in time, if regarded, not personally, but rather as a result of a life of struggles and suffering.

Use of two therapists is advisable for several reasons, namely, the continuation of the group, the representation of parental figures, and the initial dialogue between the two needed to set an example of free discussion, which then will stimulate others to join in. Many people from the lowest socioeconomic class, in their lives, have had few, if any, examples of regular attendance, whether in school or at work. Since this is a prerequisite for being an exemplary employee—which was the goal for all our members—we made it a point to attend all sessions possible. Having two therapists enabled us to continue the group, even during times of illness or vacation.

Most of our group members came from shattered families, in which there was only one parent, thus giving them little experience of healthy interaction and sharing between father and mother figures. The therapists' goal was to give them a bit of this experience, while offering an experienced placement counselor knowing all the facilities for the blind and a motherly, firm, but supporting psychiatrist who attempted to deal with their emotional needs.

Since all the members were either totally blind or seriously visually handicapped, visual cues could not be used during the therapy session. Silence is poorly tolerated, as it enhances anxiety, paranoid thinking, and isolation. The conversation has to flow and can easily be maintained by the two cotherapists until the members of the group feel more comfortable. Language has to be adjusted to the expressions used by the participants, in their respective homes or neighborhoods. It will be exaggerated at the onset of such therapy as an expression of their hostility and their difference. If the therapists make it a point to understand what they are saying and do not hesitate to use the same words, they will soon be dropped and replaced by language more socially acceptable.

Questions of blindness, poverty, and race should not be avoided but dealt with at the earliest possible opening. As one of our group members stated: A rich, educated, white, and sighted therapist cannot possibly understand the misery of the poor, blind, uneducated Negro. Our one-year group therapy proved that this is not so. Meaningful therapy can be achieved if the questions of blindness, poverty, and race are dealt with, making room for more personal problems, which are often disguised, under the cover of the above three. Out of a highly unmotivated, uneducated, and unsophisticated group of whites and Negroes from the lowest socioeconomic class, all blind and living marginal existences, grew a highly homogeneous group of involved people who shared the problems of their daily existence and their concerns, frustrations, and hopes for the future. What appeared to be unsurmountable social problems often proved to be basically human conflicts, which could be dealt with by any human being regardless of his visual ability, skin color, or social background.

WE thus encourage more counselors and therapists to bring such groups together, to tolerate the initial frustrations, and not to allow themselves to be impressed by lack of motivation. Where the need is great, the gains to be made are equally promising. Therapy with our group has been an enriching experience in spite of, or perhaps because of, all the odds against it.

Dr. Ross, assistant professor of psychiatry at the University of Chicago Hospitals and clinics, and assistant director of the psychiatric consultation and liaison service at the University's School of Medicine, has been psychiatric consultant for the Lighthouse for the Blind in Chicago.

James Anderson, placement counselor for the Chicago Lighthouse for the Blind, has been a cotherapist with psychiatric consultants in group therapy.

_____ 21

The Use of Encounter Microlabs with a Group of Visually Handicapped Rehabilitation Clients
—HERBERT GOLDMAN, Ph.D.

THE present paper is an attempt to define, illustrate and clinically assess the use of a relatively new grouping of psychotherapeutic techniques with a select group of clients. Very few articles dealing with the use of group psychotherapeutic techniques as used with visually impaired clients have appeared in the literature.[1] The present article is therefore in large part an attempt to rectify the dearth of information presently available.

Table 1 describes the clients on which the material of the present article is based, and from it, the following is indicated: 1) there were five males and three females which provided for a fairly even distribution of the sexes; 2) The average age per client was 22 years; 3) Three of the clients were totally blind and five were partially sighted. This fortuitous grouping provided for maximal interaction of the differing visual impairment groups; 4) Five of the clients were in college, one was in vocational school, and two were in high school. The educational level of this particular group was, therefore, fairly high. This group of clients met at the Missouri Bureau for the Blind, St. Louis, for a total of 10 two-hour sessions. The average number of clients at each session was five, with a range extending from a minimum of three clients to a maximum of eight. The group was led by a clinical psychologist and two co-therapists.

Reprinted by permission of the *New Outlook for the Blind* 64 (7): 219–226, 1970, published by American Foundation for the Blind, Inc.

TABLE 1. *Description of Rehabilitation Clients by Sex,*
          Age, Degree of Visual Impairment, and Present Educational
          Status

Client	Sex	Age	Degree of Vision	Present Educational Status
1	M	18	TB	Special School District
2	M	20	TB	Public High School
3	M	23	PS	Junior College
4	M	22	TB	Junior College
5	M	28	PS	Junior College
6	F	20	PS	Secretarial School
7	F	21	PS	College
8	F	20	PS	College

TB = Totally Blind   PS = Partially Sighted

WHAT IS ENCOUNTER?

The word "encounter" itself is a relatively new concept in the field of psychology and is as yet only broadly and vaguely defined. For a more extensive discussion of the development and usage of encounter techniques, the reader is referred to an excellent article by Murphy[3] and a book by Schutz.[4]

For the purposes of this presentation, encounter is defined by the following set of statements: 1) Encounter is action. Verbal as well as non-verbal techniques are utilized; 2) Encounter deals with the whole person. Cognition, sensory awareness, and resultant interactions are dealt with; 3) Encounter is a blending of technique and philosophy; 4) Encounter encourages awareness. Self-awareness and other-awareness are repeatedly emphasized; 5) Encounter is invested with growth and self-realization.

Although encounter is, therefore, a multi-faceted concept, the foregoing definition has been derived from this author's own personal experience and other therapists may envision it somewhat differently. Furthermore, many of the elements in encounter are not new and have been utilized for many, many years in various aspects of psychological endeavor, for example, Gestalt therapy, client-centered therapy, existential psychology, psychodrama, sensitivity and training groups (T-Group), etc.

WHY ENCOUNTER FOR THE VISUALLY HANDICAPPED?

After working with visually handicapped school-aged clients for a number of years, this author has reached the conclusion that "talking" therapies, when used in isolation, are quite ineffectual in producing behavioral change. Because these individuals cannot, after all, directly experience or come into actual contact with the reality of many concepts that they use appropriately, it became apparent that such concepts are really quite meaningless to them. In addition, such individuals not only receive much so-called "second-hand" experience from sighted interpreters, but they are very often from overly protective environments that further deprive them of direct experience.

Since encounter is *"action"* therapy, the visually handicapped individual is encouraged to come into direct contact with the meanings of the concepts that he often uses. He is encouraged to feel real feelings, to feel others' real feelings (empathy), to become aware of his body and to become aware of others' bodies. In essence, the visually handicapped client is asked to focus on the sensory modalities available to him and, thereby, to really experience the meanings of many of his "second-hand" concepts first-hand.

THE ENCOUNTER MICROLAB

The procedure used by this author is called a microlab because of the shortness of the sessions and the element of experimentation involved. The prefix "micro-" refers to the two-hour session; encounter weekends and longer time periods are usually called workshops. The suffix "-lab" refers to the laboratory nature of the experience wherein new behaviors are experimented with. Incorporation or rejection of these new behaviors is often based on the feedback evidence gathered in the session.

The following discussion centers on the encounter techniques themselves which are based in large part on the work of Williams.[6] They are grouped under five separate headings primarily for explanatory purposes; in reality they are not mutually exclusive. Within each grouping, where possible hierarchies of involvement or threat (minimal to maximal) are to be inferred.

REDUCING INITIAL ANXIETY

TECHNIQUES USED FOR REDUCTION OF INITIAL ANXIETY

This particular group of techniques has as its primary objective the reduction of anxiety brought about by the novelty of the procedure and environment. The opening exercises often include:

Deep Breathing. In this exercise the client is told to lie down on the floor and to make himself as comfortable as possible. Pillows and blankets are helpful here. The client is then instructed to exhale as completely as possible and then to slowly inhale through the mouth, drawing air in evenly and without sudden jerks. The client is asked to pay particular attention to the feelings of bodily calmness and relaxation which ensue.

Progressive Relaxation. In this exercise the client is instructed to make himself as comfortable as possible and then told to alternately tense and relax various muscle groups starting with the feet and ending with the facial muscles. Attention in this procedure is focused on the difference in feeling between the act of tenseness and the act of relaxation.

Corpse Posture. Here the client is told to lie on the floor and to let go. Arms are stretched above the head with legs and feet also stretched out. Clients are told to allow their heads to roll to one side and their hands to flop to one side or where they will, and to imagine that their bodies have no bones. Suggestions that their bodies are sinking into the floor or that they are floating on a cloud have also been helpful.

INITIATION OF INTERACTION

The techniques used for having people meet each other, for the initial coming together, follow a hierarchy of minimal interaction to maximal interaction and often include the following:

Milling Exercises. Here the clients are asked to randomly mill around the room following a specified sequence. They are asked to mill non-verbally and without touching and finally verbally and touching. The clients are then asked to share their experiences regarding differences between touching versus not touching as well as the differences between verbal versus non-verbal interaction.

The Go-Around. In this encounter exercise each client is instructed to go around to every client, touch him, and make an "I feel" statement followed by either "I like it" or "I don't like it." This is a potent technique which brings individuals into direct, and often intimate, contact with each other. This is an especially relevant technique for the visually handicapped individual who must come to know much of his world through the sense of touch. Many of the clients were initially quite frightened and hesitant with regard to touching another human being, but most ultimately found this to be a very rewarding experience.

First Impressions. This exercise is usually placed at the end of the second. Each client is asked to give his first impressions of every other client including any modifications which may have been made over the session. This was a totally new experience for all of the clients as they had never before been in a situation in which they had been responded to with such directness and honesty.

TECHNIQUES USED FOR TRUST BUILDING

Before individuals can begin to share meaningful problems, frustrations, and conflicts, they must be able to trust those individuals with whom they are to share them. These encounter techniques, therefore, have as their primary goal the initiation of real trust. Some of the exercises in this category are:

Fall and Catch. Each client is asked to fold his arms, lock his knees, and to fall backwards into the arms of another person. Partially sighted clients and the therapists did most of the catching in this exercise while clients with detached retinas were excluded. Only one client was unable to trust anyone to catch him.

Lifting. In this exercise each client is asked to lie on the floor, to fold his arms on his stomach, and then to be lifted up from the ground by the other clients who are equally distributed on both sides of his body. Many clients noted the pleasantness of this experience and stated that a single mass appeared to be holding them in the air rather than a number of separate and distinct individuals.

The "Blind" Walk. In this technique clients are paired off with one individual designated as the "sighted" guide and the other as the "blind" person. Clients are assigned to these roles irrespective of the degree of vision which they actually have. The instructions tell the "sighted" guides to help their "blind" partners explore the environment as completely as possible including as great a variety of sensory experiences as possible. After 15 minutes, roles are reversed and another 15 minutes are spent in the exercises. This encounter procedure proved to be one of the most effective ones used. It was quite surprising to see a totally blind client with especially poor mobility become an excellent "sighted" guide. He later noted that never before had he been given the responsibility for another person's welfare; it was a real reversal of roles as far as he was concerned.

TECHNIQUES USED FOR PROBLEM ELICITATION AND WORKING THROUGH

These encounter techniques are really the culmination of all that goes on before; i.e., the techniques discussed this far have hopefully brought the clients to a level at which meaningful problems can be shared with the group and at which an environment to foster problem solution has been established. Illustrations of these procedures are:

Leveling and Feedback. This encounter procedure is broken down into a short lecturette and an exercise. The lecturette was found to be necessary with this particular group for which psychological jargon had little associative value. The lecturette ran as follows, "Leveling with a group is saying what you really think when you feel it should be expressed. Leveling is really a form of feedback in which people feel free to express their true thoughts without fear of punishment, ridicule, or rejection. In leveling, the aims are to help the other person by being honest and open with your impressions of him—that is, how he comes across to you. Leveling is a two-way process, for you should learn to level with others and at the same time become the type of person with whom others can level as well." In the demonstrative exercise, the clients are divided into pairs in which each client tries to give feedback that is as open and as honest as is tolerable for him. The entire exercise is then discussed in a group setting.

Lecturette on Honesty, Openness, and Directness.   The values and inherent difficulties in each of these three interpersonal constructs is elaborated upon and given meaning in all exercises in which the clients participate.

Lecturette on the Here and Now.   The importance of dealing with problems, feelings, people, etc., in the *here and now* as contrasted to the *there and then* is emphasized throughout all of these exercises. Many clients avoid dealing with problems by sticking to other places and other times.

Secret Pool.   Instructions given to the group are as follows, "This is a very serious exercise which deals with empathy. One at a time, I would like you to go over to the desk where Jan (a co-therapist) is sitting and tell her a secret which she will write down on a three-by-five card. This secret should be something that is very hard to share and it must be described in no more than two sentences. No person's name will be written on the card and each member will be given someone else's card with which to deal." After the co-therapist has written down the secrets, the cards are then passed out to the clients making sure that no client receives his own card. The instructions then continue. "If any of you can read the secret on the card then he should do it. If you cannot read the card, then Jan will come over and read it for you. After you read the card (or have it read), try to say how that person who has the secret must feel. Try to get inside of his skin and be as open, honest, and direct as possible. Each member of the group may now add his own feelings as regards this particular secret." Each participant then takes his turn in reading a secret. This is an extremely potent technique for problem presentation and feedback as the client may share an extremely meaningful problem and still remain anonymous. The client may add further dimension to his own secret by being anonymously empathetic when it is read.

Magic Shop.   In this procedure the clients are told that the therapist is going to pretend that he is the shopkeeper of a Magic Shop which has anything in it that anyone could possibly desire. Each client is then requested to interact with the therapist in terms of buying *anything* that he wants. This is an extremely useful projective device which allows the individual to share his most coveted desires and at the same time allows for an approximation of how much the client is willing to give for this wish. The shopkeeper may request any number of things for payment such as money, time, work, honesty, openness, etc. It was quite interesting to note *none* of the clients requested vision. One of the clients, during discussion, noted with surprise that other wishes and desires had now become more important to him than the return of his vision.

Sharing of Positive and Negative Feelings with Regard to the Self.   Clients are encouraged to share with the entire group elements of the self which they regard as positive as well as elements which they regard as negative. Feedback is then given to each client regarding his positive and negative qualities. This type of sharing provides catharsis and allows each client to evaluate the effect that this particular quality has on others.

Statement of Goals.   At the end of the first meeting clients are requested to bring a list of goals to the next meeting. This statement of goals gives the therapist some feeling for the direction of the group and allows the client to have a constant evaluation of himself with regard to the achievement of his stated goals.

GUIDED FANTASY TECHNIQUES

These techniques are really adjunctive to those just discussed, for they deal with conflicts, conflict resolution, goals, etc. Some of the fantasy techniques which have been utilized are:

Body Image Improvement.   In this encounter procedure clients are asked to stretch out and relax utilizing some of the relaxation procedures already mentioned. Clients are then given these instructions, "In fantasy, I would like you to enter your body in any way that you want. I'd like you to explore all of your internal body parts and to make special note of those parts which you liked best as well as those parts which you liked least. When you have done this (approximately five minutes), I'd like you to come out of your body and explore the outside of your body as completely as possible. I'd like you to again make special note of those parts liked the most and those parts liked the least. (Five minutes is allowed for this.) Now I would like you to return to those parts which you liked the least, internal as well as external, and correct them." This guided fantasy technique is again especially relevant for the visually impaired individual who has many conflicts regarding his body image.

Significant Others.   The therapist instructs the group as follows, "Fantasy four or five significant figures in your life— that is, persons who have had the greatest influence on you as a person. Fantasy them in a room; notice everything in the room. Notice what the people are wearing and how they look. They are talking about you; listen carefully to what is being said and how it makes you feel. Now you enter the room. You talk to each of the people and they respond to you. What do you say? What does each of them say to you? How are you feeling about them? What do you think they are feeling about you?" These fantasies are then shared with the group. The vividness, frankness, and spontaneity of many of the fantasies shared in this therapist's particular group were indeed astounding. Many of the clients registered astonishment at many of their own fantasy productions.

Future Projection.   In this fantasy technique clients are asked to imagine what they will be doing in 10, in 20, and in 30 years. This technique is especially useful in elucidating goal orientation.

CLINICAL IMPRESSIONS

Before the first meeting of the encounter group discussed in this paper, some effort was made to objectively assess the clients who were to enter the group; i.e., pre-test as well as post-test measures were planned. A rating scale instrument[2] was selected for this purpose and was used by the counselors to rate each of their clients in the areas of social competence, social interest, personal neatness, irritability, manifest psychosis, and retardation. Each of these six categories was defined by a selected set of statements. This rating scale proved to be non-discriminating in that many of the clients were rated high in the positive qualities and low in the negative qualities. This effect may have been due to a large number of factors, including social desirability factors, the chance that this was an above average group of visually impaired clients, or the high probability that the rating scale which was selected was inappropriate for this type of rehabilitation client. The discussion which follows is, therefore, based on clinical impression and is admittedly quite subjective.

AREAS OF GROWTH

One of the primary areas of growth which appeared during the group sessions was an increase in self-assertiveness and independence. Individuals who had long sat silent began to make their needs known not only to the rest of the group but also to the therapist and cotherapist. Various clients reported that they had been able to tell their parents and teachers many things that had been bothering them for a long time, things that they had not been able to say for fear of reprisal. The type of assertiveness exhibited appears to have been of the constructive variety, as these clients reported that their efforts had been positively reinforced.

INCREASED SELF-AWARENESS

Concomitant with the above changes was an increase in self-awareness and other-awareness (empathy). Some clients reported that they had allowed themselves to feel certain feelings which they had never allowed themselves to feel before because of the tremendous guilt which had thereby ensued. Individuals began to verbalize the feelings which they had for themselves, for other group members, and for significant others. This verbalization was carried on in a direct and straightforward manner which at times led to hurt feelings but these were in turn handled within the context of the group. Certain of the clients developed an amazing capacity for empathy and were really able to feel with another person.

Through these group sessions most of the clients developed their ability to give and to receive feedback in a direct, open, and honest fashion. This was an extremely difficult endeavor for all involved. Individuals began to tell other group members how they really "came off" to them, how these other group members really made them feel. No area was sacred. Feedback themes included dress, speech, sexual attractiveness, directness, etc. One client soon learned that his use of vulgar language was really only an attention-getting device and that it was extremely self-defeating. Another client was given feedback regarding his empty verbiage. Females in the group were given realistic feedback regarding their femininity while some of the males were made aware of their effeminate behaviors.

AN EXAMPLE OF CHANGE

One of the most outstanding examples of change involved a partially sighted, female client who was an attractive albino. When she first entered the group, she was extremely fearful and close to tears. During one of the early sessions the group was asked to reveal some body "hang-up" in order to receive feedback about this physical problem from other group members. This individual was totally unable to admit her albinism and dropped out of the group. Through the efforts of one particular male client, she was brought back to the group meetings. As she became more trusting, she began to relate many of her frustrations and, at a later session, announced that she had become engaged. She noted that previously she had never entertained the possibility of marriage because of her albinism, a fact which she had never been able to admit openly. She explained that, because of her group experience, she had been able to tell her suitor of her albinism. His response was, "Is that all that's wrong? I thought it was something really serious."

CONCLUSIONS

One feeling which almost all of the participants, but especially the partially sighted participants, seemed to share was of belonging to the group. The partially sighted clients had formerly felt that they were not really a part of the "sighted" world and not really a part of the "blind" world. These particular clients reacted quite favorably to being an integral part of a group that cared for and accepted them without regard to their visual acuity.

QUALITIES OF A GROUP LEADER

Being a member or a leader of an encounter group is definitely not something to be lightly undertaken. The factors to be considered before entering an encounter group have been amply described by Shostrom.[5] Some of the warnings to be observed by the therapist are: 1) be experienced; encounter techniques are powerful and can lead to serious, undesirable consequences unless properly handled; 2) exclude psychotics and borderline psychotics; 3) as a group therapist, always be available for resolving any conflicts left unresolved in the group; 4) as a group therapist, do not be afraid to tighten the reins on a group when a client is being unmercifully crucified; and, most of all, 5) be open, honest, and direct; you are, after all, the group model.

REFERENCES

Dr. Goldman is a clinical psychologist at the Jefferson Barracks Veterans Administration Hospital and a consultant to the Missouri Bureau for the Blind and the Missouri School for the Blind, all in St. Louis.

1. Cholden, Louis S. *A psychiatrist works with blindness,* New York: American Foundation for the Blind, 1958.
2. Honingfeld, G., and Klett, C. J. The nurses' observation scale for inpatient evaluation: A scale for measuring improvement in chronic schizophrenia, *Journal of Clinical Psychology* 21 (1965): 65–71.
3. Murphy, Michael. Esalen—where it's at, *Psychology Today* I (December, 1967): 34–39.
4. Schutz, W. C. *Joy: Expanding human awareness,* New York: Grove Press, 1967.
5. Shostrom, Everett L. Group Therapy: Let the buyer beware, *Psychology Today* 2 (May, 1969): 36–40.
6. Williams, R. L. *Manual on encounter techniques.* Unpublished manuscript, Jefferson Barracks Veterans Administration Hospital, 1968.

22

Some Observations on Group Therapy with the Blind —SOL HERMAN, M.D.

Loss of vision is a severe blow to the personality and is not easily overcome. Not only is the loss of sight a perceptual handicap, but the psychological meanings of blindness to those so afflicted wreak havoc with their ability to deal effectively with life. A certain cluster of symptoms and attitudes seems to develop which may appear unrelated to the patient's particular life experiences.

The author has had the opportunity of treating briefly, in group psychotherapy, two selected populations of blind patients. As the group process unfolded, certain features not usually prominent in other patient groups were observed. This brief report will endeavor to delineate those differences, offer some explanation of the dynamic roots, and describe some differences in technique in group psychotherapy with the blind.

Reprinted by permission of the American Group Psychotherapy Association from the *International Journal of Group Psychotherapy* 16 (3): 367–372, 1966.

SELECTION OF THE GROUP

Two groups, consisting of 8 members each, were seen once weekly for a total of 14 to 16 sessions. The patients were residents at a State Rehabilitation Center for the Blind where techniques of ordinary living were taught, such as the use of a cane in ambulation, self-feeding technique, the cooking and preparing of meals, etc. The group members were selected by the staff on the basis of the patients' inability to make use of the training center as evidenced by not learning techniques, not following directions, and exhibiting irritability and depression.

Five of the 16 patients were congenitally blind or had lost their vision before the age of one. Eleven of the patients were men, one of whom was a Negro. The patients' ages ranged from 18 to 74, with a mean age of 33 years. Their intellectual levels ranged from an I.Q. of 95 to that of 140.

CLINICAL OBSERVATIONS OF PSYCHODYNAMIC THEMES

In the course of treatment the group members appeared to focus on several specific areas. The remainder of this report will describe these dynamic themes and attempt to explain their occurrence.

DENIAL AND ITS EFFECTS

As is true of the reaction to most losses, a tendency to deny the injury was a common operant within each group. Denial of the fact of blindness, however, was but one small parameter of the patients' use of this mental mechanism as a defense. Not only did they tend to minimize their blindness, they also denied most internal feelings or thoughts related to being blind. They would not admit to envy toward those with intact vision, nor would they express anger related to frustration. There was even an avoidance of the use of the word "blind," and such euphemisms as "handicapped" or "lack of vision" were substituted. One patient reported that he had refused to use a cane walking in his home town because he did not want others to know that he was blind. In the therapy sessions, group cohesion occurred only after each member verbally acknowledged to the others that he could not see. Similarly, they had to acknowledge the permanency and severity of their blindness before they could begin to deal effectively with their limitations and their feelings. This confirms Cholden's (1958) observation that the patient must recognize and mourn his loss before he can progress.

DEPRESSION AND DESPAIR

Most group members described a similar kind of depressive response to being blind, though the response was colored by the individual's unique style of life. "A terrible blow"; "You aren't a whole person"; "I felt a moody depression"; "I had to learn to gradually reinvolve myself in life," were some of the statements of the patients. Very little irritation or resentment about their loss of vision was voiced by the patients.

THE DANGERS OF DEPENDENCY

It was with feelings related to dependency and low self-esteem that these people were constantly plagued. To be or not to be dependent was a constant question, even though all recognized, to some degree, their inability to care for themselves completely. An example was a bright, charming young woman who had diabetes mellitus and who could no longer see well enough to draw up the correct amount of insulin for her daily injection but could not accept with equanimity someone else doing it for her. Being self-sufficient had always been an important goal for her, and part of her despair over her blindness was related to this lost capacity to treat herself without help.

After the group had begun to come to grips with their need for being dependent upon others, fears of being vulnerable arose. Sighted people were spoken of as "untrustworthy." It was claimed, for example, that cab drivers were prone to give insufficient change and that people who attempted to lead the blind through traffic took their arms improperly. One member contended that if he let himself depend upon someone he would only be "left in the lurch in the end."

DEVALUATION OF THE SELF AND GUILT

While each group member experienced his loss of vision in a highly characteristic fashion predicated upon his own previous life experience and orientation to his environment, a common denominator was present in their devaluation of self and devastatingly low self-esteem. In both groups, this was highlighted by spontaneous verbalizations concerning "blind beggars," about whom they spoke with contempt and ridicule. In one group session, in the midst of a heated discussion about blind beggars, one patient turned to another and requested a cigarette. He was jokingly called a beggar by the others, and after a moment of anxious laughter, the group fell silent. The members then revealed that they considered themselves no better than blind beggars. They spoke about not being able to fathom why their sighted spouses still lived with them, and they questioned the motives of their instructors.

Exquisite sensitivity to the reactions of others toward their blindness was exhibited. A wish not to be seen, avoidance of social gatherings, and denial of poor vision were some of the themes elaborated. They deprecated their own assets and regarded themselves as being as immature and helpless as "seven-year-old children." One member described his refusal to wear tinted glasses to hide his severe nystagmus even though he knew it was disconcerting to others. The group members interpreted his behavior as an attempt to rationalize expected rejection for being blind. They indicated that he gave people an excuse not to like him for having eyes that twitched rather than eyes that did not see.

Hyper-religiosity, musings as to why God had inflicted blindness upon them, and expressions of having had insufficient "true faith" were elaborated as attempts to explain their affliction. To the group members, blindness was not only a handicap but a punishment for unknown or known sins, and they felt that they had no right to be angry about it. Misfortune was their accepted lot. Believing that they deserved their "fate," they resisted attempts by the rehabilitation staff to alleviate their distress.

THERAPEUTIC INTERACTION WITHIN THE GROUP

Because of the group members' blindness, it proved necessary to employ several techniques different from those used in treatment with sighted patients. Primarily, the departures had to do with communication. Because the patients were unable to register visual cues, the therapist had to be more active and use words where, with another group, he would customarily have smiled or nodded encouragement. This increased verbal communication hindered the rapid development of transference phenomena, but this did not prove a drawback since, in this brief therapy, transference phenomena tended to disrupt the group process, and the therapy progressed faster if transference was minimized. If there was silence on the part of the therapist, this led to resentment, which the members often expressed through metaphors about instructors disappointing them and strangers disliking them. Although this kind of ventilation was initially helpful, later it appeared to be utilized primarily as a defense against the members recognizing their feelings about the realistic problems of being blind.

Concerning the patients' ways of verbalizing, they spoke rapidly and often interrupted each other. While this would have a different interpretation in a sighted group, in a group of blind patients it appeared to have no significance beyond the fact that the patients could not see that a member was not finished talking or wanted to talk. Speaking while another person was talking was a device to let the others know that a member was ready to contribute verbally. The therapist himself found that it was necessary to interrupt when he wished to comment on or interpret the group interaction.

Interestingly enough, the blind patient often revealed in behavior feelings which went unverbalized in the group sessions, as if unaware that the therapist could see. For example, two members with mutual amorous feelings, which they avoided discussing openly, held hands in the group. When a member was irritated, it was often expressed by the act of trimming fingernails or punching out braille lessons.

With the exception of the above-noted differences, the therapeutic work with these blind patients was conducted along the same lines as with sighted people.

CONCLUSIONS

Reports from the rehabilitation instructors confirmed the patients' belief that group therapy was beneficial to them. From the patients' point of view, group therapy had the advantage of allowing them to develop a feeling of closeness through learning that they shared similar experiences, thoughts, and emotions, and the mere ventilation of feelings was a relief to them. Some patients expressed the thought that they had come to a crossroads in their lives which therapy had helped them to negotiate successfully; they now felt capable of making rational decisions about their future endeavors. Although at first, as the group members themselves stripped away the façade of cheerfulness from each other in terms of their loss, their depressions became more intense, these depressive reactions were generally much lightened by the time therapy was terminated.

SUMMARY

Experience in brief group psychotherapy with emotionally handicapped blind patients at a State Rehabilitation Center revealed common experiential and emotional blocks to the patients' ability to utilize rehabilitation training. Denial, depression, dependency conflicts, and low self-esteem were prominent themes. A core conflict was the unconscious equation of blindness and devaluation of self. The need for the therapist to be much more verbally active with blind patients than with sighted patients was noted.

REFERENCES

Dr. Herman is a Consultant in Psychiatry in the Mental Health Section, Region II, of the Mental Health Career Development Program at the National Institute of Mental Health.

Cholden, L.S. (1958), *A psychiatrist works with blindness.* New York: American Foundation for the Blind.

23

The Theragnostic Group in a Rehabilitation Center for Visually Handicapped Persons
—AL MANASTER

WHILE group psychotherapy is now in rather wide use in many areas and guises, it has traditionally been used as a long-term therapeutic process, usually with "mentally disturbed" patients. Its applicability for other than a "psychiatric" population in a "psychiatric" setting, however, has become much more evident of late, there being an ever widening variety of methods, goals, and techniques subsumed under the generic heading of "group process" or "psychotherapy." These methods of group interaction have been used with executives, teachers, psychologists, etc., through "sensitivity" training in "T" groups (as found in human relations labs)[1,5] and psychodrama to help work out "normal" problems;[9] in family groups;[2] and in action and play with adults,[8] the physically handicapped,[4] and geriatric populations in rehabilitation settings.[7] In many of these situations, the emphasis appears to be less on long-range, "depth" therapy or personality reorganization than on helping the participants work through some present stress situation. Also, the prime emphasis seems to be on working with the "normal" or basically healthy, integrated individual who is undergoing some form of existential crisis.

THE CONCEPT OF THE THERAGNOSTIC GROUP

In any such group, one of the major goals, of course, is that the interaction of the group and the therapist will be therapeutic, that it will effect a change in perception, a decrease in disabling anxiety with a concomitant increase in the participant's potentials and capacities for effective coping and interaction with the world, and an increase in reality testing. In any form of group interaction (regardless of the method used or the goals), there is a certain amount of projection—the group members "telling" of their strengths, weaknesses, and values. It would seem, therefore, that there are really two facets of any group psychotherapy setting—the therapeutic and the diagnostic or informational. What would seem to be a rather logical combination of these factors is to be found in the "theragnostic admission group" which was designed specifically to perform these two functions. Pratt and DeLauge describe it as follows:

> The "gnostic," that is the knowing or understanding function of these admis-

Reprinted by permission of the *New Outlook for the Blind* 65 (8): 261–264, 1971, published by American Foundation for the Blind, Inc.

sion groups is an integral part of the therapeutic process, and of the wider treatment program. This structure provides for the occurrence of interpersonal transactions that operationally result in several types of increased understanding to be optimally exploited.

These troubled people discuss their life situation, their problems, and each other in currently oriented ongoing process. . . .

Staff participants use this increased understanding in furthering the group process itself, but also use this knowledge of the patient as a person in relation to his involvement in other types of group therapy. . . .

We purposely stress the "gnostic" understanding, knowing about the person—his assets, problems, and style of life—as opposed to "diagnostic," per se. We want to exchange esoteric techniques, that serve only to reduce troubled people to *nothing but* their symptoms (label "disease entities") for transactional evaluative procedures that will present the person within a living context. . . .[6]

THERAGNOSTIC GROUPS AT IVHI

A few years ago, over an 11-month period, "theragnostic" groups were conducted at the Illinois Visually Handicapped Institute in Chicago, a state rehabilitation center for the legally blind. It was felt that as people came into the Institute for a one-week rehabilitation evaluation, they would find themselves in the rather stressful position of being tested, examined, investigated, looked at, diagnosed, and discussed by many staff members. They were not regular students or clients, were not in a regular program, did not belong, did not have any friends, and, in general, had been stripped of privacy and responsibility. Being in this sort of a situation, even for a short time, without having a chance to express their feelings (anger, anxiety, frustration, fear) and reactions to what was happening to them would intensify the reactions to visual disability that they were already probably experiencing. The clinical staff, therefore, felt that through the use of a time-limited, problem-oriented "theragnostic" group, many previously noted negative reactions of evaluees might be prevented or lessened by offering them a chance to handle their problems and reactions in what could be a relatively positive experience. It was hoped that evaluees who participated in such a group might also evidence a more positive response to the institution and to the training program that was to follow and be able to ". . . experience from the first that the expected, rewarded . . . role is *not* passive-receptive, but active, self-reliant, helping oneself and each other."[6]

Organizing the Groups

The program was initiated in September 1966, and continued through July 1967, at which time the whole evaluation procedure at the Institute was revised. Every second week during this period, the staff of the Institute would evaluate six individuals to determine their needs and skills in functioning as visually handicapped persons in the community. As a part of this week-long evaluation program, group sessions of approximately one hour each were scheduled for Tuesday, Wednesday, and Thursday. The two co-leaders for each group were drawn not only from the clinical services staff but also included members of the teaching staff who had been trained in group therapy techniques.[3] Several of the co-leaders were themselves visually handicapped which, at times, was helpful to the clients when discussing their feelings of helplessness and their reactions to blindness.

ATTENDANCE

The evaluees were informed on the first day of evaluation (Monday) that there would be group meetings in which they could air some of their feelings and reactions to the Institute and to their disability. Although attendance at the groups was not mandatory, the evaluees were strongly encouraged to attend. Most evaluees seemed to look forward to the sessions and to freely discussing what had happened to them during the day. Once admitted as students, many of these individuals would, in the regular, ongoing group counseling program, comment on things that happened during the theragnostic group sessions.

CONDUCTING GROUP SESSIONS

Using a relatively non-directive or group-centered approach, the co-leaders encouraged the expression and discussion of feelings. Although the sessions were just three in number, a definite process of development could be observed. In the first session, the evaluees would usually deal with their feelings about being at the Institute. The discussion would be rather superficial in nature with a lot of joking and kidding around and only a little discussion of actual problems and deeper feelings. They would mention some of the things that were happening in the evaluation and would touch upon the subject of stereotypes of blindness. It appeared that they were testing the situation. In the second session, their real problems and feelings would begin to emerge: their fears, anxieties, feelings of helplessness or anger, and their reactions to the institution and to the evaluation process. During this session, a great deal of corrective interaction often occurred, with staff or another evaluee correcting misperceptions and offering new ideas and ways of looking at the situation. In the third and final session, resolutions were sought for many of the problems that had been brought up, usually involving the realization that this is the way life is, that there are positive things that can be done, and that the Institute was one way in which they could work towards the future. They also learned that they were really not alone, but that there were others who shared their problems and who were concerned with them.

BENEFITS FOR THE CLIENTS

Throughout the sessions, the emphasis was on the "here and now" situation and the strengths of the client, his ability to handle situations, his having made the choice to enter the Institute for rehabilitation services, and the example of others who had achieved some success in their lives. At the same time, there was a realistic appraisal of the desire for a miracle and the hopes that somehow or other the person would be able to see again. With this marked increase in openness and honesty, anxiety concerning the training program was lessened, with a subsequent carryover to the regular rehabilitation program. The evaluees had an opportunity to see the staff as people who were interested in them as human beings, not merely as objects to be evaluated, diagnosed, and looked at as if they were under a microscope. The interactions between the evaluees and the staff in the sessions allowed for immediate awareness and the sharing and handling of problems that might otherwise have become quite disruptive to the individual's progress, not only during evaluation, but perhaps later in the program.

In general, this kind of extremely short term, highly intense, group process was useful for both therapeutic and diagnostic purposes. It enabled the clinical staff to observe the evaluees functioning in a situation less structured than the usual diagnostic and testing type of program. The sessions were tape recorded with the permission of the group members and after each session the co-therapists were able to discuss their interpretations and impressions. At the regular staff conferences, held at the end of the evaluation week, clinical services staff would give their impressions, obtained from observations during the theragnostic group sessions as well as the information received from more formal test procedures, to help the total staff in interpreting the client's needs and potentials and planning an individual program for him.

CONCLUSIONS

The theragnostic group process appears to afford marked therapeutic benefits to evaluees who are able to develop more positive feelings about themselves and others in relation to their disability, to the rehabilitation center, and to the future. The interactions offer many insights into personality dynamics and the potentials of the visually handicapped evaluee for successful participation in a total rehabilitation program. Most importantly, the evaluee is able to find himself as a human being who has a right to be himself and to be heard and who is not an object to be evaluated, diagnosed, put into a pigeonhole, and forgotten.

REFERENCES

Mr. Manaster is staff psychologist in the Chicago Area Office of the Illinois State Employment Service and visiting professor in the behavioral sciences, College of DuPage, Glen Ellyn, Illinois.

This article is based on a paper originally presented at the 12th Golden Gate Group Psychotherapy Conference held in San Francisco, June 1969.

The author wishes to acknowledge the contributions of Illinois Visually Handicapped Institute staff who collaborated in initiating the program described in this paper: Mrs. Robert Adams (formerly staff psychologist), Miss Dorothy Dykema (formerly rehabilitation counselor), Miss Alice Drell (director of education), Larry Ginensky (clinical director), and Fred Bixby (rehabilitative counselor).

1. Clark, J. V. and Clark, F. C. Notes on the conduct of married couples group, *Human Relations Training News* 12 (No. 3, 1968): 1–3.
2. Derman, S. and Manaster, A. Family counseling with relatives of aphasic patients at Schwab Rehabilitation Hospital, *American Speech and Hearing Association Journal* 9 (1967): 175–77.
3. Manaster, A.; Pillar, J.; Drell, A.; and Dykema, D. Training of 'non-clinical' professionals in group therapy techniques, *New Outlook for the Blind* 61 (1967): 16–20.
4. Mardis, G.; Manaster, A.; Bonnici, P.; and Pearson, L. Crisis group psychotherapy in a physical rehabilitation setting. A paper presented at the American Psychological Association, Chicago, September 7, 1965.
5. Mills, Robert B. Use of diagnostic small groups in police recruit selection and training. Mimeographed. Cincinnati: University of Cincinnati, Department of Psychology, n.d.
6. Pratt, S. and DeLauge, W. Theragnostic admissions groups: For the mental hospital, a psychotherapeutic treatment of choice, *Mental Hospitals* 14 (1963): 222–24.
7. Rustin, S. L. and Wolk, R. L. The use of specialized group psychotherapy techniques in a home for the aged. In *Group Psychotherapy,* vol. 16, edited by J. L. Moreno. Beacon, N.Y.: Beacon House, 1963.
8. Saltman, Marion. New adventures thru adult play. A paper presented at the American Association of Humanistic Psychology, San Francisco, August 28, 1968.
9. Starr, Adaline. Role playing: An efficient technique at a business conference, *Group Psychotherapy* 12 (1959): 166–68.

24

Para-Analytic Group Therapy with Adolescent Multi-Handicapped Blind
—CONSTANCE AVERY

THERE appears to be a paucity of literature on group psychotherapeutic practice with the blind and especially on group psychotherapy with the multi-handicapped blind. The only reference in the literature is Cholden's (1958) paper on group therapy with blind adults.[1] This is a gap that needs to be filled. Group psychotherapy can serve many purposes. The goals and methods of operation depend upon the ages of the populations that make up the groups, the types of problems the members of the groups encounter,

Reprinted by permission of the *New Outlook for the Blind* 68 (3): 65–72, 1968, published by American Foundation for the Blind, Inc.

their academic, social, emotional, and vocational limitations and prospects.

A Vehicle for General Interpersonal Interchange and Communication

At Oak Hill School, a residential school from kindergarten through high school, conducted by The Connecticut Institute for the Blind, group psychotherapy sessions have been conducted for two and a half years with groups of blind and multi-handicapped adolescent boys and girls. Group psychotherapy sessions were started to give adolescents an opportunity to ask questions about sexual matters that their parents or housemothers might have been reluctant to answer, and to express emotional difficulties in an atmosphere where their feelings could be reflected and interpreted. The sessions also aimed to provide a vehicle for general interpersonal interchange and communication among youngsters experiencing similar adjustment difficulties at the critical period of adolescence. The boys' group was conducted by a male therapist, the consulting psychiatrist. The girls' group met with the author for forty-minute sessions weekly, from September to the end of the school year in June—amounting to about sixty-eight sessions for two years. In the two years of working with the two different multi-handicapped groups of adolescent blind girls, many similarities were found among groups, but each of the group interactions took on a different form depending upon its configuration, the personalities of its members, the social judgment and sophistication of the participating members, and the nature of the problems that were uncovered. Slavson noted that in both group psychotherapy and in individual treatment individuation of approach and process is essential.[2] He felt the fusing of analytic group psychotherapy with guidance, counseling, advice, and "teaching," as indicated, is the cardinal principle of para-analytic group psychotherapy.[2]

THE ROLE OF THE THERAPIST

The therapist's role with these multi-handicapped groups of adolescent girls was a multifaceted one depending upon the needs of the individual group members and the direction the discussion itself took. Basically the therapist's role was analytical—reflecting the feelings of the group members, clarifying the reality aspects of their thinking and behavior, and interpreting their feelings and actions. There were, however, times when her role was more that of a counselor, proferring answers to questions on matters such as sex, reproduction, and child care. The therapist encouraged group discussion but, in the presence of imperfect or incomplete knowledge on factual matters concerning such subjects as sex and reproduction, she supplemented this information by supplying accurate factual information. However, she also reflected the emotional content behind the questioning. The therapist tried to keep the direct question and answer aspect of the sessions to a minimum, leaving the sessions more non-directive and less structured.

In the first therapy session conducted at Oak Hill the therapist led the group to establish some ground rules. It was suggested that whatever was discussed during the session be kept in confidence and confined to the group itself. The therapist said that the group meetings would be an opportunity for the girls to talk over any problems they had and to discuss personal difficulties. The girls seemed to relish the opportunity to talk about problems they had kept suppressed and contained within themselves.

DESCRIPTION OF FIRST GROUP

The first group had seven members who ranged in age from fourteen to nineteen. A description of a few of the members and the course of their participation and progress in the psychotherapy sessions follows.

"M" was eighteen years of age and had limited reading vision. She wore thick glasses and traveled independently. She was in the "special" class, which consists of those with a dull normal to mentally retarded intelligence along with some other psychological or neurological limitation that caused them to function subnormally academically. Besides blindness, "M" was handicapped by defective speech and neurotic and character problems, as diagnosed by the consulting psychiatrist. At home she was greatly overprotected and sheltered, and at school she appeared to have no close friends. She was cooperative, quiet in class, and a careful worker. She seemed to have made an adequate adjustment to the "special" class. At age thirteen she was in a state mental hospital for one month, but the diagnosis and progress of her illness were unknown as no records were transferred to the school due to denial of parental permission. Her parents made an unsuccessful attempt to readmit her to the hospital a short time after her discharge.

"J" was eighteen years old and had no useful vision. She had a current average intelligence, which had risen from a previous dull normal level. Her electroencephalogram was consistent with diffuse encephalopathy. She was considerably overweight and troubled by a moderate congenital deafness. Besides these handicaps, she had character problems partially resulting from an overprotective home environment. Her emotional tolerance was low so that her behavior was explosive, impulsive, distractible, irritable, and lacking in control. She had a short attention span, her general manner was negative, and she was a compulsive talker. She was in the "special" class because of her psychogenically and organically originated behavior problems. According to her teacher she could get things done when she had the desire. Her work habits were acceptable and she was a fluent reader with good comprehension.

"E" was fifteen years old and had no useful vision. Her I.Q. was average, having risen from the borderline range in nine years. She was excessively loquacious and engaged in rocking movements, eye poking, and rigid extension of her fingers. Her illusional material bordered on delusion and ideas of reference were prominent. Her grades were mainly fair and good.

PROCESS AND APPARENT OUTCOME OF
FIRST YEAR GROUP MEMBERS

"M" had been having difficulty with her speech, which was gradually improving under the aegis of the speech therapist. "M" was getting quite discouraged because of the limited progress she was making. She seemed heartened by the group's encouragement that changes were gradually taking place, even though she couldn't see dramatic differences. She "tightened up" and was not able to speak well when she became particularly anxious. It was not until the twelfth group session that she could reveal herself sufficiently to talk about personal things that were troubling her. She finally felt comfortable enough to express confidential family and emotional problems. Her usual method of coping was to keep her feelings within herself and not communicate them. This mode of operation was encouraged by explosive and volatile parents who were always ready to launch a verbal attack on her. She felt that a catharsis afforded by the group experience of talking about family problems enabled her to express herself more openly with them and express her discontent with the general pattern of operation. Having the opportunity to talk about the turmoil may have given her the chance to reorient her ideas and feeling and present a more direct front to family members.

"J" initially recited a list of grievances against certain boys and girls in school. She felt that the boys abused her. They tried to knock her down and made depreciatory remarks to her because of her obesity. She was also concerned because the boys touched her "in private areas." She exhibited a lot of zealous religiosity and preoccupation with getting into sexual difficulties and being injured by boys. She related stories of teenagers who had sex experiences, which she considered sinful, and "against moral and civil laws." During the sessions she interrupted with various irrelevancies and continued with her private monologue unless the therapist interrupted to give the other group members a chance to speak. She revealed problems with handling her own anger as well as being aggressed against and rejected by others. Of paramount concern were her troubles in the classroom with certain teachers. She liked to air grievances against her housemother, the school curricula, and the school menus. On occasion the group became annoyed with her over-exaggerated and emotional deliveries, and directly informed her to stop acting "so badly." The girls censured her intrusive behavior and reflected the inappropriateness of her nonsequiturs.

PROPER HANDLING OF AGGRESSION A COMMON PROBLEM

After a time "J" was able to see that the other girls also had problems with handling aggression. The group experience may have helped her to see that, because a particular mode of living was a way of life for her, it could not be imposed on the other members of the group, who had their own equally valid methods of conducting their lives. Her experience in group psychotherapy gave her an opportunity to see herself in the eyes of her peers, which might have contributed to or brought about changes in her attitude and manner. She appeared to gain some insight into her problems. Her behavior became more socially acceptable and her attitude more open and tolerant.

"E," in spite of her own suspiciousness, hostility, and cynicism, assumed the role of a co-therapist in clarifying reality, reflecting the feelings of other members of the group, and in validly interpreting the behavior of other members of the group. It was particularly "J's" feelings that "E" interpreted. When "J" became particularly irrational or constricted in her thinking, "E" clarified the other point of view. "E" reflected the differences among people and their varying ways of expressing their feelings. She emphasized the necessity for mutual respect of attitudes and feelings.

INABILITY TO ESTABLISH CLOSE FRIENDSHIPS

"E" showed flagrant paranoid attitudes about having her privacy invaded, where "welfare people" read her mail and watched her home. She was unable to establish close friendships with any of the girls or boys at school, but continuously persevered in her old relationship with one of the students who had left school several years before and whom she had not seen since and from whom she had received but one written communication. "E" would persist in telling people about this friend and in asking for definitions for words such as "fresh," which had been used to describe the girl. "E" used the mechanism of denial of hostility towards her family and repression of her own anger as primary defenses. She expressed fear of getting too close to people and held grudges against many classmates and staff. She felt she could trust no one. She exhibited a strong transference relationship to the therapist and tried to involve her in displays of affection towards one of the other girls. The therapist was treating "E" in individual psychotherapy sessions also, so that the problems she revealed in the group could be handled individually too.

DESCRIPTION OF SECOND GROUP

The second group had six members whose ages ranged from thirteen to seventeen. Some of these members and their experiences in the group are described below.

"A" was in eighth grade. She was fourteen years old and had no useful vision. Her I.Q. had remained consistently in the bright normal range and she had no additional handicap. She was independent, mentally capable, and alert, but exhibited tension by biting her fingernails. She got along well with the other students. Her grades were good and excellent.

"D" was sixteen years of age and had no useful vision. Her I.Q. had risen from the mentally defective to the dull normal range in three years. An abnormal electroencephalogram suggested brain damage. Her disorganized behavior was diagnosed by the psychiatrist as neurotic. She was very anxious and hyperactive, seemingly unable to sit quietly for any length of time, and revealed tension by twisting hands, rocking movements, and continuous talking in a hurried fashion. She seemed very fearful and defensive. Her fears were related to physical harm, being overwhelmed by circumstances, and the consequences of displeasing people. She was overly moralistic, impulsive, and distractible. Her marks were all good to fair.

"H" was seventeen years old. She had enough vision to read regular first grade print. Her I.Q. had increased from the borderline to the dull normal range in just four months since a recent short stay in a mental hospital, where she had been hospitalized as a result of active hallucinatory and uncontrolled wandering, screaming, and a suicidal attempt. At that time she showed inappropriate affect and appeared moderately depressed, with "emotional deterioration." She showed no insight or judgment and her sensorium was confused. Her illness was diagnosed as a possible acute schizophrenic reaction. At the time of her admission to school her anxiety revolved mainly around failing vision but she appeared to have appropriate affect, be well-oriented, and aware of her social situation. She was quiet and controlled in the group. The staff reported, however, that she was reluctant to approach people, but was courteous and well-disciplined in the classroom, accepting all classroom responsibilities willingly and cheerfully. She was in the "special" class because of dull normal intelligence and emotional difficulties, but in this placement she completed assignments and worked well independently.

PROCESS AND APPARENT OUTCOME OF SECOND YEAR GROUP MEMBERS

"A" took the role of a co-therapist in this group. She reflected and interpreted the feelings of the other girls and proffered counsel to them. "A" felt that many of the grievances of the group were petty and that the girls should overlook and transcend them, rather than getting caught up in them. "A" expressed the feeling that all of the members of the group were there to help each other. She expounded the philosophy of individual decision and action as long as the rights of others were respected and protected.

"D" was concerned with the "double binds" that her family put her in, where her mother told her to do something in a particular way but when she did, her mother would get angry at her for doing it in that fashion. In the sessions she related to specific individuals one at a time and interacted individually with the therapist, as "J" had done the previous year.

"D" had many complaints about people who annoyed her. The girls gave her various suggestions about ignoring the criticism of others or protecting herself by countercharging verbally. "D" revealed conflicts about wanting to please others as opposed to pleasing herself. Her overt desire was to please others, but covertly she resented compromising her own desires and needs. "D" also believed that parents shold keep tight limits on young people, indicating a fear of her own uncontrollable impulses. She revealed problems in heterosexual relationships, feeling she was a misfit in not being approached for dates. The group reflected "D's" feelings and proffered advice, while the therapist interpreted her underlying feelings and motives. She seemed to want the attention of authority figures at all times and appeared quite dependent upon her teacher, mother, and the therapist. In dreams she related, "D" revealed a lot of underlying aggressive feelings towards her mother, particularly during her recent pregnancy. Her dreams also revealed considerable hostility towards her father, while abundant aggression was turned against herself in dreams of self injury. Her underlying anger towards her parents and concomitant punishment of herself was interpreted to her by the therapist, which may have enabled her to understand the hostility she harbored against her family. "D" appeared to have gained some insight into her dependency, her hostility towards her parents, and her attempt to punish herself through interpretation of her dream material.

"H" added frequent comments by way of personal appraisal and interpretation of social situations. She revealed considerable awareness and social judgment. At the same time she received needed factual information on sex, reproduction, and birth, and corrected several misconceptions that she had been harboring. "H" seemed quite alert, interested, and responsive in spite of the schizophrenic episode she had suffered several months before. She turned out to be one of the more active contributors of information on interpersonal relationships and social behavior despite considerable naiveté.

GENERAL FINDINGS

The group sessions gave the girls an opportunity to discuss matters that could not be handled or referred to in the classroom, and an opportunity for emotional release and working through of personal problems. The members shared their experiences and feelings. The group situation provided an opportunity to engage in social interaction with contemporaries and to air problems in an atmosphere of peer acceptance. The participants appeared to have gained a greater social maturity and sophistication, possibly from the recognition that many of their problems were similar to those of other adolescents. Quite significantly, they seem to have learned that no problem was so serious that it could not be aired in the group.

What Topics Should Be Discussed?

At times there was some conflict as to what topics could be discussed. In the second group certain members wanted to discuss topics such as LSD and general drug usage, whereas the rest of the group felt that these were "not appropriate." The general feeling was that they should discuss subjects of common interest rather than "way out" topics of limited interest. The first group, however, was willing to accept all material as appropriate.

Their patience became frayed only when one member persistently brought up topics that revolved around her own zealous morality and religiosity.

The girls had the opportunity to talk about particular grievances, unleash vitriolic tirades, and air grudges and grievances against family, friends, and school. They were allowed to express their anger and may have gained some adequacy in controlling it by using socially acceptable means of expression. They may have also gained insight into the unreasonability of exaggerated aggression in the light of present family realities. One general problem that concerned most members of the groups was fear that they might not be able to control their behavior. Thus they were afraid of having too much freedom and seemed to need and appreciate the firm limits of home and school. They were also in conflict as to how far they should go along with family dictates and how much they should rely on their own judgment.

GENERAL DISCUSSION TOPICS

Some of the topics brought up for discussion were boy-girl relationships, dating habits, emotional reactions of men and women, marriage, mixed-marriage, menstruation, sex, reproduction, pregnancy, labor, birth, prematurity, baby care, and death. Other topics included physical and mental illness, medical examinations, sibling rivalry, camp problems. It was suggested that in the future a discussion group be held with boys and girls together.

AREAS OF RESISTANCE

Resistance periodically came up within the group. The girls became reluctant to probe personal areas of difficulty and were silent and uncommunicative. After long periods of silence, the therapist offered topics of conversation revolving around suppresssed feelings of fear and anger. This elicited new material for discussion and opened up a renewed stream of conversational exchange and emotional ventilation. Once a topic of conversation such as family or school problems was broached by one of the girls, the rest of the group members picked it up and expressed their own feelings on that subject. The general conversation became more spontaneous and active and they talked more freely about personal difficulties.

CONFIDENTIALITY

One of the members of the second group did not respect the confidentiality of the group, and the others refused to bring out more personal material. To insure future confidentiality the group members themselves decided to censure the informer, by keeping her out of the sessions for a two-week period. This may have contributed to the maturity of the offending member when she learned to respect the limits of the group.

PROBLEMS CONCERNING BLINDNESS

Some of the general group discussion revolved around the specific problems of blindness. The girls were very concerned about the difficulties they would encounter as blind mothers in caring for their children. The group sessions afforded them an opportunity to express their trepidation and exchange their views on child care. There were many discussions revolving around blindness itself—how people got blind, what types of diseases or trauma caused blindness, and the mannerisms of the blind. They exchanged ideas and were allowed to channel feelings on mobility for the blind, and dog guides versus cane travel. There were emotional discussions on marriage to a blind man versus marriage to a sighted man. The girls were anxious to discuss how a sighted person could recognize a blind individual. They resented the pity of sighted people and their implicit rejection in considering the blind so different from themselves.

The girls felt they were disallowed from performing duties around the house that they could handle adequately. They wanted to help with cooking, cleaning, and ironing but felt their mothers either were too busy to teach them or were too fearful of the assumed hazards of allowing blind girls to participate, even though their daughters had received training in the domestic arts at school.

RELATIONS WITH SIGHTED POPULATION

The girls harbored strong resentments against people doing things for them. They felt that the sighted population outside school did not recognize their capabilities in tasks of motor coordination, dexterity, and mobility. Sighted people outside of the school milieu did not seem aware of the efficiency and skill of the blind in domestic work, certain sports, industrial arts, shop work, handcrafts, and academic studies. On the other hand, they felt that sighted people had an exaggerated view of their capabilities in other spheres, such as speed of movement, spatial conceptualization, and proficiency in self-care habits such as dressing and eating. In these areas it was difficult for them to measure up to a sighted person's expectations. They felt that sighted people didn't give them the opportunity to show what they could do, before it was assumed they could not do it.

The girls felt their families also needed a reorientation of their general attitudes and level of expectations for their blind children. Parents, they believed, were lacking in knowledge of what their blind children could do and unaware of their full capabilities. On the other hand they either pressed them to attempt more than they could handle or were intolerant when they could not participate in certain activities or measure up to levels of expectation set for the sighted. Families appeared to them to be particularly intolerant towards those children who also had neurological, intellectual, and psychological handicaps superimposed on their blindness. The resultant

problems appeared to the students to have stemmed from emotional prejudice and lack of information that caused the sighted to disallow the multi-
handicapped blind most of their remaining assets and capabilities.

REFERENCES

Mrs. Avery is a school psychologist for The Connecticut Institute for the Blind
in Hartford.

1. Cholden, L. S.: *A psychiatrist works with blindness.* American Foundation for
the Blind, New York, 1958.
2. Slavson, S. R.: Para-analytic group psychotherapy: A treatment of choice for
adolescents. *Psychotherapy Psychosomatics,* 13, 321–331, 1965.

25

Adaptation to Visual Handicap: Short-Term Group Approach
—DAVID L. KEEGAN, M.D.

INTRODUCTION

O UR present day society has an epidemic of people living with various
physical disabilities and this will continue to accelerate as our ability
to deal with life-threatening illness improves. Justifiably there is an increased interest both from medicine and government in developing better
techniques of understanding and helping people with resultant social and
psychological morbidity. Visual handicap may be looked upon as a
prototype for understanding other physical handicaps which cause multiple
major life crises and may lead to tremendous psychosocial distress and disability. The scant literature on this subject gives support to the premise that
blindness leads to significant psychosocial stress.[1,2] The reaction to loss
paradigm as a means of understanding the functional changes of visual
handicap and adjustment to it has been best discussed by Carroll, and more
recently evaluated by Fitzgerald.[3,4] Although this theoretical framework
has been criticized by some and modified by others, we have found it a
useful way of approaching people with blindness and other physical
disabilities.[5,6]

We will describe a form of short-term group therapy as a possible way
of helping the visually handicapped to understand and cope better with this
crisis and decrease damaging psychosocial sequelae.

Reprinted courtesy of *Psychosomatics* 15 (2): 76–78, 1974.

BACKGROUND

The group members were adventitiously blind adults ranging in age from twenty to fifty-five and entered the groups during their sixteen week stay in a rehabilitation center. The groups, on an average, were composed of some twelve members and were carried out on a twice-a-week basis of approximately an hour and fifteen minutes duration. The degree of visual handicap, adjustment to blindness and backgrounds of the clients varied significantly. The rehabilitation center was well known throughout the United States for its ability to handle psychological problems and thus a number of the clients who were referred there for rehabilitation training had significant disturbance including severe depression, past suicidal attempts, schizophrenia, and serious personality disorders.

GOALS AND APPROACH

The primary goal of the group was to assist members in developing a realistic understanding of functional losses suffered through visual handicap, common personal reaction patterns to these losses, and realistic rehabilitation plans. Through this process it was hoped that painful feelings would be ventilated, concerns about visual handicap expressed, and support offered by group members. The final goal was an attempt to free up emotional energy which seemed so much restricted by hostility, sadness, and anxiety so as to facilitate the rehabilitation process. The approach utilized was a short-term group dynamic with a didactic focus in which the leader would offer specific topics for discussion at the outset of each session so as to add some initial structure to the group. The topics rather loosely followed the loss prototype and the rehabilitation of these losses as discussed by Carroll in his book. It should be mentioned that although initial structure was attempted, most groups were generally quite free-wheeling discussions of many topics.

DYNAMICS AND PROCESS

The group developed a cohesiveness beyond that expected because of the trainees common residence in the rehabilitation center for the sixteen weeks of the program. This fact, along with the somewhat non-voluntary aspect of the group, produced an initial tremendous group hostility which was particularly focused on the intrusive sighted psychiatrist who was the group leader. Much of the early focus was on who is the leader, what is he all about, who sent him, and do they think we are all crazy? The common early distrust of the leader which occurs in most groups was exaggerated by tremendous visual fantasies about him, in which he might have looked like the devil himself. This early anxiety and hostility showed up in some subtle and other not so subtle comments. They spoke about how they personally had been let down by many people in their lives and how some people in the rehabilitation center were considering them emotionally sick and unstable by having them come to group sessions.

Mr. M.—"I think a person has to be blind to understand what a blind person goes through."

Miss C.—"It would surely help."

Mr. M.—"I knew of a psychiatrist who was blind and still worked."

Dr. K.—"I am a sighted psychiatrist. It certainly sounds as though many of the members of the group are worried about who I am and what I am up to and how difficult it is to be understood and to get understanding."

Mr. P.—"Just because we are blind, why do they think we are crazy."

There was early concern about confidentiality, a common development in most groups, but I think this issue took on even greater meaning because of the visual handicap and the members' inability to see the meeting room, the leader, the recorder, and other group members. A very real "who is watching us" syndrome took on neurotic reality for the members. The issue of the leader's relationship to the rehabilitation center's authority became an early focus as well. They needed the leader to assuage their anxieties about what information was confidential and whether they could attack the administration. Certainly, their hostility towards physicians, sighted people, family members could all be welded in a focus towards the authority of administration and particularly the group leader. The interpretation by the leader that the group's hostility and resentment might relate to discouragement about their handicap was broached and not surprisingly rebuffed, particularly in the early group sessions.

Dr. K.—"I wonder if some of the resentment towards each other, the center, and myself may really be discouragement and upset about your visual handicap."

Mr. B.—"My ophthalmologist ruined my one eye and then was ready to tackle the other, so I didn't let him."

Mrs. S.—"I am particularly resentful of my situation but it seems my family should be more involved, they don't seem to be interested in me anymore."

Mr. M.—"I get a lot of help from my wife, so I can't complain."

As the sessions progressed, discussion of losses and depression was encouraged but was often well defended and denied by members. However, some of those who were willing to deal with this affect received support through ventilation and encouragement from other group members. It was more common to verbalize the rehabilitative, optimistic, hopeful side than the losses, anxiety, and sadness which seemed evident to the leader.

Mr. D.—"You have been reading too much of Father Carroll's book on blindness and the death of the sighted man."

Mr. P.—"I don't feel anyone thinks they die when they are blind. I think this place has a morbid outlook."

Miss C.—"I think talking about this is good but I am not depressed and I don't think too many of us are."

Mr. P.—"The way the staff talks, it seems as though they want us all to be depressed about blindness."

Mr. D.—"It makes me feel that way as well."

The resistance and denial seemed necessary and isn't necessarily unhealthy when one considers rehabilitation as a positive ego-coping process to diminish the anxiety and depression of blindness. However, there were some magical and unrealistic expectations which were used as defenses to deal with these problems and thus much discussion evolved around the "IDEAL" blind person and the very successful blind musician, artist or professional person. These people were held up as a torch in the night and interestingly this fantasy wasn't attacked by any of the members as being unrealistic or an impossible expectation.

As termination approached, an obvious bond had arisen between members and much more support in the group was obvious. During this period denial was less, although still prevalent, and the focus was much more on the reality of rehabilitation rather than on the magical hopes. As the denial diminished and some painful affects came to the fore, some members missed sessions and a couple stopped coming entirely. The increase and openness of responses allowed more opportunity to look at the reaction of the blind person to their family, thus letting members compare reactions of their family with those of other group members. This termination phase allowed a better connection to be made between loss and separation from the group and loss of function from blindness and sadness and frustration which results.

THE LEADER

The leader had to handle the strong tendency to identify with the blind group members. This led to unrealistic withholding of interpretations, and defensiveness of the group's hostility. There was an allowance of destructive hostility initially, because it seemed to the leader that these people had the right to be hostile considering how they had been damaged through blindness. It was recognized that a care-giver may feel unrealistic pity for the members by identification with the loss of vision in himself. The leader gradually realized how unrealistic some of the hostile accusations were and how they were to a large extent projections of the extreme resentment to visual handicap by the members, and he as well as the members, had to try and understand this. It was a tremendous learning experience which the leader doesn't think would necessarily be forthcoming through leading a group of people with major psychological impairments alone.

DISCUSSION

Short-term group therapy has been used to understand diverse problems including dealing with the feelings about physical disability.[7] The variety of approaches have ranged from a rather psychoanalytic non-directive therapy to very active oriented approaches. Three other authors have reported group sessions used in blind rehabilitation, including a supportive duo-therapist type and interesting Gestalt Encounter therapy program.[8-10] Each of these reports were experiential and reported success and helpfulness to most members. I would have to say that our therapy, although helpful, could not be as optimistic as this.

It is quite obvious that a non-directive silent regression inducing technique should not be used in this setting since it is too threatening for the members and leads to significant anxiety and hostility, particularly in the early sessions. The pain of over-interpretation of feelings that people were trying to deny was also too much for some members, and even the didactic approach of discussing losses became disturbing to others. An active, fairly verbal, practical approach is needed and yet forcing a didactic approach, although adding structure and possibly decreasing anxiety, may lead to an intrusion on the part of the leader which is out of step with the group members. Certainly in our work, the pushing of discussion of losses on a number of the members I think led to a defensiveness which handicapped the openness of the group and prevented growth until quite late in the program. In groups such as this it is also important to remember that the physical focus, although threatening, tends still to be more comfortable than being considered as having a psychiatric problem or mental abnormality. In a group such as this, superficial issues must be dealt with and the deeper issues of anxiety, loss, and hostility can only be dealt with when the group is ready. The use of denial in people with blindness is evident, as has been found in people coping with any physical disorder. Denial, optimism, and hope are certainly needed to deal with a crisis such as blindness.

We found the group approach to have some positive advantages. Firstly, a small staff can be much better utilized in seeing more people. We found in people with blindness, and certainly this could be extended to people with other physical disabilities, the group dynamic allows confrontation and support by people with a similar handicap. The resistances found in individual therapy such as "I am too sick to talk" are minimized through dealing with people with similar problems. The "lonely ill" position, is decreased by group support. This is especially true when members are brought together in a rehabilitation center or hospital and a common problem and relationship allows bonds to form, and on the other hand allows discussion of significant relationship problems which can be observed in the arena of the group.[11, 12]

Group therapy of this short duration and low intensity has been questioned. Many members, however, found it to be a positive growing experience, some found it of little help, and others were quite negative and rejected the approach entirely. The members who took a negative approach, however, were taken into individual sessions to hopefully deal with any negative ramifications the group may have had. Most of the members felt important issues were looked at, some very personal, in a climate of acceptance and support. These painful reactions to blindness were seeen as natural processes of crisis adjustment and were not seen as necessarily abnormal. This allowed the trainees to better understand themselves, the program, and their family members. It would certainly seem that these verbal group techniques with support and catharsis are a useful way of decreasing the loneliness and pain of adjusting to visual handicap, and would certainly be recommended for dealing with adjustment to other physical handicaps as well.

SUMMARY

Short-term group therapy has been presented as an approach to adjustment during the very significant life crisis and the rehabilitation process of blindness. The group process, leader's reaction and certain suggestions to modify the group approach in this group of people are presented. During this time of increasing physical and psychosocial morbidity it is important to develop alternatives to handle crisis situations so that adequate solving and coping of these situations may occur. Group therapy in blindness is presented as a prototype for group therapy in other physicial disabilities.

REFERENCES

Dr. Keegan is from the Department of Psychiatry at the University of Saskatchewan, in Saskatoon, Saskatchewan. At the time of the reported work, Dr. Keegan was Fellow at the Harvard Medical School, an Assistant in Medicine (Psychiatry) at Peter Bent Brigham Hospital, Boston, Ma. and a Psychiatric Consultant for the Catholic Guild for the Blind in Newton, Ma.

The author would like to acknowledge the great assistance given him by the late Father Thomas Carroll and Dr. Thomas Gaulfield.

1. Blank, H. Robert, M.D.: Psychoanalysis and blindness, *Psychoanal. Quart.* 26:1–24, 1957.
2. Cholden, L., M.D.: Some psychiatric problems in the rehabilitation of the blind; *Bull Menninger Clinic.* 18:107–112, 1954.
3. Carroll, Father Thomas: *Blindness, what it is, what it does and how to live with it.* Boston, Little Brown and Co., 1961.
4. Fitzgerald, Roy G., M.D.: Reactions to blindness, an exploratory study of adults with recent loss of sight, *Arch. Gen. Psychiat.* 370–79, Vol. 22, April, 1970.
5. Foulkes, E., Ph.D.: The personality of the blind; A non-valid concept; *New Outlook for the Blind,* Feb., 1972.
6. Holmes, Thomas; Rahe, Richard: The social readjustment rating scale, *J. Psychosom. Res.* Vol. II, 213–218, 1967.
7. Wolf, Alexander: *Short term group psychotherapy:* Ch. VII: Short term psychotherapy, Lewis Wolberg, Ed. Grune and Stratton, New York, 1967.

8. Goldman, H., Ph.D.: The use of encounter microlabs with a group of visually handicapped rehabilitation clients, *New Outlook for the Blind,* Sept., 1970.
9. Kubler-Ross, E.; Anderson, J. R.: Psychotherapy with the least expected: Modified group therapy with blind clients, *Rehab. Lit.* 29:73, 1968.
10. Wilson, E. L.: Group therapy in a rehabilitation program (Blind Clients of N.Y. Assoc. for the Blind), *New Outlook for the Blind,* Sept., 1970.
11. Miles, B.: Social therapy for the elderly blind, *Nursing Times,* 3 March, 1967.
12. Riffenburgh, Ralph S., M.D.: The blind patient, *Arch. Opthal.* 361, Vol. 79, April, 1968.

26

An Evaluation of Personal Achievement Skills Training with the Visually Handicapped —RICHARD T. ROESSLER

To meet a need for personal-adjustment training programs for the visually handicapped, Personal Achievement Skills (PAS) training (Means & Roessler 1976; Roessler & Means 1976a,b, 1977) was adapted to verbal and braille modes of presentation through a series of pilot studies at the Criss Cole Rehabilitation Center for the Blind (Austin, Tex.) and Arkansas Enterprises for the Blind (Little Rock). An evaluation of the program's contribution to personal adjustment was then conducted at Arkansas Enterprises for the Blind.

The PAS program is a motivation and skill-building program in the area of personal adjustment (Roessler, Cook & Lillard 1977; Roessler, Means & Cook 1977). In a four-phase model focusing on group cohesion, self-exploration, self-understanding, and constructive action (Carkhuff 1969), the program teaches communication, value clarification, problem solving, and self-modification skills in a group-counseling setting. Participants in PAS groups are involved in a series of exercises and activities that enable them to become more open, to develop improved communication skills, to identify priorities and select goals, to develop systematic programs for achievement of goals, and to monitor progress toward personal goals.

The PAS program has merit for personal-adjustment training with the visually handicapped because it closely parallels a psychological understanding of coping with severe disability. For example, Adams and Lindemann (1974) emphasized that adjustment to disability requires clients no longer to see themselves as sick but rather to view themselves as different. Awareness of difference must be in terms of new needs and goals rather than a sense of being isolated or worthless.

Reprinted from the *Rehabilitation Counseling Bulletin* 21 (4): 300–305, 1978. © 1978 by American Personnel and Guidance Association. Reprinted with permission from the publisher and author.

Clients must also orient themselves in a hopeful way to the future, an attitude that several authors have discussed in terms of the development of appropriate goals (Kemp & Vash 1971; Shontz 1975). For example, one study comparing blind and sighted adolescents found no significant differences between the two groups except on the question, How do you feel about the future? Among blind clients, there was a great deal more uncertainty and concern about the meaning of the future (Bauman & Yoder 1968). Because the PAS program stresses decision making, goal identification, and program development, it may contribute to the development of a positive outlook on the future.

METHODOLOGY

PARTICIPANTS

Thirty-four clients enrolled in the personal-adjustment program at the Arkansas Enterprises for the Blind were involved in the study. Because all clients in the personal-adjustment program participate in some form of group counseling, they were randomly assigned to either of two PAS groups or to other group-counseling experiences. Of those students meeting criteria for the study (IQ > 70 and projected 12-week enrollment), 16 were in the experimental group (8 in each PAS group), and 18 were in the control group. Clients participating in the study were males (56%), females (44%), young (average age of 29), single (56%), and white (82%), with an average of 12 years of education.

INSTRUMENTS

Cantril's self-anchoring striving scale (Cantril 1965; Kilpatrick & Cantril 1960) gathers subjective, self-report responses regarding best and worst possible life on an 11-point scale. These estimates are relative to a 10-year span of past, present, and future. Life-perspective measures, such as the self-anchoring striving scale, are reported to have test-retest reliability coefficients ranging from .43 to .70 (Robinson & Shaver 1969). All students completed the striving scale as a pre- and post-test measure.

The Rotter (1966) internal-external locus-of-control scale was administered to determine whether participants perceived themselves in control of their lives. Administered before and after the training, the Rotter scale indicates whether individuals attribute changes in their lives to luck, fate, powerful others, or to their own efforts. College students' scores on the scale range from 10 to 14.

To measure self-worth, Rosenberg's (1965) self-esteem scale was administered before and after training. Test-retest reliability for the scale was .85 for a group of college students tested after 2 weeks (Robinson & Shaver 1969).

Goal-attainment scaling (Kiresuk & Sherman 1968) was used to evaluate the impact of PAS training. Clients in experimental groups selected a personal-adjustment goal and developed five outcome levels (worst to best possible) to be used to estimate progress in goal attainment.

Through a counseling interview, clients in the control groups selected from a predetermined list a goal to be accomplished during the next 10 weeks. After developing a goal-attainment scale, these clients indicated their level of goal attainment at pretesting. Without reference to their pretest level of attainment, control clients provided a posttest estimate of goal attainment using the same set of attainment levels.

Research in mental-health settings (Jones & Garwick 1973) has shown the reliability of the goal-attainment scaling procedure to range from .70 to .75. Evidence exists to suggest that goal-attainment scaling is a valid measure of client change as a result of rehabilitation services (Goodyear & Bitter 1974).

PROCEDURE

In addition to daily-living-skills training at Arkansas Enterprises for the Blind, all clients in the study participated in some form of group counseling that tended to equate factors such as grouping, special attention, and counseling assistance between experimental and control groups. For 10 weeks, control participants were involved in group counseling 45 minutes a day for 2 days a week. Experimental clients were involved in PAS training 90 minutes a day for 3 days a week for 10 weeks. Each group was led by a counselor trained in PAS; other members of the counseling staff conducted group counseling focusing on personal feelings and adjustment to disability for the control clients. Statistical analyses of the data included tests of proportions and analysis of covariance.

RESULTS

Results are presented in terms of a pretest profile of visually handicapped clients and a posttest comparison of significant outcome variables, for example, goal attainment, life perspective, internal-external control, and self-esteem.

PRETEST PROFILE

Both groups began at low levels of goal attainment, that is, at approximately worst-possible to less-than-expected outcomes. Indicating that they were moving toward their best possible life, both groups reported an optimistic life perspective. Although the experimental group reported a higher rating of the present, both groups reported high ratings of the future. In fact, life-outlook ratings tended to be higher for this group of visually handicapped clients than for a younger group of clients in work adjustment at a comprehensive rehabilitation center (Roessler & Boone 1977).

Interestingly enough, both groups reported a strong internal-control orientation toward life; they felt that they, rather than fate or luck, controlled their lives. Finally, self-esteem scores in both groups were slightly above the midrange score, which indicates a positive valuing of self.

POSTTEST COMPARISONS

Goal Attainment.   Based on post-minus pretest rating scores on the goal-attainment scale, clients in the experimental and control groups were divided into no gain–low gain (one-step gain or less) or high-gain (two-step gain or more) groups. In the experimental group, 10 (71%) were in the no gain–low gain group and 4 (29%) in the high-gain group. All control-group clients were in the no gain–low gain group. The statistical test comparing these proportions was significant at the .06 level. Hence, a trend developed for more high gainers to be in PAS.

Life Perspective.   Analyses of the proportions of experimental and control clients in change or no-change categories on life perspective revealed no differences between groups. For example, 7 of 14 experimental clients rated now more positively at the end of the study, whereas 8 of 14 control clients did so. Similarly, no difference appeared in proportions of clients reporting a more positive view of the future. In both groups, 6 of 14 rated future as closer to best-possible life at the end of the study. High ratings given to future by both groups and to now by the experimental group lessened the possibility for upward movement of ratings. Examination of sample proportions indicated a trend for past to be reevaluated somewhat by the two groups but in different directions. For example, past was rated higher at posttesting by the control clients and lower by the experimental clients.

Internal-external Control and Self-esteem.   Using a one-way analysis of covariance with the pretest as a covariate, changes on internal-external control (Rotter 1966) and self-esteem (Rosenberg 1965) were examined (Huck & McLean 1975). Adjusted posttest means are reported in Table 1. Although internal-external control perceptions were not affected by participation in PAS, self-esteem increased significantly for the experimental clients.

DISCUSSION

Experimental clients tended to report a somewhat higher level of goal attainment than did control clients. Several clients in both groups reported some degree of goal attainment, however, which may be indicative of the

TABLE 1.   *Comparison of Adjusted Posttest Means
Internal-External Control and Self-Esteem*

Measure	Experimental (n=14)	Control (n=14)	F	df	Probability
Internal-external	8.00	7.85	.02	1,25	ns
Self-esteem	31.18	28.18	9.96	1,25	.004

fact that all clients were involved in group counseling during the course of their study. Although we might have expected a greater divergence between experimental and control groups on goal attainment, the results are in the predicted direction.

Unlike results of a previous study on PAS (Roessler, Cook & Lillard 1977), life-perspective changes were not found in this study. Clients reported an exceptionally optimistic view of the present and future (Roessler & Boone 1977), which might be related to the skills they are acquiring in personal adjustment, mobility, and daily-living training at the center. In terms of past ratings, the most that can be said is that the control group seemed to say by posttesting, The past wasn't really as bad as we thought, and the experimental group, On second thought, the past was actually worse than we first rated it.

Since both groups reported a definite internal locus-of-control at the beginning of the study, it was probable that they would not change much on the scale of beliefs (Rotter 1966) during the course of the training. Pre- and postratings indicated that both groups believed that they, rather than fate or chance, controlled events in their lives.

Earlier theoretical statements regarding PAS's potential to improve the self-image of visually handicapped clients were supported in the data. Myriad factors may have contributed to the enhancement of self-esteem for experimental clients, for example, the positive aspects of group support and cohesion, the learning of new functional skills, and the greater acceptance of self and disability gained through sharing and feedback in the PAS group.

When contrasted with the other modes of group counseling for the visually handicapped, PAS contributed to increases in goal attainment and self-esteem. The value of the other group models was also apparent, however, in that control clients reported some goal attainment and comparable changes in life perspective. Overall, the fact that PAS clients had as good or better outcomes as other clients was extremely significant in that PAS is a structured, easily learned, and easily replicated approach to group counseling with visually handicapped rehabilitation clients.

REFERENCES

Richard Roessler is an Associate Professor of Rehabilitation Education at the Arkansas Rehabilitation Research and Training Center, University of Arkansas, Fayetteville.

The support and expertise of the administrative and counseling staff members of the Arkansas Enterprises for the Blind (Little Rock) and the Criss Cole Rehabilitation Center for the Blind (Austin, Tex.) were essential to the completion of the study. The research was supported in part by a grant (16–P–56812,RT–13) from the Rehabilitation Services Administration, Office of Human Development, U.S. Department of Health, Education and Welfare.

Adams, J., and Lindemann, E. Coping with long term disability. In G. Coelho, D.

Hamburg, and J. Adams (Eds.), *Coping and adaptation.* New York: Basic Books, 1974. Pp. 127–138.

Bauman, M., and Yoder, N. *Adjustment to blindness reviewed.* Springfield, Ill.: Charles C. Thomas, 1968.

Cantril, H. *The pattern of human concerns.* New Brunswick, N.J.: Rutgers University, 1965.

Carkhuff, R. *Helping and human relations* (Vol. II). New York: Holt, Rinehart & Winston, 1969.

Goodyear, D., and Bitter, J. Goal attainment scaling as a program evaluation measure in rehabilitation. *Journal of Applied Rehabilitation Counseling,* 1974, 5, 19–26.

Huck, S., and McLean, R. Using repeated measures ANOVA to analyze the data from a pretest-posttest design: A potentially confusing task. *Psychological Bulletin,* 1975, 82, 511–518.

Jones, S., and Garwick, G. New feasibility and reliability study for goal attainment scaling. *Program Evaluation Project Newsletter,* 1973, 4, 6–7.

Kemp, G., and Vash, C. Productivity after injury in a sample of spinal cord injured persons: A pilot study. *Journal of Chronic Disorders,* 1971, 24, 259–275.

Kilpatrick, F., and Cantril, H. Self-anchoring scale: A measure of the individual's unique reality world. *Journal of Individual Psychology,* 1960, 16, 158–173.

Kiresuk, T., and Sherman, R. Goal attainment scaling: A general method for evaluating comprehensive community mental health programs. *Community Mental Health Journal,* 1968, 4, 443–453.

Means, B., and Roessler, R. *Personal achievement skills leader's manual and participant's workbook.* Fayetteville: Arkansas Rehabilitation Research and Training Center, 1976.

Robinson, J., and Shaver, P. *Measures of social psychological attitudes.* Ann Arbor: University of Michigan, Institute of Social Research, 1969.

Roessler, R., and Boone, S. Life outlook of rehabilitation clients: A comparative analysis. *Journal of Applied Rehabilitation Counseling,* 1977, 8, 89–98.

Roessler, R.; Cook, D.; and Lillard, D. The effects of systematic group counseling with work adjustment clients. *Journal of Counseling Psychology,* 1977, 24, 313–317.

Roessler, R., and Means, B. *Instructor's supplement: Program development and evaluation guidelines.* Fayetteville: Arkansas Rehabilitation Research and Training Center, 1976. (a)

Roessler, R., and Means, B. *Personal achievement skills: An introduction.* Fayetteville: Arkansas Rehabilitation Research and Training Center, 1976. (b)

Roessler, R., and Means, B. *Personal achievement skills training for the visually handicapped: Instructor's manual.* Fayetteville: Arkansas Rehabilitation Research and Training Center, 1977.

Roessler, R.; Means, B.; and Cook, D. A structured group counseling format for rehabilitation settings. *Rehabilitation Literature,* 1977, 38, 193–195.

Rosenberg, M. *Society and the adolescent self-image.* Princeton, N.J.: Princeton University, 1965.

Rotter, J. Generalized expectancies for internal versus external control of reinforcement. *Psychological Monographs,* 1966, 80 (1, Whole No. 309).

Shontz, F. *The psychological aspects of physical illness and disability.* New York: Macmillan, 1975.

Personal Awareness:
Individual Exercises

1. Have a friend blindfold you* and then attempt to carry out some normal daily activities: (a) sit in a public place; i.e., a restaurant or a movie theater for three hours; (b) have a friend assist you in buying your weekly groceries; (c) spend two complete work or school days blindfolded. Carry a tape recorder to record your reactions to being deprived of your vision.

2. Write your own rehabilitation plan as if you were blind today.

3. Have you donated your eyes for transplant after your death? If no, why not? Explore implications of such an action and make a decision after you have all the facts.

4. Would you consider donating one of your eyes to a totally blind person if there were a chance he or she might see again? What if this person were someone you loved very much? Discuss the reasons for your choices.

5. Visit a mobility training program and participate in the training.

---

*In doing active simulation tasks, be sure to have a companion to help you avoid danger. A blind person is trained in mobility and is usually more skilled in survival skills than a sighted person who is attempting to experience blindness.

Structured Group Experience in Disability
—The Setting Sun*

The sense of sight is frequently taken for granted. In order to provide students with a perspective on their personal values related to sight, this experience focuses upon the impact of visual loss from a personal frame of reference.

GOALS

1. To heighten awareness of the role sight plays in a person's life.

2. To stress the importance and temporality of a person's visual resources.

3. To put into perspective the values of people faced with limited time frames regarding visual functioning.

PRELIMINARY CONSIDERATIONS

1. *Level of Intensity:* Medium to high

2. *Group Size:* 6–12 participants

3. *Time Required:* 2 hours

4. *Materials Needed:* Pencils and paper, time cards

PROCEDURE

1. Begin the session by discussing reactions to the readings in chapter 4.

2. The leader makes a transition from the readings by asking "Have you ever considered what a loss of vision would mean to *you*?"

3. Time cards are distributed to each member. They contain one of

---

*See Appendices A and B for detailed information on use of the structured group experiences in disability.

the following statements: "You have just been informed that you have a degenerative eye disease and you will be blind in: a) five years b) one year c) 6 months d) 3 months e) 1 month f) 1 week g) 1 day h) 1 hour i) 1 minute.

4. Participants are instructed to write what they would do for each of these time frames. (Time: 10 minutes)

5. When completed, one person is asked to read his response for a specific time frame. This is done until each time frame is covered. (Note the time frames may be adjusted to correspond with the number of people in the group.)

LEADERSHIP SUGGESTIONS

1. Focus upon the quantitative and qualitative aspects of the responses, i.e., does a respondent stress doing for self or for another?

2. Is the main emphasis upon hedonism vs. preparation for functioning? Respond to the implications of both.

3. Stress the differentiating effect of time and relate this to the reality that some people do not have the opportunity to be aware of a degenerative condition and must deal with a traumatic event, such as immediate sight loss due to an accident.

VARIATIONS

1. Distribute cards having the same time frame so each group member will be responding to the same time dimensions.

2. Introduce various degrees of sight loss, e.g., one eye, blurred vision, tunnel vision.

3. Explore the group's reaction to the loss of sight of a spouse or child. What would be the impact upon their relationship?

CHAPTER FIVE

Group Approaches with Persons Having Coronary Heart Disease

Overview

Cardiac patients often experience emotional stress caused by fears of a subsequent coronary attack. Such fears and related stress may become intense enough to actually provoke emotional distress or further coronary difficulties. This chapter focuses on group therapy procedures that have been used to help cardiac patients minimize emotional difficulties often experienced following myocardial infarctions and other coronary problems.

Short-term group psychotherapy is viewed by Mone as one way to help cardiac patients cope with concerns such as fear of death, fear of sexual activity, and depressive feelings imposed by a sense of helplessness. Hypochondriacal difficulties frequently associated with postcardiac patients were often overcome through the group therapy process. Also, defense mechanisms, such as denial and flight into illness, that often interfere with postcardiac care, were found to be amenable to the confrontive forces of group members. Mone's article reveals that postcardiac patients become more realistic about assets and limitations imposed by coronary difficulties through participation in the group process.

Bilodeau and Hackett, in their article entitled "Issues Raised in a Group Setting by Patients Recovering from Myocardial Infarction," identify twelve such issues, including the nature of the illness, sexual concerns, and work. Each of these is discussed in detail to offer the reader insights to consider when conducting a group with cardiac patients. Bilodeau and Hackett report that emotional difficulties such as fear, anxiety, and anger were frequent topics discussed in the group context. The authors point out the value of having a nurse, rather than a mental health practitioner, lead such groups. Nurses can provide medical information about heart disease that helps the patient in understanding his illness. The opportunity to share common concerns was seen as a therapeutic benefit of this group experience.

Few controlled experimental studies have been conducted which evaluate the impact of group therapy with cardiac patients. Such a study has been undertaken by Rahe et al, and preliminary findings are reported in "Group Therapy in the Outpatient Management of Post-Myocardial Infarction Patients." Problem areas that the authors discuss and demonstrate by case analysis include work-related difficulties, family problems, and significant life changes. The authors support the use of group therapy as a means to educate patients about their disease and provide support during the readjustment period following hospitalization.

Adsett and Bruhn's article "Short-Term Group Psychotherapy for Post-Myocardial Infarction Patients and Their Wives" focuses on the adjustment to coronary disease of patients and their wives. Adsett and Bruhn discuss group therapy themes, conflicts, and solutions related to group involvement with this population. Their findings strongly support the use of group therapy as an important post-coronary rehabilitation component. Coronary patients and their wives were frequently shown to have diverse and conflicting reactions in adjusting to postcoronary marital relationships; however, such differences can be resolved through skillful guidance of the group process.

Each of the articles in this section emphasizes the debilitating effects of emotional stress for persons who experience coronary difficulties. This stress is particularly accentuated following a myocardial infarction since the stricken person becomes highly sensitized to the reality that the next attack may be terminal. Unfortunately, few systematic attempts have been made to help cardiac patients cope more effectively with the heightened emotional stress that frequently follows hospital discharge. This section focuses on group approaches designed to reduce anxiety and speed the return to functional life and living.

27

Short-Term Group Psychotherapy with Postcardiac Patients —LOUIS C. MONE, M.S.W.

CARDIAC patients are subject to emotional stress by the nature of their illness. It is widely known, for example, that patients who have had a myocardial infarction, initially and often for a year or more, have such severe anxiety that it interferes with a return to adequate functioning as defined by a resumption of personal responsibilities (Adsett and Bruhn, 1968). The cardiac surgical patient's stress and his reactions to it are seemingly even more severe. These patients postoperatively have a high incidence of suicidal attempts and psychotic episodes (McMahon, 1966; Zaks, 1959).

If the patient's adaptation to coronary heart disease is unsuccessful, the stressful situation continues. Some authors (Bruhn et al., 1968; Schneider, 1967) assert that this may cause further damage to the cardiovascular system which may result in death.

In their attempt to adjust to their condition, postcardiac patients must deal with pronounced feelings of the fear of death, helplessness, uselessness, depression, and apprehension about being able to return to work and resume personal responsibilities. Zaks and Boshes (1964), after studying approximately 130 cardiac patients of various types, classified patient reactions into two groups: "flight into health" and "flight into illness." These categories were described as follows:

Flight into health is often encountered in the beginning stages of heart disease, although it can occur in all stages. It is essentially a form of denial. It is characterized by an attempt to deny either the existence of the disease itself or its consequences, by means of excessive physical activity. Such patients frequently do things which they consciously know they should not do and which they know are dangerous or detrimental to their state of health.

Flight into illness . . . is often associated with general tendencies to withdraw under stress, as is found in schizoid and related conditions. It is also sometimes found in severe anxiety reactions, particularly when it occurs in the early stages of heart disease; that is, at a time when the patient's

Reprinted by permission of the American Group Psychotherapy Association from the *International Journal of Group Psychotherapy* 20 (1): 98–108, 1970.

actual activity potential is still more or less within normal limits. Not infrequently, it accompanies depressive states. It is closely related to the patient's fears of possible complete dependency, helplessness, or abandonment at moments of crisis, such as so-called "heart attacks." It is a means of conquering anxiety which permits a person to feel better at the time of stress. We therefore must assume that what is really intended is an attempt to deny [Zaks and Boshes, 1964].

Thus, it is evident that the cardiac patient's reaction to his disability may delay or interfere with the normal rehabilitative process and cause further medical complications. The focus of this paper will be on the use of short-term group psychotherapy as a method of rehabilitating postcardiac patients.

PROCEDURE

SELECTION OF PATIENTS

A letter outlining the program was sent to 171 physicians, general practitioners or internists, practicing in a county-wide area. Thirty-nine physicians returned the enclosed postal card indicating that they were interested and willing to refer myocardial infarction patients to the Middlesex County Heart Association, the sponsor of the project. Due to the small number of patients referred, the program was expanded to include not only myocardial infarction patients but the broad spectrum of heart-diseased patients. Also, the heads of social service departments in the four general hospitals in the area and the County Rehabilitation Commission were advised of the program.

The criteria for referring a patient to the group were the following:

1. That the patient had been diagnosed by a physician as a cardiac-diseased patient.
2. That he had recently [1] been discharged from a hospital.
3. That the patient was believed to anticipate or actually presented problems in adjustment to his cardiac condition.
4. That the patient was not functioning adequately in his usual role as head of the family, wage earner, homemaker, etc.

The author interviewed the candidates for group individually. The interview was approximately forty-five minutes in length and was devoted to taking a history of the patient's illness and essential background material. The author used this time to evaluate the patient's suitability for the group. If the therapist felt that the patient could benefit from group therapy, the therapeutic aims, research goals, and rules (confidentiality, first names, etc.) were explained to the patient, and he was given the choice of entering the group. If the therapist felt that the patient was not a suitable candidate for the program or would not benefit from the group experience, an appropriate referral or recommendation was made.

[1]Less than one year.

Structure and Setting of the Group

The group consisted of both male and female patients, and it met weekly for ten consecutive ninety-minute sessions.The group was open-ended, with new patients entering the group as they were referred. It was hoped that the older members of the group would be supportive to the newer ones and would serve, by nature of their own rehabilitative progress, as models motivating them toward rehabilitation.

The group met in a private conference room at the Heart Association office. The author led the group, tape-recorded each session, analyzed the recordings, and made brief notes after each meeting about the main themes of the session. He conferred with a consulting cardiologist primarily for clarification of medical aspects of cardiac disease in its various forms. Originally, the plan had been to include the cardiologist as co-leader, but this idea was abandoned for two main reasons: one, that the presence of a cardiologist might contaminate the aims of the group in that the discussion might become predominantly medical, and, two, if this did occur, the answers to medical questions might conflict with the referring physician's handling of the case.

Following the tenth session, whether or not the patient had attended every meeting, the therapist saw the patient individually for an assessment of progress or lack of it. This final interview was also utilized to make appropriate referrals to other agencies or practitioners if indicated.

Since this was a Heart Association project, a maximum fee of $15.00 was charged to those patients who could afford it and waived for those who could not. The fee was primarily an attempt to insure some commitment on the part of the patient to the program.

Measures of Assessment

Preceding the patient's entry into the group and following the tenth session, the patient was given the Minnesota Multiphasic Personality Inventory test (MMPI), Form R. The therapist was specifically interested in objective measurement and comparison test scores with respect to levels of dependency, denial, depression, anxiety, hypochrondriasis, and ego strength. A questionnaire prepared by the author was also given to each patient to be completed during the final individual interview. A different form of the same questionnaire was completed by the referring agent and by the group therapist.

Aims of the Group

The following goals of this short-term group psychotherapy project were:

1. To gain more specific knowledge of the psychosocial problems confronting the cardiac patient.

2. To observe how these patients attempted to cope with their cardiac-related problems.
3. To provide an atmosphere for ventilation and sharing of problems.

The therapist directed his efforts toward enabling the patient to resolve his problems, using support, appeals to the patient's ego, and encouraging the patient to draw upon his own resources. The focus was on current adaptive problems rather than on long-standing, deep psychic problems. Directions and intervention by the therapist were more common than would be true in traditional long-term group psychotherapy.

RESULTS

CHARACTERISTICS

Fourteen patients entered and completed the program. There were twelve men and two women. The mean age for all 14 was 44.9 years. The mean age for the women was considerably higher, 57.0, while for the men it was 42.0. The educational mean for the whole group was 11.5. The men were somewhat higher, achieving a mean score of 11.9, as compared to the women's 8.5. Thirteen out of the 14 patients were unemployed at the time of entry into the program.

In terms of the patient's immediate cardiac condition, nine had suffered myocardial infarctions, eight men and one woman; three were cardiac surgical patients, two men and one woman; and two male patients had coronary insufficiency.

The dynamics evident in this group were those common to other therapy groups; only the content differed. Resistance and group cohesiveness were apparent from the start and continued throughout in varying degrees. For example, during an early segment of the first session, one member said, "We don't want to think of the heart." The resistance was also evident in such comments as, "Couldn't we meet just one hour a week or maybe every other week. We will run out of things to talk about." In point of fact, there were never any prolonged silences and the group never seemed lost for words. In some instances resistance was acted out in lateness and absenteeism. Since the resistance of any group or individual is an unconscious process and must be made conscious if there is to be any therapeutic gain, the therapist played a very active role in interpreting the resistances as they arose, endeavoring to make the members of the group aware that they did not want to talk about their condition and how it made them feel because it was emotionally painful. During the initial phases of the group, the therapist was concerned about how far to probe. It was felt that too much exploration might impose too great a strain upon the patient, perhaps giving impetus to another heart attack during the session, a feeling shared by Adsett and Bruhn (1968) in their work with myocardial infarction patients. As the therapist became more comfortable in the group, however, and realized that the patients were not as vulnerable as he had originally thought, he played a more active role. Probing was mainly directed to conscious and preconscious thoughts and feelings, with unconscious material handled to a lesser extent. The leader interpreted the latter as it arose in regard to resistance and when it interfered with the patient's rehabilitation.

COMMON GROUP THEMES

The main theme that prevailed during the first three sessions, and continued throughout the sessions but to a lesser degree, was fear of death. One woman, even though her doctor had given her permission to walk and ride in a car, was hesitant about traveling to and from the group meetings for fear she would have another heart attack. Self-imposed limitations were true even of surgical patients; not walking as much as the doctor prescribed, refusal to leave their homes unless absolutely necessary, and avoidance of intercourse with spouses were examples. This hesitancy about engaging in physician-sanctioned activity had to do with the patients' acute sensitivity to body function and minor aches and pains. All of them were keenly aware of their heart beat, and many were sensitive to their pulse rate. For example, the woman mentioned above was in the habit of frequently checking her pulse. Almost invariably pain and increased heart and pulse rate were consciously or unconsciously associated with the onset of another "heart attack." Those feeling were quite pronounced during the early phase of therapy, but with encouragement from the therapist to express these feelings and fantasies, the distortions diminished. This resulted in freeing the patients to participate in prescribed and sanctioned activities, aiding in the rehabilitative process.

Feelings and concerns about sexual activity were raised by members of the group themselves in approximately the fifth session. This was of particular concern for the men, for it stirred up feelings of impotency. Some attempted to cope with these feelings by avoiding contact with their spouses that might be conducive to sexual relations, while others denied having any sexual desires. The therapist interpreted this behavior and denial to the group as an attempt to defend against their fear of being impotent. The nonsurgical heart patients tended more toward avoiding sexual relations than the surgical heart patients. One patient unconsciously felt his heart attack as an assault on his penis; in talking about his heart attack, he said, "I feel I have been hit below the belt." Schneider (1967), in his analysis of a cardiac victim, found that his patient regarded his heart attack as "a direct castration."

Associated with the fear of death was a moderate feeling of depression related to a sense of helplessness and uselessness. Such feelings were due in part to the limitations imposed by their illness. Spouses and relatives would say, "You can't do this," such as driving the car, lifting the garage door, taking out the garbage, etc. With respect to the male patient, these were tasks formerly performed by him, and not to be able to do them led not only to his feeling helpless and useless but to fears of becoming a burden and dependent on others. Some patients attempted to deny these feelings by engaging in certain activities against the doctor's orders in a "flight into health." Others endeavored to compensate for such feelings by doing light housework and cooking.

Helplessness accompanied by feelings of abandonment were felt by a number of patients when someone important to them was not close at hand. This was especially true during the early phase of group therapy. The fantasy behind this feeling was, "If I have another heart attack, no one will be around to get the necessary help to revive me and I will die." As these feelings were verbalized, the members of the group supported and encouraged each other, enhancing the therapeutic goals and the rehabilitative process. The therapist also tended to be supportive, but directed his support to the healthy part of the patient's ego. It was necessary for the therapist actively to lead the group to discuss relevant concerns and feelings in regard to their condition. As the group sessions progressed, there was a considerable reduction in the feelings mentioned above, and in the main patients functioned at a much higher level when compared to their functioning prior to entering the program. All 14 patients have resumed some if not all of their usual activities performed prior to the onset of illness. For example, ten patients reported a return to usual sexual activity and one of them reported increased sexual relations. Of the four remaining patients, two did not return to usual sexual activity and with the other two it was unascertained. Ten patients are gainfully employed, one patient is currently seeking employment, and the remaining three have not been given sanction by their physician to resume employment. It should be noted, however, that all patients experienced anxiety over returning to work. They were anxious in relation to how they would be received by their co-workers and concerned about their ability to perform on their job. There was also a considerable amount of anxiety about whether or not they would be returning to their previously held positions.

ASSESSMENT OF FINDINGS

Due to the incomplete returns of the referring agents' response to the questionnaire, it is difficult to evaluate their judgments and compare them to the therapist's and the patients' own assessments. Therefore, I shall only report the patients' response to the questionnaire. With regard to anxiety, eight felt less anxiety, one felt more anxiety, and five felt no change. Ten patients felt less depressed, and four felt no change. Seven felt more independent, three more dependent, and four no change. Thirteen had a more realistic attitude about their heart condition, and one had no opinion. Ten were less hypochondriacal, and four felt more hypochondriacal. With respect to the final question, ten patients felt their group experience had been helpful to them in resuming usual duties of provider, homemaker, etc. In short, the six-question questionnaire indicated a relatively positive patient response to their group experience.

In the main, the individual patient's MMPI pregroup test, when compared to the postgroup response, showed favorable results, but the differences with respect to the level of dependency, denial, and ego strength were small and not significant. However, with regard to hypochondriasis and depression, there was a significant decline. There is a high correlation of these two areas when compared to the questionnaire results.

CONCLUSION

In view of the seemingly overwhelming psychosocial problems the cardiac patient is confronted with during his recovery, it is a wonder that many adapt to their condition without psychotherapeutic intervention. Perhaps there are fewer such cases than physicians are aware of or care to admit. In weighing what has been reported and my own observation of cardiac patients, the author is of the opinion that all heart-diseased patients who are subjected to sudden cardiac disability, however temporary it may be, need psychotherapeutic help in securing a reasonable level of functioning.

The patients who have completed this program thus far are functioning at a much higher level now than prior to their entering the group. More specifically, their feelings and attitudes about their condition are more realistic and there is less concern over minor aches and pains. This decrease in hypochondriasis and depression is a seemingly significant factor in the rehabilitative process, since it leads to an adequate level of functioning and to behavioral change. It is my impression that this reduction of hypochondriasis and depression frees the patient's psychic energy, formerly directed to this area, allowing it to be employed by the patient's ego in performing its various functions. Perhaps depression is most significant, since any depressed person has a retarded motivational capacity which tends to inhibit all areas of functioning.

In passing, it is interesting to note that despite the strong hypochondriacal features in all of these patients, this was the clinical area in which a significant number benefited most. This result seems in contradiction to Slavson's (1964) statements on the criteria for group selection in which he indicates that the hypochondriacal patients are inaccessible to group therapy. The group process is particularly helpful in keeping hypochondriacal feelings in the foreground where they can be worked through. As soon as one member of the group begins discussing his anxiety about aches and pains, it spreads to the other members of the group (identification) and they begin verbalizing their feelings. The group method is also of significant value in dealing with the patient who wants to deny everything related to his illness. The group discussion reminds him of his condition, and if he attempts to deny it verbally, the other members of the group and the therapist confront him with this denial. Confrontation is also of value with those patients who attempt to use their illness for secondary gain. Challenged by both the group and the therapist, it is difficult for the patient to maintain this maladaptive defense.

From the evidence thus far gathered, it seems reasonable to conclude that short-term group psychotherapy facilitates the rehabilitation of the postcardiac patient.

REFERENCES

Louis Mone is the Chief Psychiatric Social Worker at the American Foundation of Religion and Psychiatry in New York.

Adsett, C. A., and Bruhn, J. G. (1968), Short-term group psychotherapy for post-myocardial infarction patients and their wives. *Canad. Med. Assn. J.,* 99:577–584.

Bruhn, J. G.; McCrady, K. E.; and Du Plessis, A. (1968), Evidence of "emotional drain" preceding death from myocardial infarction. *Psychiat. Digest,* 29:34–40.

McMahon, A. W. (1966), Some emotional aspects of rehabilitation in cardiac disease. Symposium on *Rehabilitation in Cardiac Disease,* Tufts University School of Medicine, March 3–4.

Schneider, D. E. (1967), *Psychoanalysis of heart attack.* New York: Dial Press.

Slavson, S. R. (1964), *A testbook in analytic group psychotherapy.* New York: International Universities Press.

Zaks, M. S. (1959), Disturbances in psychologic functions and neuropsychiatric complications in heart surgery. In: *Cardiology: An encyclopedia of the cardiovascular system,* Volume III, ed. Blakiston. New York: McGraw-Hill, ch. 19.

——, and Boshes, B. (1964), Psychological aspects of heart disease. Paper presented at the Illinois Heart Association's Fourth Annual Seminar for Nurses. Joliet, Illinois, May 24.

28

Issues Raised in a Group Setting by Patients Recovering from Myocardial Infarction —CAROLYN BASCOM

BILODEAU, R.N. and THOMAS P. HACKETT, M.D.

R ECENT studies have confirmed the common knowledge that a patient's emotional reactions to myocardial infarction continue long after hospitalization. The successful adjustment achieved by most patients in the hospital seems to be shaken when the patient faces the stresses of life following discharge. Worries about changes in physical activity and work

Reprinted from the *American Journal of Psychiatry,* vol. 128, pp. 73–78, 1971. Copyright 1971, the American Psychiatric Association. Reprinted by permission.

capability,[1-7] acceptance by the family,[2,3,7] sexual adequacy,[2,3] modifications in smoking and drinking habits,[2-4,6,7] and recurrent heart attack with possible death[2,3,7] may become overwhelming. Attempts to master these concerns through repression, denial, and other defensive measures are seldom successful.

In order to examine the psychological problems of coronary convalescence and to test the value of group meetings in resolving them, an approach was devised that used the techniques of small group therapy. These techniques provided the investigator (C.B.B.) with an organizational format already tested in a medical setting[8-10] and allowed her to gather data from a number of patients simultaneously. At the time this project was started, the literature contained no study on the use of group therapy with patients recovering from myocardial infarction. Since then, Adsett and Bruhn have published findings that indicate an "improved psychosocial adaptation" in patients and their wives as a result of group therapy.[3]

This study was undertaken not only to gain information about the emotional component in coronary heart disease, but also to determine whether a group of postcoronary men would be willing to meet 12 times with a nurse as their leader. If such sessions proved valuable to the patients, it would be profitable to incorporate such meetings into a coronary convalescence program.

METHODS

Our sample consisted of English-speaking male patients under 55 years of age who were admitted to the coronary care unit on the ward medical service with their first myocardial infarction. To establish rapport with potential group members and to provide an orientation to group process, the nurse (C.B.B.) conducted five taped interviews with each patient during hospitalization. In the fourth interview she introduced the idea of a "heart club" where men could share their concerns and feelings about heart disease. The meetings would also provide nurses and doctors with coronary convalescence data.

Of the ten patients randomly selected, five could not attend because of distance or severity of illness. The five participants ranged in age from 35 to 53. One was divorced; four were married. Their jobs involved strenuous physical activity frequently complicated by tension or pressure.

The nurse maintained biweekly telephone contact with each patient from day of discharge until the first group meeting. These calls maintained their interest and provided for expression of concerns and questions.

Weekly evening meetings lasted 75 minutes. With members' permission, sessions were taped.

FINDINGS

Four members came regularly, and a fifth attended irregularly.

TABLE 1. *The 15 Most Frequently Expressed Issues*

Issue	Percent of All Issues Raised	Time Consumed Percent	Rank
Leader	10.7	6.8	5
Group cohesiveness	7.7	4.2	10
Current state of physical health	7.3	5.0	8
Medical care after discharge	6.3	7.1	4
Work	5.7	8.5	2
Medications	5.1	6.0	6
Smoking	4.8	8.7	1
Current state of emotional health	4.5	2.3	14
Death	4.1	3.3	12
Attitude of others	3.5	3.5	11
Nature of illness	3.5	2.2	15
Nutrition	3.2	7.5	3
Illness and death of others	3.2	2.7	13
Family, home, friends	3.1	4.3	9
Finances	3.0	5.2	7

ANALYSIS OF DATA

Thirty-four issues were identified from transcriptions of the taped sessions. Issues were introduced by members and generally reflected group concerns. Each meeting was analyzed to obtain: 1) the number of different times an issue was raised, 2) the amount of time spent on each issue, and 3) the number of different issues introduced. A Spearman rank order correlation coefficient applied to the total number of times each issue was expressed in the 12 meetings and the total amount of time spent on each issue showed a high positive correlation ($r = .85$) that is significant at less than the .01 level.

The 15 most frequently expressed issues are listed in table 1. Ten of these were raised in every meeting. These 15 issues comprised 75.5 percent of all issues expressed and consumed 77.3 percent of the discussion time. "Leader" refers to all comments made concerning the group leader, including requests for her opinion on medical or social matters, comments on her appearance and role, and expressions of positive or negative feelings toward her. "Group cohesiveness" refers to comments reflecting the growing bond of unity within the group. The following is an example: "We're charter members. When my grandchildren get older they might see a plaque listing the names of the charter members of the heart club up on the wall of the hospital lobby and say, 'There he is.' "

The number of different issues raised in each meeting dropped steadily from 29 in the first meeting to 19 in the 12th meeting. This progressive decrease may indicate that some of the issues expressed at earlier meetings had been resolved.

To provide a broader view of the issues raised by group members, the 34 issues were grouped into seven general categories. The number of times that issues within each category were raised was totaled. Issues concerned with group process ranked first, indicating members' acceptance of and involvement in the weekly meetings. Second were issues concerned with current and future states of health.

Ranking third were issues concerned with effects of illness on one's life. The number of times issues in these first three categories were raised increased in the last six meetings. Ranking fourth were issues concerned with treatment of illness; issues concerned with the role of patient and its effect on the family ranked fifth. Ranking sixth were issues concerning history of illness; in last place were issues related to hospital care. The last four categories were raised more frequently in the first six meetings.

COMMONLY RAISED ISSUES

1. Nature of Illness.   Competition was high as members graphically described and compared the severity, course, and symptoms of their heart attacks. Nearly 70 percent of the times this issue was raised occurred in the first three meetings. A constant struggle to understand and accept the illness and its implications was obvious as members alternately voiced doubt and asserted belief in the diagnosis. "I still don't know what the hell kind of heart attack I had." "How bad was my heart attack. . . . Is it good, bad, medium, half-medium?" "I don't know what I've had yet, whether I had a heart attack or whether I ran out of wind." "Is his worse than mine, or is mine worse than his?"

2. Medications.   Not only the name and type of medication, but also the color, number, and dosage of pills were compared. The greater the number of pills per day and/or the need for nitroglycerin, the further a member was "on the way out." A decrease in number indicated improvement. Members exhibited excellent knowledge of anticoagulants, but viewed tranquilizers as "crutches" on which no real man ought to depend. None recalled having had the importance of sedation explained or emphasized by his doctor.

3. Nutrition.   Members discussed with considerable feeling the problems involved in adhering to diets, e.g., weight gain, watching others eating foods they were deprived of, and family vigilance. "My granddaughter, she's only a little thing, she looks at everything I eat during the day, and at night she tells the old lady everything I've eaten." Misconceptions and questions concerning foods allowed on the diets were repeatedly raised even though members had received written diet instructions before discharge. Although members recognized the importance of weight control, four out of five found this task difficult and blamed having cut down or stopped smoking for their increased appetites.

4. Medical Care after Discharge.   Each member was followed in the medical clinic by a house officer who cared for him in the hospital and was keenly aware of his doctor's response to his progress. The longer the time between appointments, the better the members felt they were.

5. Smoking.   All members viewed smoking as a direct road to a second heart attack, and willpower was stressed as an important factor in stopping. Three members stopped smoking completely, while two resumed smoking cigarettes, but less frequently than before their heart attacks.

6. Work and Activities.   Members varied in the degree of anxiety they experienced with increased activity and the return to work. Two were given less strenuous jobs, but were unhappy performing them. Two returned to their previous work; this violated one member's medical restrictions. The fifth member received a disability pension.

7. Sex.   All members directly or indirectly admitted diminished libido and fear of death during intercourse, a fear that was shared by their spouses. "Your heart's weak yet, man . . . sex life alone can kill you right now." Two members who attempted intercourse and were impotent blamed tranquilizers. Two others stated that they were in no hurry to commence sexual activity, while the fifth was reluctant to ask his doctor because "he might say I have to wait a year." No member had discussed these concerns with his doctor, and no doctor had introduced the subject.

8. Illness and Death of Others.   Patients were interested in comparing or finding differences in symptoms, course, treatment, and survival rate of others with the diagnosis of heart attack. Disregarding medical advice was held responsible for recurrent heart attacks and death in others. Identification with long-term survivors increased as the group members progressed in convalescence.

9. Attitude of Family.   From the third meeting on, members described being closely supervised by their families on activities, diet, smoking, medication, and naps. Aggravation, frustration, humiliation, and anger in reaction to this surveillance were vividly expressed. "When you get out of here with a heart attack, it's a pain in the ass to go home because everybody's on your back." At the same time, members interpreted their spouses' behavior as necessary for their continued well-being and as a manifestation of concern. They recommended a separate "heart club" for wives, but specifically stated that the two clubs should not hold joint meetings.

10. Current States of Health.   All members experienced increased body awareness. They repeatedly commented on the presence or absence of symptoms and immediately associated them with a recurrent heart attack. "You know, as soon as you feel lousy you say, 'Oh, oh, it's the ticker.' " They described themselves as generally more grouchy and irritable with diminished tolerance for aggravation, tension, and noise.

11. Future States of Health. Two members felt certain they would have second heart attacks—one because he found adhering to restrictions so difficult and the other because his tolerance for activity was low. One member denied concern about the future. Two admitted that fear of another coronary made them comply with the limitations of a cardiac regimen. The subject of death was raised in the form of direct comments or questions, veiled observations, and jokes. "For Christ's sake, she's talking to four mummies. She's getting us here every week to get all the information she can, and then she'll probably go to our funerals." Four of the five agreed that the thought of death came to mind frequently, and one of these found his sleep affected by these thoughts.

12. Group Process. Although the group was presented to the patients as a club, the process of growing into and becoming a cohesive group was a dynamic and prominent feature. Members were generally talkative and assertive and grew in their ability to share with and give support to others. As they became comfortable in the group setting they used slang and profanity, joked and teased, and expressed feelings freely. "All right, John, you haven't said a word for five minutes. Get your name on this tape or you don't get credit for showing up." "I enjoy talking to you because I can get more information from you than anybody I know. We can sit down relaxed and talk to you." "If we didn't come in, the club wouldn't run. . . . Even if I have to come in on a stretcher they're going to bring me in on Tuesday nights."

ROLE OF THE NURSE

In the hospital and in telephone contacts, the nurse listened to the patient, provided information as he was able to assimilate it, and encouraged him to communicate with his doctor when necessary. If the patient's spouse answered the telephone, the nurse talked with her about the patient and asked for her responses to his illness. Most frequently the spouse felt guilty that she was not doing enough, feared that her husband would have another heart attack, and was angry that he would not adhere to restrictions or demanded special attention. Occasionally the nurse suggested modifications in approach so that the patient would not feel so helpless and dependent.

In the group sessions the nurse was relatively nondirective and gave little interpretation to the material discussed. She attempted to create an atmosphere in which the members could interact easily with her and with other members.

PATIENT REACTIONS

All participants reacted positively to the hospital visits, telephone calls, and group meetings. They regarded the nurse's efforts in their behalf as evidence that the hospital was interested in them. They appreciated the opportunity to talk and commented on feeling better after doing so. The telephone calls were seen as a bridge between the security of the hospital and home, with its many sources of anxiety and frustration. Knowing that the nurse would call diminished members' feelings of helplessness and isolation.

Patients saw the nurse as someone they could "bother" even with "silly" questions. She helped them to avoid disturbing the doctor who was "busy" and often inaccessible; they trusted that she would advise them to contact the doctor when necessary. As medical appointments became more infrequent, members saw the club as the main place for them to ask questions, voice concerns, and find support.

The predominant feelings expressed were fear and anxiety. To cope with these and other feelings of aggravation, anger, dependency, sadness, inadequacy, and shame the members used various observable techniques: joking, changing the subject, displacement, projection, denial, rationalization, and identification. As the meetings progressed, the use of some of these mechanisms diminished, and members could express more of their feelings directly.

No patient experienced angina, dyspnea, or any other untoward physical or emotional symptom during these meetings. Rather, the meetings were described as the most relaxing time of the week, a time when members were accepted for just being themselves. Because of their positive response to the group, members requested continuation of the meetings. They were continued for 12 more weeks and thereafter on a monthly basis.

DISCUSSION

Our findings agreed with those of others that convalescence is a period riddled with emotional difficulties. Furthermore, many of the concerns and conflicts experienced by patients after discharge center around issues that could be resolved in part through explanations and clarification by the doctor. An uneven pattern of communication emerged in which some areas were meticulously covered, while others were hardly touched. Thus each patient knew a great deal about his cardiac and anticoagulant medication, yet had serious questions about the type of sexual activity that was permissible.

All were told they must be relaxed and get sufficient rest, but none had been encouraged to use tranquilizers and hypnotics to attain this state of mind should their own efforts fail. "Avoid overexertion" was advice that each remembered, but all were vexed with the question of what constitutes too much activity. Although each patient realized that he had had a myocardial infarction, there was a constant reassessment of the experience that ranged from considering it to have been mild, on the one hand, to lethal, on the other. These fluctuations were largely the function of the defense of denial, but they also betrayed a lack of information.

The following points, although obvious, emerged as suggestions for the discharge preparation of similar patients:

1. Patients will benefit from learning that the adjustment to a myocardial infarction is an ongoing process that continues long after hospitalization ends. Telling patients that during this period the majority of patients experience feelings of fear and depression might make these responses more endurable.

2. Anticipating the anxiety that occurs when the patient leaves the hospital, starts to increase his activities, and returns to work might reduce apprehension at these critical points. The use of tranquilizers should be advocated by the physician as an aid to relaxation. Specific sanction of the use of sedatives and hypnotics is necessary in order to overcome the moral stigma that is so often attached to their use.

3. Clear, written instructions on medications, diet, sex, activities, and the return to work, as well as discussions of these issues with both the patient and his spouse, should minimize conflicts at home after discharge.

4. Since so many pleasures are stripped from the patient recovering from myocardial infarction, it is well to remind him that many of the restrictions are temporary and that some substitutes are available.

CONCLUSIONS

Male patients recovering from myocardial infarctions joined and had positive feelings toward this group experience. The regularity and frequency of the meetings gave patients an opportunity to express fears before they blossomed. The nurse could review or reinforce old teaching and help patients find more effective ways of coping with frustration.

This study merely opens the door to an area that urgently requires investigation. Does the use of groups conducted by a nurse significantly affect the recovery process of coronary patients during three months of convalescence? If so, what type of group is apt to be most effective? What is the optimal size? Does the sex and profession of the leader make a difference? How long should group activity persist? Will patients cared for on the private service have a need for such a group?

Since coronary heart disease is one of the most serious threats to this nation's health and exacts an immeasurable economic toll, any remedial device deserves attention, particularly if it is as simple and inexpensive as the formation and maintenance of heart clubs.

REFERENCES

At the time this study was conducted, Mrs. Bilodeau was studying for the degree of master of science at Boston University School of Nursing; she is currently Psychiatric Nurse Clinician, Massachusetts General Hospital Department of Nursing, Boston, Mass. Dr. Hackett is Associate Psychiatrist, Massachusetts General Hospital and Assistant Professor of Psychiatry, Harvard Medical School.

This work was supported in part by Public Health Service training grant

MH–5018–21 from the National Institute of Mental Health and by Public Health Service contract 43–67–1443 with the National Institutes of Health.

1. Wynn, A.: Unwarranted emotional distress in men with ischemic heart disease (IHD). *Med. J. Aust.* 2:847–851, 1967.
2. Druss, R. G., Kornfeld, D. S.: The survivors of cardiac arrest. *JAMA* 201:291–296, 1967.
3. Adsett, C. A., Bruhn, J. G.: Short-term group psychotherapy for myocardial patients and their wives. *Canad. Med. Ass. J.* 99:577–584, 1968.
4. Willis, F. N., Dunsmore, N. M.: Work orientation, health attitudes, and compliance with therapeutic advice. *Nurs. Res.* 16:22–25, 1967.
5. Nite, G., Willis, F. N.: *The coronary patient: Hospital care and rehabilitation.* New York, Macmillan Co. 1964, pp. 269–270.
6. Roth, O.; Berki, A.; Wolff, G. D.: Long-range observations in fifty-three young patients with myocardial infarction. *Amer. J. Cardiol.* 19:331–338, 1967.
7. Hackett, T. P., Cassem, N. H.: Psychological reactions to life-threatening illness: a study of acute myocardial infarction, in *Psychological aspects of stress.* Edited by Abram, H. S. Springfield, Ill., Charles C. Thomas, 1970, pp. 29–43.
8. Linden, M. E.: The use of group psychotherapy in psychosomatic medicine, in *Psychosomatic medicine: The first hahnemann symposium.* Edited by Nodine, J. H., Moyer, J. H., Philadelphia, Lea & Febiger, 1962, pp. 757–758.
9. Schoenberg, B., Senescu, R.: Group psychotherapy for patients with chronic multiple somatic complaints. *J. Chronic Dis.* 19:649–657, 1966.
10. Deutsch, A. C., Lippman, A.: Group psychotherapy for patients with psychosomatic illnesses. *Psychosomatics* 5:14–20, 1964.

29

Group Therapy in the Outpatient Management of Post-Myocardial Infarction Patients

—Cdr. RICHARD H. RAHE, MC, USNR, Lt. CHARLES F. TUFFLI, Jr., MC, USNR, Lt. RAYMOND J. SUCHOR, Jr., MC, USNR, and Capt. RANSOM J. ARTHUR, MC, USN

INTRODUCTION

A post-myocardial infarction follow-up clinic was established at the U.S. Naval Hospital, San Diego, California, to evaluate all survivors of myocardial infarction (MI) regularly over the years following their infarctions. Aside from periodic cardiologic evaluations (every three months for the first year, and every six months for the following years) subjects are also counseled regarding their individualized diets, recommended body

Reprinted by permission from the *International Journal of Psychiatry in Medicine* 4 (1): 77–88, 1973.© 1973, Baywood Publishing Co., Inc.

weights and physical activity, and, if smokers, are given anti-smoking advice.

To assess the utility of group therapy as an adjunct to the above outpatient management of post-MI patients, half of all subjects under 60 years of age with demonstrable evidence of having suffered their first transmural myocardial infarction were randomly assigned to attend a series of six every-other-week one-and-one-half-hour group therapy sessions during the first few months following hospital discharge. The remaining half comprised the control group. Our long-range research goals are to evaluate comparisons between group therapy subjects and control subjects in terms of their job rehabilitation rates, prevalence of angina pectoris, nitroglycerin use, rehospitalizations, reinfarction and mortality rates. This initial report, however, was prompted by our early findings with the group therapy experience.

Over the past two decades numerous reports have appeared in the medical literature dealing with social, psychological, and behavioral characteristics of subjects who experience myocardial infarction.[1-12] A brief summary of important findings is presented to illustrate the information upon which much of our group therapy subject matter was based.

Recent studies of the distribution of coronary heart disease (CHD) among social classes in the United States and other western countries indicate that it is equally distributed among all social classes.[1,2] In addition, incidence of myocardial infarction seems to be rather equally distributed throughout industry, regardless of an individual's managerial level.[3] Of other social variables, level of education appears to discriminate between high and low risk subjects in the development of CHD. In one large industry, where men with only high school educations competed with college-educated men for various job positions, the high school graduates consistently showed significantly higher prevalence for CHD than did the college men.[3] Recent social changes have also been reported as characteristic of subjects' lives shortly prior to their MI. A significant increase in subjects' life changes, primarily those occurring within six months prior to their infarctions, has been seen in MI subjects compared to that seen for control subjects.[4,5]

Psychologic studies of MI patients have indicated that these individuals are not prone to focus upon, or even report, most illness symptoms—including symptoms of infarction.[6,7] Psychological and behavioral characteristics of MI subjects have included a life-long pattern of many hours of overwork, burdensome and self-imposed job responsibilities, a high personal drive and competitiveness, and intolerance to delay—often manifest by their rushing against time deadlines.[8-11] A striking feature of these patients' personality characteristics is the frequent lack of personal satisfactions resultant from this style of life.[12]

It seemed to us that the logical next step to be taken following documentation of such social, psychological, and behavioral characteristics of subjects developing MI was a trial of the usefulness of such information in the clinical management of MI survivors. Therefore, in our group therapy sessions we explored the above outlined areas of our subjects' previous life experience, personality, and behavior, as they progressed through the early phases of rehabilitation.

METHODS AND MATERIALS

THE GROUP THERAPY FORMAT

The 90-minute group therapy sessions were held every other week between 6:30 and 8:00 P.M. in the conference room at the "Heart Station" of the Naval Hospital. These evening hours allowed most participants ample time to drive there from work or after an early dinner. The chairs were arranged in a circle with doctors (from one to three in number) interspersed among the patients. A blackboard was kept nearby for outlining various aspects of the discussions. Group composition was allowed to vary according to hospital census; some sessions had only two patients, some had as many as seven. Subjects were requested to attend a minimum of four sessions, and a maximum of six sessions. In two cases patients were allowed to continue attendance after their sixth session due to unresolved situational difficulties. Sessions were tape recorded.

LIFE CHANGES EVALUATION METHODOLOGY

As an aid to estimate an individual's current state of psychological and environmental upheaval, the life change unit (LCU) system, previously devised by the senior author, was used.[13] This is helpful in rehabilitation as it represents an approximation of the psychological stress the patient was under at the time of his MI, and what he must contend with upon his recovery. Previous studies have indicated that the average yearly LCU score for healthy young Americans is 150 LCU.[13] The mean LCU score for our treatment patients was 203 LCU for the year prior to their MI. The mean LCU total for the controls for the year prior to MI was 231 LCU. This difference in mean LCU totals between treatment and control subjects was not statistically significant.

Both group therapy and control group subjects completed the recent life changes questionnaire—the Schedule of Recent Experience (SRE), designed to measure subjects' recent life changes over the recent few years as presented in previous publications.[5,13] Examples of life changes are: recent residential move; recent promotion at work; recent divorce; and so forth. A total of forty-two life changes comprise the questionnaire and cover work, family, personal and interpersonal areas of subjects' recent life adjustment. As in previous studies with this questionnaire, subjects' recent life changes were given "weights" to indicate the relative degrees of significance for each life change compared with other life changes in the SRE.[13] Thus, each subject could be assigned recent yearly life change magnitudes, expressed in LCU. Examples of this method of estimating subjects' recent life changes over the year prior to infarctions will be presented in the following case histories.

DEMOGRAPHIC DATA

To date, twenty-three patients have completed the group therapy treatment program and twenty-one additional patients are being followed in the control group. The mean age of treatment patients was forty-seven years, compared to fifty years for controls. Treatment patients included twenty males and three females, compared to twenty males and one female in the control group. Ninety percent of treatment patients were married; eighty-eight percent of controls were married. In none of the above parameters did the treatment group differ significantly from controls.

RESULTS

Several insights were gained in the group therapy sessions as to what the convalescing post-infarction patient experiences over the first three to six months following his MI. For convenience and brevity, these have been categorized and given the following headings: subjects' retrospective view of their life changes prior to infarction, memories of the hospitalization experience, the return home, resumption of physical activity, and return to work.

SUBJECTS' RETROSPECTIVE VIEW OF LIFE CHANGES PRIOR TO INFARCTION

It was often the case that during the first or second group therapy session patients performed a "psychological post-mortem" upon their life changes encountered over the year or so prior to infarction. They appeared to be psychologically ready to inspect their previous life change pattern and to evaluate whether they were pursuing a course of action leading to fulfillment in their work and their life in general or, more commonly, whether they were pursuing unrealistic and ultimately frustrating life demands.

An appraisal of their recent life changes was in some subjects accompanied by a mild to moderate depressive reaction. The depression appeared to be due to perceptions that they were partially responsible for their infarction through "allowing" their recent life events to accumulate to a high level. A subject exemplifying this phenomenon is presented below.

Case 1. A 41-year-old father of two and retired Chief Petty Officer, until the time of his infarction, had worked up to twenty hours a day as an electronics technician, a welder, a machinist, a volunteer worker for retarded children, a magician, a clown, and during Christmastime—a Santa Claus. During his younger days he had been a football player and a wrestler and had always prided himself on his enormous strength. During the year prior to his infarction, especially during the prior three months, he experienced several job changes (due to the difficult economy of the time) (89 LCU), and had taken correspondence courses to help him with new work possibilities (26 LCU). His lack of steady vocation had led to financial difficulties (38 LCU). Approximately nine months prior to his infarction, the subject had taken on some minor purchases (17 LCU), preparing to buy a new home (40 LCU). Finance companies threatened legal action for back payments due (30 LCU). Finally, three weeks prior to his infarction, his daughter abruptly married and left home (29 LCU). His LCU total for the year prior to infarction was 269.

After an uneventful hospital course, the patient returned home and noted a rather abrupt onset of moderately severe depressive reaction. He reported difficulties in disciplining his two sons, both of whom were strong like himself, without resorting to his prior physically threatening behavior. He had particular difficulty achieving a prescribed weight loss in a household where all family members ate large amounts of food. He blamed himself for worsening the family's already dire financial state through his recent unemployment resulting from his MI. He returned to work earlier than was medically recommended—within two months following hospital discharge. Aside from some initial angina upon exertion, the subject did well and found that in working eight hours a day he still did "twice the work of the average man." Although difficult for him, the subject dropped many of his avocational pursuits. He discovered that he could turn his previous welding experience into a hobby (modern sculpture). His sons began to contribute to the family's income and after the patient adjusted to his psychological loss of stature, his depression began to improve.

MEMORIES OF HOSPITALIZATION EXPERIENCE

Psychological reactions of MI patients to their first few days in the coronary care unit, especially in regard to significant anxiety and depression, have been described in detail by other researchers.[14] Once MI patients leave the hospital, however, they frequently look back upon their experience with greatly minimized accounts of the seriousness of their illness.[15]

The tendency for MI patients to deny and repress the seriousness of their illness was repeatedly seen in our group sessions. Comments made about the hospital experience focused upon what patients saw as a rather boring second and third week of recuperation, rather than upon their sometimes critical life and death situations in the coronary care unit.

Our patients proved to be persons who liked to take on responsibilities, and capable of carrying out self-education. It was during the second and third weeks of hospitalization that patients frequently expressed a readiness to learn about their disease, as well as to learn about their ideal post-hospitalization management. This readiness to learn about MI was generally underestimated by the ward staff, at least as judged by the patients' ignorance regarding CHD upon their arrival at the group sessions. One patient actually voiced the wish that he could have been assigned reading material regarding his heart disease by his physician when he saw him on rounds each day. He then suggested that on rounds the following day his physician could quiz him on what he had learned—to be sure that he properly understood his reading assignments. An exception to this general finding is presented in the case history below.

Case 2. A 38-year-old father of three and Chief Petty Officer experienced his infarction eight months prior to his retirement from active duty in the Navy. During the year prior to his MI he had been working up to eighteen hours per day on three different jobs. His recent life changes were the following. The year prior to his infarction he had begun training as an electronics technician, the job he planned to continue after his retirement (26 LCU); he reported concern over the health of his youngest son (44 LCU); he registered more than the usual number of arguments with his wife (35 LCU); he had received recent awards for outstanding work (28 LCU); a relative had moved into the home (39 LCU); he had recently bought a new home (31 LCU); and he had begun to make major improvements upon this home (25 LCU). His total LCU reported for the year prior to infarction was 228.

During the second week of his hospital course, the ward physician noticed the patient's high anxiety level and poor frustration tolerance. The physician took him aside and discussed his disease and its management with him. The physician emphasized both physical and mental adjustments the patient should attempt to make. At the time he appeared for his first outpatient group therapy session, the patient had already stopped smoking, had lost twenty pounds, and had begun his exercise (walking) program. He had experienced some family (disciplinary) problems which he resolved shortly after his return home. Partly as a result of this single discussion with his doctor, and partly from the group therapy sessions, the subject managed to develop a slower pace of life, increased his frustration tolerance, and augmented his life satisfactions. As an example, he stated: "I now drive my car ten to fifteen miles an hour *slower* than the speed limit. I'm the guy now I used to honk at before."

THE RETURN HOME

Convalescence provided most of our male patients with their first experience of living at home all day and involved them, often unwillingly, with their wives and children in the management of the home. Children's disciplinary problems, in many cases previously ignored by the patient prior to his MI, now rose to the patients' attention. Wives, too, had to adjust themselves to having their husbands home all day, especially as "an invalid."

A commonly described reaction of the spouse to a patient's return home from the hospital was one of over-solicitousness. This attitude, seemingly a combination of a wife's realistic fears of the possible death of her mate, along with subconscious resentment about having been left alone to handle the family affairs over the preceding three to four weeks, appeared to lead to insistence on performing even the most menial tasks for the patient.

Patient-family confusion regarding the subject's diet was perhaps the most commonly reported difficulty upon his return home. Wives were frequently ill-informed as to how to prepare low fat or low carbohydrate meals. Alternatively, the wife might prepare dietarily correct meals, but with an unsavory result. Almost all of our patients were instructed to lose weight, and if the family continued to eat its previous diet while he was to reduce in weight, the patient realistically felt unsupported in his weight reduction efforts.

Disciplining the children often posed a particular problem for the post-MI patient after his first few days at home. Almost to a man, our patients were not long-suffering types. Many of our patients resumed their habitual, pre-infarction behavior and adopted a physically threatening posture toward the children. Although some older children could well have called their father's "bluff," generally order was restored to the household with little more than a verbal confrontation. Interpersonal conflicts, though often dramatic, were usually resolved within two to four weeks following hospital discharge. The following case history illustrates such a conflict.

Case 3.   A 41-year-old father of three, Chief Medical Corpsman, over the year prior to his infarction had undergone a residential move (from Scotland to California) (20 LCU), a change in responsibilities at his work (29 LCU), a purchase of a new home (31 LCU), a change in his work hours and conditions (20 LCU), a change in his social activities (18 LCU), a change in his church activities (19 LCU), a change in his recreation (19 LCU), recent concern over the behavior of a child (44 LCU), an increase in his usual number of arguments with his wife (35 LCU), and change in family get-togethers (15 LCU). The patient's total life changes score for the year prior to his infarction was 250 LCU.

It was during this year of frequent social transitions that the patient recalls becoming more involved in his work, ignoring home problems, and becoming frequently irritated by minor transgressions perpetrated in his home and by his neighbors. During his first few weeks at home, the patient was amazed by the "lack of discipline" in his children. One child actually taunted the subject by running out of the house to avoid punishment. The subject was afraid to run after him so soon after his infarction, so he locked the child out until the early hours of the morning. A "serious talk" followed the readmittance of the son into the house. No resurgence of problems at home was reported throughout the remainder of the group therapy sessions.

RESUMPTION OF PHYSICAL ACTIVITY

A common finding in group sessions was that while the patients were in hospital, minimal attention apparently was given by physicians and nursing personnel to counseling them as to when they might resume physical (including sexual) activities. We found it necessary to frequently repeat instructions as to how subjects should begin a graduated, regularized, physical activities program—not only to attain their previous physical condition, but to achieve (sometimes for the first time) bona fide physical conditioning. A good deal of our discussions, originally planned to cover psychological aspects of CHD, were spent in instructing patients how to take their own pulse rates, regulate their exercise, use nitroglycerin when first attempts at physical activity lead to angina, and so forth. This illustrates how extremely beneficial "psychotherapy" is performed by simply providing intelligible and practical answers for patients' medical concerns.

The beginning of a physical fitness program (walking from one to three miles per day over the second and third month following hospital discharge) often served an important psychological function in that it gave the patients a reassuring "measure" of their physical recovery. Immediately post-hospitalization, the patients were generally surprised by their weakness and easy fatigability. Previous to their infarctions they had often maintained physically grueling schedules. As patients developed their physical conditioning after MI's, significant self-confidence returned.

The acceptance of and adherence to an exercise program has approximated 100 per cent among our patients. Of all post-infarction management dictums, this one appears to be the best accepted. Perhaps because this program has such a high degree of face validity (to condition the heart), patients rarely missed their daily walks.

RETURN TO WORK

As patients, in the group sessions, planned their return to work, it was the ideal time to discuss their previous work patterns and behaviors. We focused on whether or not they previously took on excessive overtime work, how much importance they placed on doing their work perfectly, their concern with meeting time deadlines, their competition with fellow workers for work output, promotions, bonuses, and so forth. We also assessed their work satisfactions, or, more commonly, the lack of them.

Patients uniformly reported excessive overtime work and frequently had intense job dissatisfactions and/or irritations with co-workers. One of the more noticeable benefits of the group therapy sessions was having patients reflect upon these dimensions of their work behavior in the midst of others quite similarly inclined. Excuses for overwork were rapidly "debunked" by others, and when one patient made appropriate plans for adjustments in his work patterns, it served as a good example for several other group members.

When patients became involved in their return to work, they sometimes commenced smoking again or began to gain weight. This period of backsliding was tolerated during the first week or so back on the job, but if it continued longer than this, it was pointed out in the group sessions. The admonitions of others struggling with these same temptations usually supported the "offending" patient's efforts to take concrete steps to cut out smoking altogether, to achieve a weight reduction, or to solidify his physical training program. At times like this, an awareness of an individual patient's psychological traits and emotional problems was of critical importance in order to appreciate the often immense efforts certain patients had to make in adhering to their diet, exercise, and so forth.

This same group process also helped subjects in modifying their overwork behavior. It was pointed out by other patients as often as by the doctors when a patient had pursued unrealistic work patterns and life goals. Often, to a patient's surprise, his work efficiency increased when he reduced his energies devoted to work. He also began to enjoy out-of-work activities—notably those with his family. The focus of patients' hobbies often changed from one of strict, self-imposed demands (often in order to make extra money) to having fun.

Case 4. A 49-year-old father of two and airfield crash chief worked a schedule of twenty-four hours on-duty alternating with twenty-four hours off-duty. On his days off, he would work out of his garage as an electronics technician, specializing in TV repairs. The subject worked during his day off for increased financial gain and also because he felt too restless to "just relax" on his day off. The subject reported a stable life during the year prior to his infarction. He had experienced a recent illness (accident) (53 LCU), a change in his sleeping habits (16 LCU), a change in his recreational activities (19 LCU), and recent awards for excellent work performance (28 LCU), and his wife had begun working outside the home (26 LCU). His total life changes for the year prior to infarction was just 142 LCU.

On the day of his heart attack the subject was racing toward a burning airplane when his own vehicle caught fire. "I stopped to put out the fire in my truck and the fire started in my chest."

The subject had an uncomplicated hospital course and over his six group therapy sessions managed to lose weight, stop smoking, and start an exercise program. His greatest difficulty, however, was in changing his work behavior.

He had always prided himself on being the first person to arrive at a fire and often took on the responsibility usually delegated to junior firefighters, by being the first one inside a burning plane. He found it extremely difficult to delegate responsibilities, and this was a major focus of attention during several of his group sessions. Between the group therapy sessions and the subject's superiors at work, it was decided that upon his return to work, one of his men would be assigned to look after him during fire alarms. This man would try to prevent the patient from becoming too wrapped up in his work, and physically stop him from running into a burning plane. Although the patient did not like this arrangement, he did agree to the need for it.

COMMENT

We frequently used the term "psychological risk factors" in an attempt to convey to our subjects that overwork, job dissatisfactions, home problems, rushing against time deadlines, and so forth, might be considered alongside diet, exercise, and smoking in their rehabilitation program. For most patients, the presentation of such a spectrum of psychological and physical risk factors helped by affording them several arenas in which they might concentrate their rehabilitation efforts. If one or two areas (characteristically weight reduction and stopping smoking) were difficult to change right away, they could take satisfaction from their progress with the other risk factors.

Psychologically, a key issue for post-infarction patients was whether or not they considered themselves to have a physical liability. Most patients stated that previously they had thought of themselves as masculine, reliable, strong, almost invulnerable to illness. Their myocardial infarctions revealed to them that they were indeed vulnerable to illness, but after their hospitalization they tended to revert to their previous attitudes regarding their health. Unless they periodically reminded themselves of their coronary disease, they saw little reason to pursue dietary, exercise, and anti-smoking regimens or to change previous attitudes and behaviors.

A note should be made in regard to the use of humor during these group sessions. Whereas humor is generally not accepted in conventional psychotherapy, or at least is spoken of with severe admonitions, humor appeared to be of considerable importance in allowing expression of the patients' realizations of the possible fatal outcome from their disease. Also, patients' feelings of diminished sense of worth upon the revelation of a previously unsuspected life-threatening disease can often best be expressed with humor.[16] An example of this use of humor in our group sessions was given by a patient whose father and older brother had both died in their mid-fifties from coronary disease. In introducing himself to the group, he stated, "I was prepared to die around the same age as my kin, but I must admit I was somewhat disappointed in myself when I developed my heart attack ten years early."

The lack of patient knowledge regarding their disease and its management, even with the sustained doctor-patient contact afforded by hospitalization, was obvious. The patients in both control and intervention groups were frequently characterized by total ignorance about causes of this disease, its effects on their life adjustment, and its management. As pointed out by Weed, "Any patient with a chronic illness must be his own physician; his lack of knowledge concerning his disease and of the necessities and details of therapeutic intervention cannot be compensated for by a stern, two-minute reprimand delivered at three- to six-month intervals."[17]

This brief presentation of selected clinical findings from our group therapy sessions is intended to support the use of group therapy in the early outpatient management of post-myocardial infarction subjects. Crucial items too often omitted in post-discharge care, such as basic correct information about recuperating hearts, is simple to provide. Our study is still in its early stages, and similar projects have been started elsewhere with encouraging early results.[18] Whether or not any long-term benefits will accrue to these patients, in terms of higher percentages of return to work, fewer cardiac symptoms, lower reinfarction and death rates, and so forth, remains to be seen after years of follow-up. However, several short-term benefits of group therapy have become so apparent that the teaching value alone of our sessions has attracted occasional Navy cardiologists away from their time-urgent pursuits to attend a few of the group sessions.

REFERENCES

The authors are affiliated with the U.S. Navy Medical Neuropsychiatric Research Unit in San Diego, California, where Commander Rahe is the Head of the Biochemical Correlates Division, Lieutenant Tuffli is a research physician, Lieutenant Suchor is a research physician, and Captain Arthur is Commanding Officer.

The authors wish to acknowledge that LCDR Kirk Prindle, MC, USNR, and E. N. Landry, R.N., were instrumental in setting up the coronary disease aftercare clinic, along with the cooperation of Captain R. Morgan, MC, USN, Head of Cardiology, U.S. Naval Hospital (Balboa), San Diego, California.

The article is report No. 72-20, supported by the Bureau of Medicine and Surgery, Department of the Navy, under Research Work Unit MR011. O1-61101N. Opinions expressed are those of the authors and are not to be construed as necessarily reflecting the official view or endorsement of the Department of the Navy.

1. Antonovsky, A: Social class and the major cardiovascular diseases. *J. Chron. Dis.* 21:65–106, 1968.
2. Wardwell, W.; Hyman, M. M.; Bahnson, C.: Socio-environmental antecedents to CHD in 87 white males. *Soc. Sci. Med.* 2:165–83, 1968.
3. Hinkle, L. E., Jr.; Whitney, L. H.; Lehman, E. W., et al: Occupation, education, and coronary heart disease. *Science* 161:238, 1968.
4. Syme, S. L.; Hyman, M. M.; Enterline, P. E.: Some social and cultural factors associated with the occurrence of coronary heart disease. *J. Chron. Dis.* 17:277, 1968.
5. Theorell, T., Rahe, R. H.: Psychosocial factors and myocardial infarction: I. An inpatient study in Sweden. *J. Psychosom. Res.* 15:25–31, 1971.
6. Ostfeld, A.; Lebovits, B. Z.; Shekelle, R. B., et al: A prospective study of the relationship between personality and CHD. *J. Chron. Dis.* 17:265–76, 1964.
7. Wikland, B.: Medically unattended fatal cases of ischemic heart disease in a defined population. *Acta. Med. Scand.,* Suppl:524, 1971.
8. Brozek, J.; Keys, A.; Blackburn, H.: Personality differences between potential coronary and non-coronary subjects. *Ann. N.Y. Acad. Sci.* 134:1057–64, 1966.
9. Jenkins, C. D.: Psychologic and social precursors of coronary disease (two parts). *N. Engl. J. Med.* 284:244–55 and 307–17, 1971.
10. Friedman, N., Rosenman, R. H.: Association of specific overt behavior pattern with blood and cardiovascular findings. *JAMA* 169:1286–96, 1959.
11. Rosenman, R. H.: Emotional factors in coronary heart disease. *Postgrad. Med.* 42:165–72, 1967.
12. Liljefors, I., Rahe, R. H.: An identical twin study of psychosocial factors in coronary heart disease in Sweden. *Psychosom. Med.* 32:523–42, 1970.
13. Rahe, R. H.: Life crisis and health change, *Psychotropic drug response: Advances in prediction.* Edited by May PRA, Wittenborn JR. Springfield, Ill., Charles C. Thomas, 1969, pp 92–125.
14. Cassem, N., Hackett, T. P.: Psychiatric consultation in a coronary care unit. *Ann. Intern. Med.* 75:9–14, 1971.

15. Croog, S. H.; Shapiro, D. S.; Levine, S.: Denial among male heart patients. *Psychosom. Med.* 33:385–97, 1971.
16. Bilodeau, C. B., Hackett, T. P.: Issues raised in a group setting by patients recovering from myocardial infarction. *Amer. J. Psychiat.* 128:73, 1971.
17. Weed, L. L.: *Medical records, medical education, and patient care.* Cleveland, The Press of Case Western Reserve University, 1969.
18. Ibrahim, M. A.; Feldman, J. B.; Sultz, H. A., et al: The management of myocardial infarction: a controlled study of the effects of group therapy upon prognosis. Presented at the Conference on Cardiovascular Epidemiology, Tampa, 1972.

30

Short-Term Group Psychotherapy for Post-Myocardial Infarction Patients and Their Wives —C. ALEX ADSETT, M.D., F. R.C.P.[C] and JOHN G. BRUHN, Ph.D.

THE psychological condition of the patient who has experienced a myocardial infarction is the result of the interaction of many factors operating before, during, and after the occurrence of the infarction. Some of these factors include age, duration of the illness, personality characteristics and patterns of emotional expression, the nature of the familial and work situation and the attitudes of friends and, in particular, the attitudes of the physician.[1] These factors greatly influence the patient's understanding and acceptance of his illness throughout his recovery, although psychological reactions such as depression may be more apparent during the acute episode.[2] The attitudes of both the physician and the spouse are of special importance in influencing the nature of the patient's emotional adaptation and subsequent clinical course. The involvement of the spouse in discussions of the patient's illness, and of the meaning of symptoms and subsequent modifications in his way of life, helps to minimize the extremes of either lack of concern or overconcern and determines how realistic and hopeful the patient is about his future.[3] It has been shown that when the helpers are not in agreement about the patient's capabilities, the patient has more difficulty in adjusting.[4]

The services of the psychiatrist are becoming integral parts of the rehabilitative regimen for coronary patients, especially for those patients who appear to have greater difficulty in adjusting to their illness.[5] Our impression, derived from a longitudinal study of coronary patients over seven years, has been that patients who lack closely knit familial relationships and support from friends and colleagues have greater difficulty in adjustment

Reprinted by permission from the *Canadian Medical Association Journal* 99: 577–584, 1968.

than patients who have support from others.[6] Therefore, it was decided to institute a group therapy program for patients who seemed to be having adjustment difficulties. Since the patient's spouse was usually involved in the problems of adapting, the spouse was also included in the therapy program.

Among questions implicit in the goals of group therapy were those concerned with possible changes in physiological factors during and after therapy, including the possibility of prolonging life. Therefore, it was proposed to follow the therapy patients longitudinally to determine their long-term adaptation compared to a matched group of coronary patients who were not included in the therapy program.

METHOD

SUBJECT SELECTION

From a group of 65 post-infarction patients in the University of Oklahoma Neurocardiology Research Project,[7] 10 men with the following characteristics were invited to join the therapy program: those who

1. Had had at least one severe well-documented myocardial infarction, one year or more before the initiation of group therapy.
2. Were under the age of 55 at the time of their initial heart attack.
3. Were married.
4. Possessed the characteristics of high drive and intense frustration, and had more than usual psychological difficulty adapting to their cardiac disability.

The presence of these characteristics was assessed by psychiatric and sociologic interviews and psychological tests.

The 10 couples were seen separately for a half-hour interview with the two authors, in order to discuss the concept of group therapy, outline its therapeutic and research goals, and elicit the couple's feelings about participating. Two couples were unwilling to take part, and two more couples dropped out of the program almost at the beginning. Thus, the final therapy group was composed of six patients and their wives. These six patients were then matched for age, sex, and race with six coronary patients from the Neurocardiology Program who were not asked to join the therapy group.

Before the first therapy meeting each of the six patients and his wife had an initial individual semi-structured psychiatric interview to delineate basic individual strengths and weaknesses and for a more detailed personality assessment.

GROUP STRUCTURE

We considered two alternatives for including the wives in the group therapy: either to have a joint group or to have separate husband-and-wife groups. After discussions with the couples and subsequently among ourselves, we decided on separate groups. We felt that separate groups over a short-time period might minimize inhibitions and that the two groups could be brought together for a joint session later.

The groups met for 75 minutes on alternate Saturday mornings over a period of six months for a total of 10 meetings for each group. The group meetings were attended by both therapist (C.A.A.) and co-therapist (J.G.B.) and were tape-recorded. Each taped session was analyzed by the authors after the meeting, by selecting the main theme, the group focal conflict and the group solution to the conflict, similar to the technique outlined by Whitman and Stock.[8]

PHYSIOLOGICAL MEASUREMENTS

Since all patients were participants in the Neurocardiology Research program and were clinically evaluated by their respective project physicians at approximately six- to eight-week intervals, and in addition underwent numerous physiological and psychological tests at each visit, it was possible to obtain a wide variety of data on the patients before, during and after the six-month period of therapy. In addition, during several of the group sessions, individual patients wore a one-lead portable electrocardiogram apparatus.

The physiological measurements that were of special interest to the group therapy study were blood pressure, pulse rate, serum cholesterol and serum uric acid. Anxiety and depression subscales from the Minnesota Multiphasic Personality Inventory were also determined in the patients at each clinic visit.

GOALS OF THERAPY

The goals of the group therapy program were:

1. To observe how the patients and their wives were coping with the patient's handicap and how much support they were able to give and accept in their relationship with each other and with the other group members.

2. To help the patients and their wives with their feelings and problems generated by the patients' heart disease. The therapy was focused on this specific task using the technique of short-term focal therapy in which the therapist assists the group members in expressing feelings and finding solutions to the problems associated with the patients' disability. The therapists were active participants at times, but during much of the sessions a modified non-directive technique was employed. A great deal of support was provided by the therapists, and the group members were encouraged to support each other. The therapists did not attempt to deal with many long-standing psychological problems in the subjects' lives, but attempted to work with current problems related to, or activated by, the heart disorder.[9]

3. To observe any concurrent physiological changes during the period of group therapy.

4. To observe the long-term adaptation and clinical course of mem-

bers of the group compared with a matched sample of patients not participating in group therapy.

RESULTS

CHARACTERISTICS OF THE THERAPY AND COMPARISON GROUPS

The therapy patients did not differ significantly from their matched
"controls" or from the patients who refused to participate in group therapy
with respect to age. The mean age of the therapy patients was 47.5 years,
for the matched "controls" 49.0 years, and for the refusals 51.5 years. The
three groups also did not differ significantly in education. The therapy
group had a mean education of 13.0 years, the matched "controls" 13.3
years and the refusals 13.0 years. In addition, the three groups were not
statistically different on I.Q., 117.5 for the therapy group, 109.3 for the
matched "controls" and 112.8 for the refusals.

On the Minnesota Multiphasic Personality Inventory, however, the
matched "controls" had significantly higher scores on he Hypomania scale
(Ma) than the therapy patients. The refusals differed from both the therapy
group and the matched "controls," having higher scores on the Psychopathic (Pd), Paranoia (Pa), and Hypomania (Ma) scales on the
M.M.P.I.

GENERAL OBSERVATIONS

The six coronary patients showed a variety of personalties, conflicts
and defences. Although all of the men shared the common concern of their
heart condition and its influence on their style of life, the younger patients
were more concerned than the older patients. The threat of further disability or death, although pre-conscious, was activated into a conscious fear
by various life situations. For example, reading or hearing about a death
from heart disease stirred up intense anxiety; particularly when the death
was associated with physical activity, it led to a fear of their own activity.
The men were talkative and aggressive, and developed at least the beginning of group cohesiveness, although there was moderate absenteeism (13
incidents). In general, the men developed a concern for others in the group
and made genuine efforts to help group members with their problems. They
talked about the reasons why they thought they had a coronary attack and
about how they could prevent a recurrence. Each of them emotionally
relived the traumatic experience of his heart attack. They openly discussed
the threat of death, funerals, sexual difficulties, and hostility and anger
towards loved ones. Tension and anxiety were relieved by sharing feelings,
by much humour and joking, and at times by rationalizing that a heart attack is beneficial because it makes one face up to one's self. The patients
also dealt with the feelings of shame and loss of self-esteem, e.g. "I am not
the man I used to be." Mild depressive features were noted at times, but no
severe depressed mood was evident. A recurrent conflict was the desire to

be mothered and given sympathy by their wives as opposed to the need to be manly and independent.

The wives were quieter, more dependent and wanted more direction and structure from the therapists. They saw themselves in the role of "feeders," for cooking food for their husbands and watching their husbands' diets. They seemed overly protective of their husbands and afraid to make many demands on them. There was much concern about hurting or upsetting the men; and the women were strikingly inhibited in expressing aggressive or sexual feelings. Many of the wives tended to avoid facing the possibility that the husband might have a future fatal heart attack. They rationalized that the fact of having had a heart attack might have changed their husbands' ways of life in such a way that now they were less likely to have trouble than other men. The wives' group had a high degree of absenteeism (19 incidents) and never developed a cohesive group with as much concern and closeness toward one another as was present among the men. While the men dealt predominantly with the loss of self-esteem, the women were concerned with guilt feelings. They questioned what they might have done to contribute to their husband's heart attack and felt that they were greatly responsible as protectors of their husband's future health. The wives were anxious, but in addition showed as much as or more depressive feelings than their husbands.

There was a significant carry-over of information between the two groups. Material from one group was occasionally brought into the other group, which indicated at least partial sharing of group experiences in the home. The wives, however, complained that their husbands did not share much information with them. The one final joint session was more tense than those with separate groups, but one meeting is insufficient to evaluate this therapy structure. The subjects suggested in the final joint meeting that it would have been preferable, in retrospect, to have one or two joint meetings at the beginning as well as at the end of the separate group sessions. Their rationale was that an early introduction to the spouses of fellow group members would help them understand each other's problems better.

SEPARATE PATIENT-WIFE SESSIONS

The themes, group conflicts and group solutions of the separate sessions are outlined in Tables I and II. The one joint group session is outlined in Table III.

Because the method used in analyzing the group sessions does not convey the feelings of the individuals involved, a few comments are quoted from both groups.

One of the men when talking about the period shortly before the onset of his acute myocardial infarction said: "When I came under strain and a little bit of stress I couldn't find my way out. I didn't have anybody to talk to. I was in a different environment. I didn't know who I wanted to open up to. If I had someone to whom I possibly could have conveyed my thoughts it would have been different, I think. I think it's just a matter of holding on to things inside of you, not wanting to tell anybody what's really wrong. It's getting that explosive feeling outside of you and then you can sit down and really relax."

One of the patients expressed the effects of emotions on his symptoms of angina pectoris as follows. "You know I can run a mile and my chest wall will go to hurting. But I can sit right here and start arguing with you and my chest wall will go to hurting a whole lot worse than if I run a mile."

The restless need for activity and inability to relax that these patients characteristically showed were illustrated by the following remark: "I have got to have something to do, so I go to Toastmasters on Tuesday night, on Thursday nights I go to the lodge and I have O.U. on Monday and Wednesday nights. But I can't come home and work and piddle around the house and watch TV. I'd go crazy."

The men's difficulty in becoming deeply involved with others, particularly with their wives, whom they saw as not only providing love and sympathy but also as dominating and controlling, is illustrated by this quote:

"On week-ends I'm glad when I can just get away from her for three or four hours and go out to the lake and try to catch bass. I just need to get away from her for just a little bit because she hounds me to death. But yet, if she wouldn't hound me to death I'd say I was neglected."

The intense feeling of shame, sense of inadequacy and failure, and their attempts to maintain self-esteem by proving they are as good as they used to be, came out strikingly among the men. One patient, in responding to another patient, who was trying to perform inapproriate feats of strength, said: "It looks like you and I are trying to do the same thing, trying to prove to ourselves that we are still capable of doing the things that we did before, but we have to find a limit to it."

Another patient expressed his feelings of shame and inferiority in this way: "Regardless of what business you're in, if you have to turn something down when you're not used to saying 'no' you're always saying 'yes, I can do it'; but it comes to the point now that you have to say 'no' and that's what bothers us more than anything."

The wives expressed feelings about needing to control their husbands, being responsible for them, and somehow preventing them from having future heart trouble. One woman expressed her burden thus: "I try to shield him from the possibility of another one through stress or something that I can control, but there are many things I can't control, but still I like to think that I can."

Many of the wives felt very guilty about past negative, aggressive feelings and behaviour that they had expressed to their husbands and were therefore inhibited in expressing their feelings since the husband's heart attack. One woman stated: "I had it in my head, if I said anything cross to him in any way, that he could die, and I didn't want that on my mind." Another expressed her conflict thus: "If we know what irritates them and deliberately disregard it, should something happen I would feel terribly conscience-stricken for the rest of my life. But you're not exactly normal sometimes, not to express what you want even when you know it may affect

TABLE I. *Separate Patient Meetings*

	Theme	Group Conflict	Group Solution
1	Reliving experience of acute heart attack and speculation as to why it happened	Death anxiety vs. Need to understand and work through	Share frightening experience with others and noting positive effects of heart attack on life style
2	Four members absent. Passive, quiet meeting with difficulty expressing feelings	Anger at absentees and therapists vs. Anxiety and guilt about expressing negative feelings	Angry feelings modified to feeling disappointed and subdued
3	Discussion of heart attacks, their cause and how to avoid further trouble	Concern about a future heart attack vs. Avoidance and denial of the threat	Avoid feelings and look for intellectual answer in diet, physical activity, emotions
4	Angry feelings may get out of hand and hurt others or selves	Anger at wives and others vs. Fear of injury to others or selves	Discussion of anger and angry incidents in counterphobic way with denial of anxiety
5	The heart patients' state of helplessness and dependency	Desire to be taken care of vs. Shame	Each person should find own solution—a need for love and sympathy but also need for action by oneself
6	Change in sex life since heart attack	Need to play male role vs. Fear of injury from sex activity	Much joking. Sex not too important as one gets older. Wives not interested
7	Two members absent because of death of relatives. Need for others and concern for others	Need to be selves and express feelings vs. Concern about hurting others	People are different but can improve relationships by better communication
8	Four members absent. Two members gradually brought out individual problems	Desire for help vs. Shame over inadequacies	Everyone has problems—better to get help working them out
9	Recent cardiac deaths. Search for "Why?"	Need to explore and understand vs. Death anxiety	Ventilate anxiety but reduce tension with jokes and intellectualizing
10	Mixed feelings about terminating group. How far can one go in expressing feelings?	Desire to express feelings vs. Need to maintain control	Expression of feelings demanding on individual but something to work toward

TABLE II. *Separate Spouse Meetings*

	Theme	Group Conflict	Group Solution
1	Need to assume responsibility to feed and protect husband	Concern for husband vs. Irritation at husband's poor co-operation	Accept role of feeder and protector patiently
2	A heavy burden put on wives by husband's cardiac disability	Anger at husband's demands vs. Guilt over anger	Wives owe husbands special privileges but there is a limit to wives' giving
3	Review of husband's heart attack and wife's helpless fright	Anxiety and helplessness vs. Need to be strong and protective	Life not so bad—others worse off. Wives can control many pressures
4	Husbands not as good as before—easily upset. Wives need to be prepared for emergency	Need to express feelings vs. Fear of upsetting and hurting husband	Avoid strong feelings and be on guard for a blow-up
5	Trivial talk and difficulty talking with therapists who are men	Dependency and attraction to doctors vs. Fear of overinvolvement	Avoid involvement and dependency on doctors by keeping feelings to self
6	Anxiety about husbands and need to depend on doctor yet no right to burden others	Wish to be taken care of vs. Need to be strong and maintain control	Deny own needs in favour of husband's needs
7	Difficulty talking in the group. Is it better to forget unpleasant realities or discuss them?	Need to share anxiety about losing husband vs. Wish to avoid unpleasant feelings	Conflict handled by talking about losing husband but then denying it and forgetting about it
8	Anxiety about the future and what plans should be made in case husband dies	Desire to work through plans for future vs. Desire to escape unpleasantness	Some deny the dangers; others have completed plans; no need to talk more
9	Wife feels responsible for husband and has fear of upsetting him, yet has own needs too	Need to be self vs. Fear of hurting husband	Can learn to be one's self again but still must give extra to husband
10	Desire to help husband but may not know what is happening or what to do	Need to help husband vs. Uncertainty as to the course	Wife can't take all the responsibility. Husband and physician can carry some of load.

TABLE III. *Marital Pairs' Meeting*

Theme	Group Conflict	Group Solution
Value of meetings—share feelings and find one is not alone. Learn about different ways of looking at and handling problems	Desire to take part in group sharing of feelings vs. Anxiety about self-exposure	Talk freely—joke—intellectualize. Avoid feelings which are very frightening or unacceptable

them. Because I can sort of tell from intuition the things that will irritate my husband, like you would with a child, and I try to avoid them. But there are times when I almost revolt and I would like to be able to pick at him."

One of the wives had gone through a very stressful period with intense guilt feelings and inhibitions of expression of negative feeling towards her husband. Her husband completely controlled the family until she finally came to terms with her fear of hurting him. "Well, I have found out that the more normal that I can keep the home the better off he is. Before if he came in and said, 'I am having chest pains' I would be terribly upset and say, 'Oh, dear, how do you feel?' Well, that's worse because I know that he knows when it's severe enough that he has to call the doctor. I think initially I wasn't giving my husband credit for knowing and I sure didn't know what to do. But one can only do so much and that's it."

PHYSIOLOGICAL MEASURES

The therapy group and their matched "controls" did not differ significantly from each other with respect to blood pressure, pulse, anxiety or depression when these measurements for the six months preceding therapy were compared with those for the six-month period of therapy and the six months following therapy. The therapy group, however, had significantly higher serum cholesterol levels, both during and after therapy, than their matches ($P = .03$). The therapy group also had significantly higher serum uric acid levels following therapy than their matches ($P = .03$). No significant changes occurred in the electrocardiograms of the patients while undergoing group therapy.

FOLLOW-UP OF CLINICAL COURSE

Although the follow-up period since the termination of group therapy is short, there have been no subsequent infarctions or hospitalizations for severe chest pain among either the therapy group or their matches. However, among the four patients who refused to participate in therapy, one has experienced a second myocardial infarction and one has had a mild stroke.

DISCUSSION AND CONCLUSIONS

Our observations of this group of coronary patients suggest that considerable anxiety continues at a pre-conscious level for several years after the infarction. This anxiety is rapidly mobilized by environmental events which trigger mental associations to the heart disorder. Hence, it seems reasonable to conclude that the acute life-threatening experience of a heart attack not only demands a tremendous initial pyschological adaptation, but it remains a potent factor in the future life of some individuals.

It was interesting to observe that the patients were able to deal more openly with their feelings than were their spouses, an observation we have also made in patients with other serious clinical illnesses such as incurable cancer. It seems that it is often easier for the seriously ill patient to discuss his feelings than it is for his family or relatives to talk about it. In the men's group, anxiety, hostility, shame, and desire for dependency were all freely verbalized, and there was considerable support given by the group to individual members. The men made extensive use of joking and humour to relieve tense periods. In addition to humour, overcompensation and flight into activity appeared to be common coping mechanisms in this group of patients.

The spouses of the patients, although they seemed to benefit from expressing their feelings and sharing common problems with other wives, were definitely more inhibited. They had particular difficulty in dealing with anger toward their husbands and their guilt feelings over their husbands' disabilities. They were also unable to accept and discuss their sexual and dependent needs. They tended to deny their own needs in order to take care of their husbands. They were able, however, to express freely their anxiety and feelings of helplessness about what to do for their husbands and about the uncertainty of the future.

The women's inhibition of negative affects and of their own needs most likely resulted from their sense of responsibility for their husband's disability and their need to tightly control aggressive or sexual desires that might be harmful to the male. The tendency of the wives to deny their own dependency needs in favour of mothering their husbands seemed to be their way of coping with uncertainty. The fact that the two therapists were males may also have contributed to differences in the expression of feelings in the two groups. It seemed that the wives saw the therapists as men who would side with their husbands and be critical of the woman's role in the husband's illness rather than understanding their needs and feelings. Furthermore, in the men's group there was a tendency to compete with the therapists as rival males and to feel concern about the therapists as stronger men. The women, on the other hand, were afraid of their feelings toward the therapists and of becoming involved with them in a dependent way, perhaps through fear of being disloyal to their husbands.

The lack of cohesiveness in the women's group compared with the men's group is also an interesting phenomenon. It may be that the men were drawn closer together as victims of a life-threatening experience, and also because of their shared experiences as research subjects in the heart study. Again, the presence of two male therapists may have been a factor in the difference. The men were able to joke and tease and, at times, use profane language. The women, on the other hand, made only minor use of humour and were completely unable to use uninhibited expressions or earthy language. While the men seemed to be competing with the therapists, the women seemed to compete more among themselves for the attention of the therapists and this may have reduced group cohesiveness.

The group therapy process during the ten 75-minute sessions was not a uniform development and was influenced considerably by extraneous events. For example, such coincidental happenings as a fatal heart attack in a locally prominent young football coach led to intense death anxiety and serious doubts about physical fitness programs. About the same week in the six-month period, the co-therapist's father died and a patient's brother died of a heart attack. In the session that followed, four of the six patients were absent.

The individual group sessions varied in the level of activity and affective expression. One way of viewing the process conceptually might be Piers' circular model of psychodynamic interaction with alternating periods of activity and reaction.[10] Aggression leads to guilt or anxiety which is followed by the assumption of a passive dependent position. Dependency in turn mobilizes shame which may lead to further aggression and the cycle may recur.

While the ability of individuals to use interpersonal relationships for emotional support varied, it seemed that both the men and the women were able to share some of their feelings and find the group experience helpful and supportive. Perhaps there was less threat of over-involvement or over-dependency on one person in a group situation, and it was comforting to learn that others were experiencing some of the same feelings and problems. The groups also highlighted differences in personalities, ways of life and solutions to problems, helping patients and their wives to be more flexible in adapting to their life situations.

Serum cholesterol was the only physiological variable that showed a significant increase during the period of therapy even though emotionally charged subjects were discussed. However, both serum cholesterol and serum uric acid were elevated following therapy. It is unknown, however, whether these changes are related to the process of therapy, to environmental factors occurring outside of therapy, or to both of these.

The possibility of a detrimental influence on certain physiological parameters of an expressive type of group therapy needs to be considered in view of the report by Titchener, Sheldon and Ross[11] of such an effect on blood pressure in a group of hypertensives.

However, the literature on short-term group therapy for organic disease indicates a beneficial effect on the clinical course in most cases.[12] None of our patients during the group sessions experienced angina or physical symptoms other than some anxiety symptoms such as mild restlessness, sweating and palpitations. This suggests that patients can discuss emotionally charged material in supportive atmosphere without precipitating angina or electrocardiographic changes. This observation has practical implications for the management of cardiac patients. One of the major changes in a patient's family life is that the patient tends to become the centre of the household, and often controls the family when other members are afraid to express their feelings to him for fear of producing cardiac symptoms. This leads to a tense family atmosphere undesirable for the patient's well-being.

The therapists also had some concern about imposing stress upon the patients and perhaps producing a heart attack during a meeting. Yet if physicians are to help families deal more realistically with the relative who has had a heart attack, they must learn to respond to the patient on the basis of reality factors rather than be controlled by a fear that the patient will drop dead if they stir him emotionally or encourage him to lead an active life.

Whether the morbidity and mortality of this group of six patients will differ significantly from the control group of six patients who did not experience group therapy, cannot yet be answered. All of these patients will be followed up for a number of years, and it is hoped that data will become available to indicate some trends for future investigation. However, it is extremely difficult to separate the effects of psychotherapy from the complexities of the clinical processes of the disease.

The authors' experience with this group suggests ideas for future studies in the management of patients with myocardial infarction. Since this group therapy program was a pilot study, there is a need for clinical trials using larger treatment and control groups to obtain sufficient data for statistical analysis. In addition, different therapeutic styles need to be tried, such as using joint groups rather than separate groups. Another possibility, particularly since a myocardial infarction affects not only the patient's spouse but also his children, would be to employ family group therapy focused on family interactions.

Consideration also needs to be given to the role of psychological treatment at different phases of the post-infarction period. For example, a few individual psychotherapeutic sessions focused on the acute psychological trauma of a heart attack may be appropriate toward the end of the acute stage while the patient is in the hospital. Later, during the rehabilitative phase, group psychotherapy oriented to problems of returning to work and activities would be valuable. In addition, since our observations suggest that there may be long-term adaptation problems in the post-infarction patient, short-term group sessions might be appropriate during the chronic phase. Such sessions could be helpful for those patients who are having specific adjustment problems and who need additional support beyond that provided in the usual busy practitioner's office.

Summary. Ten patients with coronary disease who were experiencing difficulty in the long-term adaptation to their heart attacks were offered focused short-term group psychotherapy. Six of these patients chose to participate in 10 biweekly group sessions while their wives met for parallel group therapy on alternate weeks.

The therapists observed that the patients readily became anxious about further heart attacks in response to certain environmental stimuli and coped with this anxiety by joking or counterphobic behaviour. The patients also expressed deep feelings of loss of self-esteem and conflict over their need to be cared for in the presence of their continuing need to be independent. The wives saw themselves as feeders and protectors of their husbands and appeared to be overly protective and non-demanding. They were anxious regarding the uncertain future and had guilt feelings about how they might have contributed to the husband's heart attack.

Physiological monitoring of the patients at six-week intervals revealed significantly higher serum cholesterol levels during and following therapy and significantly higher uric acid levels following therapy. No significant change occurred in pulse, blood pressure or electrocardiogram and no anginal attacks were experienced during therapy sessions.

As a result of the group therapy, patients and their wives appeared to achieve an improved psychosocial adaptation. The clinical follow-up has been too brief to evaluate the long-term effect. However, among the four patients refusing therapy one has had a second infarct and another a mild stroke. None of the six patients on therapy or their "matches" have shown physical deterioration. More extensive studies of this treatment modality for coronary patients appear to be indicated.

REFERENCES

Dr. Adsett is Associate Professor of Psychiatry at McMaster University in Hamilton, Ontario. Dr. Bruhn is Associate Professor of Sociology in Medicine at the University of Oklahoma in Oklahoma City, Oklahoma.

This article evolved from the Neurocardiology Research Program, University of Oklahoma Medical Center in Oklahoma City, Oklahoma. This work was supported in part by the United States Public Health Service Research Grant No. HE–06286–07 from the National Heart Institute, U.S. Public Health Service.

1. World Health Organization. Expert committee on rehabilitation of patients with cardiovascular diseases: *W.H.O. Techn. Rep. Scr.* No. 270, 1, 1964.
2. Verwoerdt, A. and Dovenmuehle, R. H.: *Geriatrics.* 19: 856, 1964.
3. Klein, R. F. et al.: *J. A. M. A.,* 194: 143, 1965.
4. New, P. K. et al.: *Social Science and Medicine,* 2: 111, 1968.
5. Kaufman, J. G. and Becker, M. C.: *Geriatrics,* 10:355, 1955.
6. Bruhn, J. G.: *J. Okla. Med. Ass.,* 60: 65, 1967.
7. Bruhn, J. G. et al.: *Amer. J. Med. Sci.* 251: 629, 1966.
8. Whitman, R. M. and Stock, D.: *Psychiatry,* 21:269, 1958.
9. Wolberg, L. R.: The technic of short-term psychotherapy. In: *Short-term psychotherapy.* edited by L. R. Wolberg, with nine contributors, Grune & Stratton Inc., New York, 1965. p. 127.
10. Piers, G. and Singer, M.B.: Shame and guilt: a psychoanalytic and a cultural

study, monograph in *American lectures in psychiatry,* Charles C. Thomas, Publisher, Springfield, Ill., 1958.

11. Titchener, J. L., Sheldon, M. B. and Ross, W. D.: *J. Psychosom. Res.,* 4: 10. 1959.

12. Wolf, A.: Short-term group psychotherapy. In: *Short-term psychotherapy,* edited by L. R. Wolberg, with nine contributors, Grune & Stratton Inc., New York. 1965. p. 219.

Personal Awareness:
Individual Exercises

1. Imagine that one week from now a severe myocardial infarction will result in your living under major limitations, e.g., no sexual activity for one year, no working, and the knowledge that your next attack could be your last. Write a paper focusing on your activities for this week.

2. List the things that would change in your life if your spouse or loved one had coronary heart disease.

3. You have been told that chances are very good that you will have a heart attack in six months unless you drastically change your life style. Develop a program designed to help you delay or avoid having a heart attack. Can you follow through with this program? What would be most difficult for you to change?

4. Volunteer your services to your community heart association in whatever way you can be of help.

5. You have just been informed by your physician that due to your heart condition you must change your occupation. What would you do?

6. Have you taken a Cardiopulmonary Resuscitation (CPR) course? If not, why not? If you have taken a CPR course enlist at least ten other persons to do so also, if you feel it is a worthwhile experience.

7. Proper diet and exercise are two primary deterrents for future coronary problems. (1) Obtain more information about these and other health-enhancing strategies; (2) develop a systematic program for implementing these strategies to improve your life style; and (3) stick with your plan for a minimum of one month.

Structured Group Experience in Disability
—Changes*

The post-myocardial infarction patient frequently experiences intense emotional conflicts which interfere with continued functioning. This group experience is designed to acquaint participants with various life changes following a myocardial infarction and to enable them to experience the effects of such changes on one's life.

GOALS

1. To sensitize participants to unique difficulties imposed by a myocardial infarction in personal and interpersonal relationships.

2. To increase personal awareness concerning preventative aspects of coronary problems.

3. To facilitatively explore and act upon ways to make life and living more meaningful.

PRELIMINARY CONSIDERATIONS

1. *Level of Intensity:*   Medium, but may progress to higher levels in some groups.

2. *Group Size:* Groups of 6–10 participants

3. *Time Required:* 2 hours

4. *Materials:* Paper and pencil

5. *Physical Setting:* Comfortable room with moveable chairs

PROCEDURE

1. Small groups are formed.

*See Appendices A and B for detailed information on the use of the structured group experiences in disability.

2. Participants are directed to imagine that within one week they will experience a severe myocardial infarction.

3. Each member lists important ways in which his or her life would change following discharge from the hospital.

4. Group members are asked to write down their perceived feelings about the difficulty in adjusting to each change which is listed.

5. Group members individually share their changes and feelings with members of the group.

6. Each group is directed to agree on the three major changes that would be most difficult to cope with.

7. The groups are challenged to devise meaningful ways to cope with these difficulties.

8. A panel made up of one member from each group is selected to present each group's concerns and coping strategies to the large group. A discussion follows the presentation.

LEADERSHIP SUGGESTIONS

1. The leader may wish to begin with a brief talk on psychosocial aspects of postcardiac functioning.

2. To heighten the anxiety and reality of the potential heart attack, the leader may wish to relax group members and involve them with a visual imagery of themselves having a heart attack and being hospitalized.

3. A film showing a heart attack occuring and subsequent reactions of the patient and staff may be shown.

4. A key factor is to go beyond the initial task and to focus upon the changes in the person's life.

VARIATIONS

1. Rather than have the group members focus on having a heart attack themselves, attention might be directed towards a significant loved one of each participant.

2. A list of common postcardiac patient issues described in this sec-

tion could be distributed with each group member directed to rank order these issues as they would affect his or her life if a heart attack were experienced.

3. The same task as above only with a significant family member experiencing the heart attack rather than the participant.

CHAPTER SIX

Group Approaches with the Families of Disabled Persons

Overview

The parents and other relatives of disabled persons represent a virtually untapped resource for vitalizing and strengthening the rehabilitation effort. While this concept is easily understood, it is not always easily implemented. Caring for a disabled child can often be a lonely and isolating process. However, this need not be the case. One way of facing the challenge is to use the resources of the group process to provide support, encouragement, and skills to those parents and family who are faced with the reality of disability. Likewise, the importance of a supportive family for disabled adults cannot be overemphasized. The usefulness of group approaches with the families of disabled persons is highlighted by the articles in this chapter.

In the opening article "Adapting to Illness Through Family Groups," Huberty discusses the importance of group counseling for medical patients and their families to help these individuals cope with emotional stress caused by hospitalization and disease. Huberty notes that despite the wide range of physical disabilities, the problems of adapting to illness are often similar. Specific information on

Huberty's experience in conducting family groups with several diverse patient populations demonstrates that such group work had benefits for participating hospital staff as well as for patients and their families.

In "Group Therapy for Parents of Handicapped Children," Wilson presents a sensitive approach to the needs of parents who must daily face the burden of disability. By using a semi-instructional approach, the group was given the opportunity to cover a spectrum of topics, including society's acceptance of the physically handicapped and parents' reactions to their own emotions. As the parent of a handicapped child, the group leader felt an advantage in sharing a common concern with the other parents. The author believes that such parent-led groups offer great potential.

In an article entitled "Mothers of Disabled Children—The Value of Weekly Group Meetings" Linder describes the importance of group meetings for discussion of problems common to parents of disabled children. The value of meeting with others undergoing similar kinds of stress was felt by the majority of mothers who participated.

Presenting the problems encountered by parents of the hemophiliac child, Mattsson and Agle, in their article "Group Therapy with Parents of Hemophiliacs," insightfully discuss the benefits of group meetings in airing concerns and fears. The main focus of this valuable article is upon successfully coping with long-term health problems.

In "Group Treatment of Families of Burn-Injured Patients," Abramson stresses the significance for burn patients of the transition period between hospitalization and outpatient rehabilitation efforts. Abramson discusses the use of group efforts to provide relatives of the patient with an opportunity to share their common concerns and learn how to cope more effectively with their disabled family member. Abramson relates critical aspects of this special group including the structure of the group and important issues related to rehabilitation planning. In conclusion Abramson provides specific recommendations for the difficulties inherent in using family groups to help cope with traumatic injury and the rehabilitation transition following hospitalization.

"Rehabilitating the Stroke Patient Through Patient-Family Groups" by D'Afflitti and Weitz stresses the importance of family understanding and support in making a successful transition from hospital to home. Special considerations including group membership problems, group organization, and group issues and reactions are explored. Seen as an opportunity to create change, the group experience enabled many participants to share, explore, and resolve a variety of issues in their lives. D'Afflitti and Weitz introduce a comprehensive examination of the importance of the family system in the rehabilitation process.

Challenging the sensitivity of traditional psychotherapy to the needs of the physically handicapped, Heisler in her article, "Dynamic Group Psychotherapy with Parents of Cerebral Palsied Children," emphasizes the necessity of having parents become more aware of their own inner functioning and the ways that their own behavior affects the behavior and development of the child. Heisler urges a humanistic rather than behavioral approach to the problems of caring for these children and facilitating their development.

"Management of Family Emotion Stress: Family Group Therapy in a Private Oncology Practice" by Wellisch, Mosher, and Van Scoy is a most timely article which responds to the needs of cancer patients as well as their families. Highlighted are many critical issues such as guilt and other powerful emotions that are related to a group process with cancer patients. Special implications regarding children and cancer-related issues are also discussed to provide the reader with important considerations for family group practice.

In this chapter a variety of articles are presented which provide the reader with a greater awareness of the importance of utilizing the family members of persons having disabilities in the group process. Persons with disabilities do not live in a vacuum and are strongly impacted by the presence or absence of family members. By integrating family members in the disabled person's treatment program there is a far greater potential for a more comprehensive rehabilitation planning.

31

Adapting to Illness Through
Family Groups —DAVID J. HUBERTY, M.S.W.

G ROUP work for behavioral problems, psychiatric disorders or family pathology is readily accepted in most social agencies or settings where a social model of treatment is the primary modality. In hospital work, however, social work is properly described as an ancillary or supportive profession which provides supportive services to the primary professions of medicine and nursing. In this secondary setting, the role of the social worker is frequently limited to those functions assigned by the medical staff or by the hospital administration. While group treatment or group therapy is an accepted function on hospital psychiatric units, the suggestion that group counseling be done on general medical floors is often met with suspicion by the nursing staff and with reluctance, apprehension, and at times refusal of permission to see the patient from the strictly medically-oriented physicians.

Prior to 1971, medical social work at St. Mary's Hospital and St. Mary's Extended Care Center was recognized as a supportive service, the primary function of which was to assist in the more traditional medical casework problems of patients, such as making referrals to nursing homes, arranging financial assistance through local welfare departments, and facilitating other referrals, such as finding a babysitter for a patient's children, arranging remedial reading for a patient's husband, or helping patients with job problems.

The counseling potential of social casework was, in fact, accomplished indirectly through counseling that necessarily related to the specifics of the referral. However, referrals by physicians rarely, if ever, were made specifically to provide psychological support or assist a family in working through the difficult emotional changes that always accompany disability and lengthy hospitalization.

During the last three years at St. Mary's, major efforts have been made to develop and implement social group work within a variety of medical diagnostic categories. This paper describes the evolution and development of five such groups: Stroke, Oncology, Diabetes, Out-Patient Tumor Clinic, and Cardiac Surgery.

PURVIEW OF SOCIAL WORK

First, it was quite natural for group work to develop out of the Social Service Department as there are three areas of expertise relevant to group work to which social workers may lay claim. While these areas of expertise

Reprinted by permission from the *International Journal of Psychiatry in Medicine* 5 (3): 231–242, 1974. © 1974, Baywood Publishing Co., Inc.

are in no way limited to social work, they are distinct areas of professional training in a master's degree curriculum in accredited schools of social work.

1. Group Work: Social group work is one of five specialized methods in the field of social work. Schools of social work provide both academic and experiential training in group dynamics and group therapy under the supervision of experienced group workers and group therapists. Therefore, the social worker does bring specialized training and developed skills to the group method of counseling.

2. Family Dynamics: The process of adapting to illness is not one that takes place within each patient in isolation but rather is an interactional process of adjustment between the patient and his spouse, his children, his parents, as well as among those significant others as they form a network of emotional and social supports. It is the family system that encounters major adjustments as a result of one member's hospitalization. Changes in employment and income, decision-making roles, and responsibility are just a few of the non-medical components that affect and complicate the patient's adaptation to his medical diagnosis and very possibly impinge upon his rehabilitation. As a result of specific training in family dynamics and family therapy along with a theoretical framework of a "systems" approach to counseling, social workers tend to view the family as a necessary component in any individual's healthy response to change.

3. Emotional and Social Components of Illness: As a profession with its training orientation balanced between sociology and psychology, social workers are oriented by training and experience to the emotional and social components of the vicissitudes of life, including illness, disability, and dying.

With these three areas of focus within the purview of social work, the Social Service Department at St. Mary's Medical Complex was available to be of broader service to the patient by working with him and his family in group counseling sessions. Also, social workers had demonstrated their group work skills on the psychiatric unit and on an adolescent drug unit. Therefore, development of the medical groups was essentially an extension and combination of two approved areas of social work practice within the hospital—psychiatric *group work* (and family counseling) and *medical* casework. While the five medical groups discussed in this paper did not begin meeting at the same time, they do have a number of elements in common, discussed here in a generic way, followed by a more specific description of each medical group with examples illustrating the development of the program and the success of a particular group session in a patient's life or that of his family.

ADAPTING TO ILLNESS

There are similarities among the broad diagnoses of cancer, stroke, heart attack, and diabetes and the group formations in these areas. First, in adapting to a major change in one's life, it is universally true that the person goes through a *process* moving towards acceptance or an adjustment to his new status in life. Accompanying long-term hospitalization, physical limitations from a chronic illness or disability may be perceived as a loss of freedom and the beginning of unwanted dependency. Whether a patient uses his illness and feelings for self-pity or for motivation for recovery will largely depend on how successfully he works through various emotional stages leading to assigning some significance of his illness to his life's goals.

Kübler-Ross identifies five stages of grief in the dying process.[1] Similar stages, which may manifest considerable overlap, may also be applied to a patient and his family who are adapting to a major medical change in their lives. There is initially some *denial* of the limitations of the disability followed by *anger* over "why me?" This is frequently followed by *bargaining* with medical personnel, family members or just within one's own mind: "If I am a good patient, I will get well quicker," or "If my surgery is successful, I'll start going to church again regularly." This phase is likely to be followed by *depression* as one realizes that the disability is permanent or that the limitations imposed by the disability are, in fact, real. The final stage in the adjustment process is an *acceptance* of the *realistic* limitations of the disability with perhaps an alteration of life goals or an incorporation of the illness into the meaning of life resulting in a calm optimism. Thus, the *process* of adapting to the illness and disability is a working premise in medical group work with the patient.

A second *common* characteristic, if not completely universal, is that families will also go through a similar kind of process. Although this is perhaps more dramatic and therefore more apparent with the family of the dying patient, it is nevertheless just as real in any serious illness. For both the patient and his family there is a great degree of psychological uncertainty. This, of necessity, results in anxiety, frustration, anger, and depression. In terms of family dynamics, it is of note that in one study where the patients were recovering from myocardial infarction, 100 per cent of the families interviewed evidenced "steady eroding conflict" and disruptive family relationships.[2] It is not unreasonable to anticipate that similar family disruption may occur in an equally high percentage of families where the patient has some other serious disability. Even the most stable marriage and family relationship are challenged if not marred by the disability. Of course, couples and families frequently will respond to the crisis of hospitalization and disability with increased sensitivity and understanding. In these cases the result is closer interpersonal ties and a deeper emotional strength. Every major crisis provides the dual opportunity for destruction or growth. It is not crisis that destroys families, marriages, or individuals, but how they choose to negotiate that crisis and deal with it.

Throughout these universal processes of adaptation to illness, it is appropriate that even very normal and emotionally healthy families experiencing such crises be assisted in this adjustment and grieving by the use of group work. Over and over again families remark on how helpful it is to talk with others experiencing similar circumstances. Sharing and comparing unfamiliar challenges and pain draw a strength previously untapped, partly achieved through giving emotional support to other patients or families who are hurting more. Families are specifically invited and encouraged to attend each of the group sessions. Although attendance by family members varied, family involvement did increase as the groups became more universally understood and accepted by the medical and nursing staff as well as the families themselves.

The group setting is unique in providing the opportunity for development of a mutual support system. Also, more advanced or experienced group members may provide assurances from their broader perspective on the disability and the adjustment process to the newer members. No other counseling context provides for this mutual support.

DEVELOPMENT OF MEDICAL COUNSELING GROUPS

All medical group work at St. Mary's follows the multidisciplinary team approach, each group co-led in some combination by a social group worker, a nurse, an occupational therapist, and chaplain. Each group evolved out of a different area within the hospital and required different administrative procedures for implementation. Each of the groups was initiated after a hospital staff member identified a need for some level of counseling for a patient and/or his family in order to help them adjust to the particular disease.

GOALS OF THE GROUP

Each group has the general goal of assisting the patient, preferably with his family, in working through the stages leading toward acceptance of disability or illness and adjusting to it as a family unit. Working with patients and their families requires sensitivity to a wide range of emotions which may interfere with a healthy adjustment and to the various ways a health crisis will be interpreted by family members. A family's interpretation of a crisis will have a great effect on how the patient responds to treatment and rehabilitation. If interpreted as a threat, the crisis will produce anxiety; if interpreted as a loss, it will produce depression; if interpreted as a challenge, both anxiety and hope will create problem-solving energy and promote motivation and individual growth as well as emotional growth within the family unit.[3] Certainly if different family members interpret the crisis in different ways, the initial goal is to help the members identify and clarify to each other the various subjective meanings of the crisis. Thus, while we may describe some specific goals for each group, the goals for an individual patient and his family within a group session may become very individualized to fit their needs at that moment.

CASE EXAMPLES

While the specific cases below are not uncommon, they have, nonetheless, been chosen to illustrate some of the more dramatic positive results of the group work process. The support of other persons in the same situation is a powerful tool in helping families cope with a difficult change in their lives. There are also case examples of people who have stayed away from the groups because they were not yet ready to face the crisis or who preferred to adapt through their own family supports or directly with the help of their physician. The groups were consciously designed to permit people the option of not attending or of freely leaving a group session if they felt uncomfortable for any reason.

STROKE GROUP

The first medical counseling group evolved out of the need for families to obtain more information about strokes in general and the rehabilitative progress of their family member in particular. After an afternoon lecture approach failed to meet these needs, a family group discussion format was initiated during evening hours. Since the stroke rehabilitation program ranges between two weeks and three months, patients and families could be expected to attend between two and twelve group sessions. In addition to helping them adapt to communication problems and the physical limitations imposed by a recent stroke, the "Family Involvement Evening," as the group was called, enabled the staff to get a better picture of the patient's family and therefore begin discharge planning earlier and more completely. The groups enabled the social worker to work with the family earlier in the rehabilitation process in an effort to help them and the patient work through the guilt, anger, and stigma[4], always present to some degree. Since these three feelings tend to get in the way of *expecting* and *allowing* maximum independence from the patient, it is extremely important that they be openly discussed and confronted.

Case Example.   The patient was a woman in her late 60's. She and her husband had been very close most of their forty years of marriage. Their daughter lived out of town and was therefore unable to attend the group; one son, age 35, the patient's favorite, sided with his mother on most issues; another son, age 29, appeared to be favored by his father and, although quiet, supported his father's point of view.

The patient's husband was completely overwhelmed by her stroke and debilitated condition. Because of his deep feelings of love and concern, he immediately made it clear to the doctors and the staff that he would spend whatever was necessary to give her the best of care: "She deserves the excellent care that she is getting here. She can stay here for the rest of her life!" The thought of ever taking his wife home with the responsibility for her care was more than he could face.

The staff soon realized that despite the patient's good potential to return home, the husband's attitude was a major rehabilitation barrier. His level of coping with the crisis was to "pay for the best of care." Counseling also needed to be done with the older son who, through his denial of the real limitations imposed by his mother's stroke, maintained that she could be *completely* independent again. The younger son's blind acceptance of his father's view of the stroke and plan for institutional care needed to be tempered too.

Each new step in rehabilitation was interpreted by the patient's husband as a set-back. When the patient was scheduled to receive a leg brace, he interpreted this as a crisis and "proof" for his belief that she would never recover. In the group setting, however, another patient who had recently received a brace announced, "This is what your wife's brace is going to do," and he stood up and began walking around the group. This well-timed demonstration helped the husband realize that a brace was progress. Within a few weeks, however, the husband had moved to the other extreme: "I look forward to the day when I can dance with Joan again." At that point a non-patient in the group strongly confronted: "You're putting your goals on her and she probably won't be able to reach them and do you know what that's going to do to her?" The husband's gradual realization that he was projecting his own unrealistic hopes was followed by depression. Because he had not really faced her disability realistically, he was still hesitant to take his wife home and only did so reluctantly on a "trial weekend." That weekend his wife proved that, although limited, she could generally function well at home *with his help*. He *experienced* that she *needed* him and that he could, in fact, assist her and provide good care. Her affect improved markedly over that weekend and only then did he begin to understand how important it was for her to return home.

Over a period of twelve weeks and twelve group sessions the patient's husband moved from a denial of rehabilitation and his role in that process, through anger and depression, and finally on to an acceptance of the realities of the stroke, including both its *limitations* and *potential*. Without this rather lengthy process in group, the patient would most likely have been institutionalized because her husband simply wanted "the best possible care," which he was convinced was expensive, long-term institutional care.

Oncology Family Group

Patients who are either weakened by the disease itself or by treatments for their cancer are hospitalized in the Extended Care Center's specialized Oncology Unit for two weeks to several months. These are patients with disseminated cancer in advanced stages. Therefore, the goals of this specialized unit are totally directed towards helping the patient increase his physical strength and achieve optimum health and independence within the confines of his disease.

The Oncology Family Group was more specifically directed towards helping the family and patient to assess on a physical, social, and psychological level what would be the best placement upon discharge; frequently this was back home, but at times nursing homes or other placements are more appropriate for all concerned. While the groups primary function is to help the patient, one of the most effective and efficient ways of helping and supporting a patient is to deal with the whole system of people involved with that patient.[5] This means a process of adjustment working its way down from the spouse, children, perhaps extended family members and also staff members who may get very involved and feel very close to the patient.[6] These are all people who *directly* affect the patient. The following case illustrates the impact of dying on other members in the family network.

Case Example. The patient, a woman age 56, with stomach cancer and metastasis to her lungs and breasts, had been in the Extended Care Center nine weeks. She was failing rapidly at the time of the group session recounted here and was too ill to attend. It was the sixth group for her husband, her two sons and the wife of the younger son.

The younger son told the group how he had always felt left out of the family process. He frequently did things contrary to his parents' preferences, including marrying against their wishes. He felt guilty about having to stand by what he felt was right and yet watch his parents grieve and hurt. Now with his mother dying he felt he wanted to be forgiven for some of his decisions. He wanted to have the opportunity to express to his mother how he really had made some mistakes and how she was right in many ways. The group accepted what he said and suggested his going to her and telling her how he felt. One nurse added her support by telling this son how his mother had expressed her desire to forgive her children of some things; the mother had said she felt bad that they had been reaching out to her for so many years and yet never really touched despite their being a close family; that because of the dying process, things had fallen into a different perspective for her and what really mattered was that they were together.

For the family this process provided a new perspective and new ways of relating: The husband of the patient really heard what his son had said and responded with the brief comment that "I've always had a hard time expressing my emotions in a physical or verbal way too." At this point, his daughter-in-law looked towards him and told him she never realized he could not express his feelings: "I've always been afraid of you, but now I feel like hugging you." Her father-in-law said nothing, but other group members encouraged her to do just that.

A death in a family is still a death and a loss but also a "rebirth" for many family members, depending on how they choose to negotiate the crisis. This family's searching into themselves allowed the patient to die a relatively peaceful and happy death and enabled the living members to become closer. As one nurse observed after the group: "He lost a wife but gained a daughter-in-law and a new kind of son he never knew existed before." This patient died four hours after the group session ended.

DIABETIC GROUP

The Diabetic Group developed from a need identified by a nurse patient-teaching coordinator who felt that the five classes which offer factual information to in-hospital diabetic patients simply did not deal with some of the emotional components of diabetes. She noted that inaccurate information about diabetes within the family network was not getting clarified because of the families' apparent emotional blocking of clarifications. On her request a social worker sat in on one of the classes each week and attempted to take the last twenty minutes of the class to discuss how patients felt about being diabetic. After a number of relatively unsuccessful weeks using this structure, a sixth hour within the diabetic class schedule was added and geared towards the feeling level of the patients.

The goals in this group were three-fold: 1) to give the patient an opportunity to share his feelings regarding his diabetes, 2) to clarify misinformation, and 3) to evaluate the patient's level of adjustment to his diabetes. This evaluation was then communicated to the attending physician by charting in the Physician's Progress Notes any concern about the progress of the patient's adjustment.

Case Example.   Mr. Stevens, a 37-year-old laborer, had, a year prior to the hospitalization, been doing a great deal of heavy lifting at his job. At that time he was promoted to foreman, which meant his work time was spent supervising rather than lifting. Despite clearly explained etiology of diabetes, Mr. Stevens in the group setting continued to blame his job promotion for his "catching diabetes." "If I had kept working hard I wouldn't have this [weakling's] disease." He further described that the disease meant a real *loss of freedom:* "Instead of being able to eat a twelve ounce steak I am now limited to a three ounce steak." Severe depression was the most accurate way to describe Mr. Stevens' reaction to his diabetes. The threat to his masculinity was hinted at in his reference to his job. With his high level of anxiety and the way in which he was interpreting his diabetes, it would not be unlikely for this patient to return home and experience temporary sexual impotence along with other manifestations of depreciated self-esteem.

Since the physician's major concern in the effective management of diabetes is the *reaction* of the individual,[7] this information was relayed to the attending physician for follow-up with the patient after discharge from the hospital. It should be added that Mr. Stevens' obvious depression was not only ignored but chastised by some well-meaning nursing personnel. Since they understood the disease process of diabetes, they were quick to try to cheer up the patient by telling him just how lucky he was not to have a more serious disease and that he "should not feel depressed." Not accepting his depression meant that he was not accepted as a person, which further confirmed his interpretation that "it is not okay to be a diabetic."

TUMOR CLINIC GROUP

In June 1973, a new chaplain joined St. Mary's staff. He questioned many hospital personnel on what they thought he might bring to hospital programming. A nurse in the emergency room mentioned that a group of outpatient cancer patients came to the hospital every Tuesday for blood analysis, medication and an examination by their physician. Since they usually had a long wait in the clinic, she thought that perhaps he could "visit" with them and therefore help their time go faster. The result was informal group discussions initiated by the chaplain and a social worker for a period of about two months during which time the group became more formalized and structured. Since the discussions repeatedly returned to the side effects of radiation and chemotherapy and the terminal possibilities of cancer, this group provided an opportunity for an exchange of experiences, thoughts, and feelings that are often avoided by relatives and friends of cancer patients. Weekly memorandums provided feedback to the attending physicians of a patient's social and psychological developments.

Since the patients in the tumor clinic have cancer in an advanced stage, many of them will be returning to the hospital as inpatients sometime in the foreseeable future (six months to three years). Usually family contact with hospital personnel ceases during periods of out patient cancer treatment. At the very time they need support the most they frequently have no one to talk with.[8] One result of the weekly group sessions has been the development of a close relationship with the chaplain who has assisted some of the patients and their families through the dying process many months later.

Case Example.   One member of the group was a 17-year-old girl with a primary tumor (fibrosarcoma) on her wrist with metastasis to the brain. She and her family and hospital personnel knew that her life expectancy was short. Also in the group that day was a 65-year-old man whose wife was being discharged from inpatient care to a "cancer home" where she would, with all certainty, soon die. He had just received that news and came to the group somewhat lost, emotionally numb, fearful of the future, and near to tears.

The young girl was able to leave that group with some hope for herself and a thanksgiving over still having a number of weeks, or months, or perhaps a few years, ahead of her in contrast to the man's wife who had a limited number of days or, at most, weeks to live. Although saddened, the older man was also able to leave the group having shared his grief with some people who could relate closely with his loss. He left feeling somewhat better that he had had many good years with his wife. There was no way of making the situation better for either of them and there was no attempt on the part of the group to do that. But it was clear that he was supported by the group and the group members were able to give of themselves and to share in his pain. He was not alone!

CARDIAC FAMILY GROUP

The Cardiac Group was the only one that grew directly out of the social workers' assumption that cardiac patients and their families likely experience emotional reactions similar to that of other chronic disease patients. Based on that assumption a review of the literature was made and a proposal written to the hospital Coronary Patient Education Committee. After several rewritings and assurances to the physicians and nursing staff, the group began under co-leadership of a head nurse, chaplain, occupational therapist, and social group worker.

A specific goal was to provide families an opportunity to discuss with staff their concerns regarding the unexpected current hospitalization of their cardiac patient and what might be expected when he returned home. Prior to the group effort, families were seeking out busy nurses on a one-to-one basis. The group setting allowed time for such questions as well as an opportunity to discuss possible changes in family life that might result from the illness.

Case Example.   At the time of this writing, the Cardiac Group has been in existence for only four weeks. While no specific case is cited here, we have noticed with this group an extension of the mutual support system that builds in all of the groups. Families have quickly gotten to know each other on a personal level surrounding the crisis of cardiac surgery.

Having met and shared their fears, guilt, and uncertainty, they continue supporting one another outside of the group sessions throughout the hospital stay. Group members help alleviate the loneliness experienced during hospitalization. They spend time together in waiting rooms, at meal time, and during evening hours, visiting one another's hospitalized family member and often continuing this concern and support after discharge.

CONCLUSION

In developing a number of medical groups, the Social Service Department has attained greater visibility and consequently increased casework referrals. More importantly, the existence of the medical family counseling groups has called widespread attention within the hospital to the emotional, social, and family components of adjusting to illness and hospitalization. As a result, the groups have served as a tool for inservice education for nursing staff, physcians, and other ancillary hospital personnel. Social group work skills have been learned well by non-social workers and leadership for some of the groups has been assumed by non-social work personnel. Nurses, occupational therapists, and chaplains co-lead in all the groups with the assistance of the social worker. This interdisciplinary approach has facilitated staff relationships.

It should be emphasized that all of the groups have worked mainly with emotionally healthy patients and families experiencing acute stress related to hospitalization. As a result, family pathology and underlying family problems have not been the focus of the groups; the groups have, however, consistently helped reduce the anxiety of patients and their families about the particular disease and prepared them for more full and independent lives while living with the disease or disability.

REFERENCES

David Huberty was formerly Director of Social Services at St. Mary's Hospital in Minneapolis, Minnesota, and is currently the Coordinator of Detoxification and Halfway House Services at The Central Minnesota Mental Health Center in St. Cloud, Minnesota.

1. Kübler-Ross, E.: *On death and dying.* New York, Macmillan, 1969.
2. Cassem, N. H., Hackett, T. P.: Psychological rehabilitation of myocardial infarction patients in the acute phase. *Heart and Lung* 2:382–88, 1973.
3. Rapoport, L.: The state of crisis: some theoretical considerations. *Crisis intervention: Selected readings.* Edited by Parad H. New York, Family Service Association of America, 1965, pp. 129–39.
4. Hyman, M.: Social psychological determinants of patients' performance in stroke rehabilitation. *Arch. Phys. Med.* 53:217–25, 1972.
5. Brennan, M. J.: The cancer gestalt. *Geriatrics* 25:96–101, 1970.
6. Carey, R. G.: Living until death. *Hosp. Prog.* 55:82–87, 1974.
7. Kimball, C. P.: Emotional and psychosocial aspects of diabetes mellitus. *Med. Clin. N. Amer.* 55:1007–1018, 1971.
8. Hertzberg, L. J.: Cancer and the dying patient. *Amer. J. Psychiat.,* 128:40–44, 1972.

32

Group Therapy for Parents
of Handicapped Children
—ARTHUR L. WILSON, M.Ed.

P ARENTS of normal children often need help in developing and maintaining a stable emotional atmosphere in their family. Parents of handicapped children have an even greater problem in creating an emotion-free atmosphere within the family, for the child's handicap acts as a disruptive factor in the normal parent-child relationship. The disabled child's emotional stability is a major factor in his ability to function as an autonomous and independent person in life, and independence is the goal of all who work with him. Often the child's emotions are a function of environmental stimuli, the most obvious of which is his family.

In most cases, the handicapped child has suffered a minimum of emotional damage since the disability has been present from birth. A constant stress, however, has been placed on the parents, who have suffered the birth trauma, continual visits to physicians for diagnosis, never-ending hospitalizations for treatment or surgery, and countless hours in conveying their child to clinics for therapy or to specialized schools. Yet few people

Reprinted by permission from *Rehabilitation Literature* 32: 332–335, 1971.

realize the tremendous emotional expense involved in years of dealing with disability. Most people see only the happy and smiling faces of mother and child in the neighborhood supermarket. Each passing person looks sympathetically at the child on crutches or in a wheelchair. Little ladies smile and pat the child on the head, while the child is unable to understand the reason for the interest. Understandably the public attention is directed toward the person who is visibly different from the others, not to the one who has endured the emotional assault.

There are literally thousands of social agencies in this country offering services to handicapped people. Many of these agencies, too often, fail to see beyond the visible handicap in offering their service to the child and do not deal with the real source of family stability, the parents. Too frequently these agencies focus on superficial services designed to make the children happy without recognizing and treating the potential emotional disability at its source.

IN an attempt to treat the needs of these parents, a series of eight group therapy sessions was conducted for parents of handicapped children under the aegis of the local Easter Seal Society and a Title VI Regional Special Education Center. This represented the first attempt, in the locality, to bring parents of handicapped children together for the purpose of discussing common problems of raising a special child. Most parents and observers felt the sessions to be successful in providing emotional outlet and group reinforcement and support. By the eighth session, many members had expressed a desire to continue to function, not only to provide support for each other but to work toward increasing the number of services for handicapped families in the area. The success of the therapy sessions demonstrated the need of parents for services administered directly to them, as well as those for their disabled child.

The group of parents who met were selected from a list of potential participants compiled from the records of the Easter Seal Society, the county health department, and specialized schools for the handicapped. Parents were contacted intially by form letter, which brought in little response. Only after the parents were contacted personally would they make a commitment to attend the sessions. The parents finally consenting to attend had children with cerebral palsy, blindness, deafness, spina bifida, mental retardation, or muscular dystrophy. They were of divergent interests and background, yet their one common interest—their child—erased the diversity of background and allowed them to discuss freely their problems and concerns. The series of eight meetings demonstrated that each parent had experienced similar traumas, disappointments, and frustrations in dealing with his child's disability. Those with older children, who had been through the trial-and-error process of raising a special child, were able to share their experiences with younger parents just beginning the arduous routine. Parents of the older children, too, verbalized their frustrations in finding suitable schools to meet the needs of their child, the problems of transportation to school once it was found, and the ever-present difficulty in maintaining normal peer social relationships.

Each session was structured to utilize a semi-instructional approach that would stimulate parent interaction. The instructional base would provide stimulus to initiate discussion from a cold group working within an hour's time limit. It could also help to salvage a session in case parent interaction failed to materialize. Topics of discussion were:

—Does Your Child Display Concern Over His Handicap? This session will focus on the handicapped child's emotions and the role that emotions play in developing independent functioning. Technics that parents may use to foster healthy emotional growth will be discussed.

—How Can Parents Deal with Their Own Frustrations and Emotions? This discussion will center around the parent-child interaction and the resulting effect on the parents.

—How To Help Your Child Learn. This session will center around basic ideas of learning and emphasize methods and technics that parents can use at home to encourage intellectual growth in their handicapped child.

—Help Your Child Get More Out of Life. Each person evaluates himself. Handicapped persons may think of themselves as being inferior. The parent must help the child to develop positive and worthwhile attitudes about himself.

—Society's Acceptance of the Physically Handicapped. A discussion of the attitudes of other people toward the crippled child, a look at the reasons behind these views, and some ideas for dealing with them.

—How To Deal with Unwanted Sympathy and Help. The problem of sympathy and pity will be discussed in terms of its insincerity and devaluation of the child.

—Guarding Against Overprotection. This session will deal with identifying interactions in the home environment that foster a dependency of the handicapped child. The goal of the parent should be to make the child as self-sufficient as possible.

—Your Important Role in the Teen Years. This final session will deal with the physical changes the adolescent child undergoes and their special significance for the child with a disability.

The group leader presented this syllabus to the parents at the first meeting. The parents were encouraged to suggest topics in addition to those listed. Interest was high in all topic areas and the group also wanted to include the problems of sibling rivalry and transportation. These two areas seemed to be of common concern to the group members irrespective of their child's age or handicap. Discussion of transportation problems consumed a great deal of time and culminated in a presentation by a representative of the Ohio Division of Special Education. Transportation seemed a problem to parents due to their child's inability to move about by ordinary means, causing a constant drain on the time and energy of the family. Sibling rivalry is severely intensified in the family with a special child. Evidently the increased attention the parent must direct to the handicapped child accents the rivalry and jealousy of siblings. Solution of this is a major challenge to parents.

TWELVE people attended the first meeting. Informality was achieved by serving coffee, arranging chairs in a circle, providing name tags, and holding the sessions in a small room. The persons' being close encouraged individual discussion before and after each session. Because most of the 12 had not previously met, personal interaction prior to the meeting was minimal. As the session began, the atmosphere in the room was cold and unyielding. The group leader opened the session by talking, which served to put the members at ease and to draw the group's attention to a common purpose.

After a few general remarks, the leader spoke of his own experience in raising a handicapped child. This included a description of the child's problem, the clinical aspects of the birth, and the frustrations in raising the child. This dialogue soon impelled each parent to recall similar experiences and feelings so that the strangeness of the situation was quickly forgotten. Comments from the members began. Eventually each parent wanted to tell of his child's handicap and the problems and emotions that he had experienced at some point in the child's life.

Later meetings were conducted similarly. The group leader initiated the discussion by speaking of the subject scheduled for that session and, invariably, the comments would create a chain of reaction from the group. Most members' remarks related to their own experience or belief. Parent talk would be greatest following a group member's account of some personal experience or frustration in raising his child. It usually involved a problem with which every other parent could directly identify.

Often the hour would pass before a subject under discussion was closed. When this happened, the group leader would use the first few minutes of the next week's session to restate comments and ideas of the previous meeting. This would ignite the same tempo of interaction until the subject had been exhausted. A scheduled topic would be sacrificed if the group demonstrated a need to pursue an idea of the previous meeting or if a new question had arisen during the week. Most sessions resulted in an entire hour's being used by parent interaction after only a few remarks by the leader at the beginning.

Once the group began interacting, the leader would withdraw from the discussion to allow free interaction. The leader did not attempt to control the direction or subject matter of the parents. The group leader would emerge only to clarify points, to interpret what was being said, or to bring closure to a subject or session.

A pattern of group behavior became apparent: After the leader had withdrawn from the discussion and the parent interaction had continued for a length of time, discussion would disintegrate so that the parents were talking to their neighbors in groups of two or three with a complete loss of central group focus. The leader would then emerge, restate the comments and thoughts prior to the group breakdown, and move the group, as a single unit, again on a discussion of this issue. There was no attempt by the leader to keep the group discussion on the topic listed for that session. The group, as a matter of fact, typically did not continue to discuss the topic presented by the leader but would, usually very quickly, move to other topics that came about as a result of the interaction. Again there was no attempt by the leader to control the direction of the group as long as the discussion was centered, with everyone participating. After the first few minutes of each session, the parents themselves became the group leaders.

DURING the last three sessions, guest speakers were invited to attend and talk on a subject of interest to the group. They were specialists in the areas of transportation, mental retardation, and social agency services. These people followed the same format used by the group leader, taking the first part of the hour to speak and then requesting questions from the group members. It was noticeable that group participation and interaction were severely delayed whenever a guest was present. The group leader usually had to ask a series of questions or to direct questions to group members before any discussion or interaction could begin.

It is interesting to note that new members who entered the group periodically after the first meeting did not have a deleterious effect on the group interaction. Evidently the entry level of the new person was the prime consideration in group interference. If the new member was an equal, acceptance was immediate. If, however, the new person was not a peer but someone attending the session to speak and inform, an outsider, acceptance was not tendered. In attempting to weigh the advantages of the information gained by the group from the guest speakers against the therapeutic value of their own interaction, the latter would have to be considered the more valuable.

THE sessions were held in a classroom adjacent to the gymnasium at a local university. Therapy groups were conducted simultaneously with a Saturday morning recreation program for handicapped children. The parents brought their child to the recreation program and went across the hall for the group session. This tandem approach was most instrumental in getting parents to attend the therapy sessions regularly. Most important in their minds, a service was being provided for their child that they would make an extra effort to make use of, yet their time was being utilized doubly by their attendance at the group session. As an added encouragement the parents were paid $5.00 expense money for each of the eight meetings they attended. Initially it was felt that the money would be a prime motivating factor. It became the opinion of most observers, however, that the parents would have attended without the money. Three considerations appear to account for their attendance: *1)* they had to bring their child to the recreation program anyway, *2)* their time and effort were doubly utilized, and *3)* they wanted to meet with other parents and discuss common experiences and the problems of raising a special child.

The group leader was a parent of a handicapped child and a trained psychologist. The fact of parenthood, however, seemed to be the outstanding qualification in determining the success of the group. The greatest degree of discussion and interaction typically occurred after the leader had revealed some emotion or insight that only a parent could have experienced. These emotions of raising a handicapped child appeared to evoke the empathy and memory of the group, which led to the interaction.

On the basis of this experience, it appears feasible that such parent groups could be formed without payment of a stipend and could be conducted by a person other than a trained psychologist. Although the leader's training in counseling and psychology certainly had an impact on the success of the group, the commonality of special parenthood appeared to be the most important consideration. It would seem that, with some guidance and instruction, parents of handicapped children could form and lead such groups. A perceptive parent with a high degree of emotional security and a minimal need for ego-reinforcement would likely be the most successful. This security would allow the parent to tolerate the criticisms and defenses of the group members and to withdraw from group discussion without trying to dominate and control it. Appropriate instruction for such parents should include technics for initiating discussion, withdrawing from the interaction, emerging to clarify, interpret, or unify the group, and then withdrawing again from the discussion.

IN summary, it appears that there is a need among parents of handicapped children to meet and discuss problems with others experiencing the same problems. Since a dearth of trained professionals may be available in various areas to conduct such groups, astute parents may be selected and instructed to conduct the groups with a minimum of training and time involved. Combining the right personality with a few basic technics could lead to a successful group experience. Providing a program for the parent and child simultaneously will insure greater attendance and regularity than if parent and child are asked to attend at different times. Maintaining group membership (introducing no new variables) would lead to the most effective interaction. When these factors are combined, a successful group experience may be expected.

REFERENCES

Arthur Wilson is a staff psychologist for the Fairborn Board of Education, Fairborn, Ohio, and has been engaged in private practice for the past two years.

Arbuckle, Dugald S. *Counseling: Philosophy, theory and practice.* Boston: Allyn and Bacon, 1965.

Ayrault, Evelyn West. *You can raise your handicapped child.* New York: G. P. Putnam's Sons, 1964.

Benjamin, Alfred. *The helping interview.* Edited by C. Gilbert Wrenn. Boston: Houghton Mifflin, 1969.

Ross, Alan O. *The exceptional child in the family; helping parents of exceptional children.* New York: Grune and Stratton, 1964.

Spock, Benjamin, and Lerrigo, Marion O. *Caring for your disabled child.* New York: Macmillan, 1965.

Tyler, Leona E. *The work of the counselor. (3rd ed.)* New York: Appleton-Century-Crofts, 1969.

Woody, Robert H. *Behavioral problem children in the schools; recognition, diagnosis, and behavioral modification.* New York: Appleton-Century-Crofts, 1969.

Wright, Beatrice A. *Physical disability—A psychological approach.* New York: Harper and Bros., 1960.

33

Mothers of Disabled Children
—the Value of Weekly Group Meetings
—RALPH LINDER

THE parents of a chronically ill or disabled child are in an obviously difficult situation, to understate the case considerably. Their situation is a totally novel and unexpected one and, paradoxically, is a direct correlate of medical progress. The chronically ill, disabled, or dying child is a rarity nowadays, whereas a half-century ago such tragedies were commonplace and it was an unusually fortunate family that did not have immediate contact with childhood morbidity and mortality.

This rarity is in itself the cause of one of the problems which parents of a disabled child must face; that of the child's behaviour. At a time when most children are healthy, popular theories of behaviour are not immediately relevant to the parents of a child afflicted with disability or disease. How, for instance, are the parents to know where sickness ends and temperament begins?

A second problem is that of relating to the medical establishment. Even the healthiest child is occasionally ill or will have routine medical contacts for check-ups and immunizations. Because of this, most parents will

Reprinted from *Developmental Medicine and Child Neurology,* vol. 12, 1970, 202–206, by permission of the Editor.

have an opportunity to compare experiences and reactions. In contrast, the chronically ill child is usually treated in a large and impersonal medical center with which neither the parents nor their friends will have had any previous contacts. Accordingly the parents have no guidelines to action.

These are only two of the dilemmas which face such parents, and to a very large extent these and other problems arise from a lack of contact with others who are in the same situation.

THE GROUP

For the past six months the author has had a weekly meeting with what is now a group of five mothers of children disabled by muscular dystrophy, cerebral palsy, or congenital cardiac anomaly. There was no clearly defined goal in mind in starting this group, except that individual contacts with such parents had demonstrated their sense of isolation and their sometimes desperate search for answers to their problems. The feeling was that perhaps these parents could help each other, and we suggested to some of them that they might like to get together and compare notes.

We started with a list of twelve parents, chosen largely because they were felt to be in need of such an experience and because they were also felt to be in tune with our vaguely defined purpose. Of this initial dozen, eight appeared for at least one session. Some dropped out immediately because they did not see how their child would gain any significant benefit from parental 'talk.' One lady, described later, stopped attending because she found the emotions aroused to be overwhelming. Finally, after some months, we arrived at our present membership of five mothers. It was attempted to recruit fathers as well, but since the meetings are held during the day this was unsuccessful.

THE FIRST STAGE

The mothers who joined our group were indeed alone. All of them have husbands and other members of the family; they have friends: they have doctors (in the plural this often means they have no doctor at all); they have therapists and they have a social worker: yet they were alone in the sense that none of them had any contact with *other* parents of disabled children.

They had all initially responded to their respective tragedies by going into a kind of mourning and at the time we began these meetings four of the mothers were still in that state. Three mothers had children whose diagnoses augured an early death and these women felt socially isolated not only because they had no heart for enjoyment of the normal diversions and preoccupations of life, but also because those of their friends and family who knew about the child felt uncomfortable in their presence. In all the women, the sense of being alone was constantly reinforced by the questions which were never answered. Does one discipline a disabled child? Does one send a dying child to school? Is it 'normal' to find oneself occasionally

wishing a chronically ill and deteriorating child already dead? What of the
healthy siblings; is it 'normal' to neglect them under the circumstances?
How does one explain what is happening both to the disabled child and to
the sibs? These and many other questions were always presenting themselves. They were occasionally asked of doctors, although the parents knew
that they were not really medical in nature and that, at best, they would
merely get another person's opinion.

When these mothers came together for the first time, there occurred a
kind of initiation rite, which was repeated in subsequent weeks as new
members joined the group. It consisted of introductions followed by descriptions of the circumstances leading to the diagnosis of their children's
conditions. It was typical for the descriptions to begin with the child's manifestation of some peculiarity, usually belittled by the pediatrician but,
because it persisted, eventually leading to the child being brought to a major medical center. In some cases the subsequent diagnosis was made
readily and in others only after prolonged investigations, but each mother
had her horror story to tell. And the stories were horrible indeed, not simply because of the facts of the illness, but also because of the manner in
which these facts were conveyed. A hospital corridor, a harassed and indif-
ferent intern or resident, the parents frantic about the child; these were the
often-reported elements in what was perhaps the most devastating event in
these parents' lives. Tears were shed each time these stories were told, tears
of anguish and anger on the part of the teller and tears of sympathy on the
part of the listener. It was strange, but understandable, that the repeated
telling and hearing of these tales never staled. Each time a new fact was
recalled, a new reaction remembered and lived through again, another
responsive chord was struck.

These introductions seemed to be both necessary and helpful to most
of the members of the group. One mother, however, after attending two
sessions, called to say that she would not return; she found herself crying
most of the time, not only for herself and for her child (a boy with muscular
dystrophy), but also for the other mothers in the group and their children.
It was perhaps a pity that she did not stay, as the temper of the group soon
changed.

THE SECOND STAGE

After the first stage of introductions and tears, there followed a period
where the mothers talked about their children, their day-to-day problems
and the manner in which these problems were being handled. The discussions still revolved about the children's disabilities, but no longer morbidly
so. They asked each other about schooling. They discussed the doctors involved in the care of their children, the frustrations encountered in dealing
with the 'medical bureaucracy,' their gratitude to some doctors and their
contempt for others, their resentment at seeing their children used as teaching material and their simultaneous sense of reassurance that the children
were receiving the best available medical care.

THE THIRD STAGE

This stage came when they began to ask such questions as 'What did you do over the week-end?' Because the question was asked by one of their own group, it was almost as if, for the first time in a long while, they had been given permission to enjoy themselves. The next time the question was asked, some of the group did have something other than household chores to report.

As they enquired into each other's lives, marital problems were aired, some of which were so serious that husband and wife had not been on speaking terms for some months and separation and divorce were being considered. Once the subject of marriage had been raised it seemed an appropriate one to discuss, although it was rather outside the initially conceived purpose of the group. The two precarious marriages have remained so but the other three have improved.

As the women talked to each other about their relationships with their husbands, common frustrations emerged. For instance, all the women reported that the subject of their children's disabilities was not spoken of at home; the husbands did not wish to discuss it. This was not only frustrating to the mothers but, in some cases, it actually interfered with the medical management of the child. The attitude of the husbands was invariably associated with active denial, so that the husbands were prone to 'doctor hopping' in the hope that a new and more hopeful diagnosis might be made. At the same time, they were usually reluctant to grant permission for further diagnostic tests and thus sabotaged in advance the very consultations they urged upon their wives. As such experiences were aired in the group, their very prevalence proved to be reassuring and led to a greater resolve on the part of the mothers in their interactions with their husbands.

If the women were intimidated by their husbands, they were even more intimidated by their doctors and this attitude, too, is beginning to change. Because they can now talk over extra-medical problems among themselves, they can approach physicians on their own terms. They have come to realize that the contemporary physician is a trained specialist; as such, he has much to offer but cannot solve all their problems. Some of the groups have recently reported that they tend to be less anxious and less emotional when talking to their children's doctors and that they are more able to organize their thinking and to press for definite answers to definite questions.

COMMENTS

As a result of these meetings, these mothers have become more relaxed and more at peace with themselves. The group has become an important reference point in their lives and merely knowing that it is there is reassuring. Some of the women have said that as problems arise between meetings they carry on an imaginary dialogue with each other and resolve the problem in this way. Others are able to lay the problem aside, knowing that there will be an opportunity to discuss it in a few days.

This is where the group stands at the moment. We plan that the meetings will continue for as long as the mothers feel it to be useful. We hope soon to be able to include in the group some mothers whose children have only recently been diagnosed as being chronically ill or disabled. One would suspect that the group could exert its most profound and positive influence during this initial acutely stressful period.

There has also been an unanticipated side-effect from these meetings which is of interest. When we first approached these mothers, some of them said that they would only be able to attend if we could provide some baby-sitting service for their pre-school youngsters, and we arranged to do so. Initially there were only one or two children requiring supervision but as the group of mothers grew larger we began to have six or eight children to watch. While this presented problems, it also had unforeseen advantages. The children, now looked after by a most sensitive secretary and a gracious administrator, have come to look forward to and enjoy their weekly get-togethers as much as their mothers do. One of the youngsters who had adamantly refused to leave his mother when she first joined the group now races off to the play area without so much as a backward glance. Another bright four-year-old, unable to participate in normal play activities because of his disability, was noted by his mother to carry on conversations with one of the other children in the group. The mother became concerned when he began carrying on this conversation when at home alone in his room but the group chose to interpret the boy's solitary conversation as a reflection of his need for and pleasure in having found a friend. This explanation not only soothed the mother, it also led to the suggestion that the children's group be formalized and perhaps expanded. We are exploring this possibility.

In conclusion, it might be thought that our group of five is not a large one, considering our much larger available pool, but perhaps, in the present context, statistics does not provide the best evidence of significance.

Ralph Linder is a Clinical Psychologist at the Division of Rehabilitative Medicine, Montefiore Hospital and Medical Center in New York.

34

Group Therapy with Parents of Hemophiliacs
—AKE MATTSSON, M.D., and DAVID P. AGLE, M.D.

Pediatricians and psychiatrists long have recognized many special emotional problems facing children with chronic diseases and have contributed numerous reports on ways to promote a good psychosocial adaptation of the chronically ill child. Less information is available as to the problems faced by the parents of these children and their methods of mental adaptation. This paper reports observations made during group therapy with parents of young hemophiliacs.

Hemophilia is a lifelong, serious illness, almost exclusively of males, characterized primarily by bleeding into the soft tissues and joints. The bleeding tendency is due to clotting defects that are transmitted as sex-linked recessive traits by carrier mother to recipient son. Most patients with hemophilia show an onset of symptoms in early childhood and are subjected to repeated bleeding episodes. These hemorrhages often cause severe pain and require immobilization, hospital admission, and various treatment procedures. Thus a constant threat of fresh bleeding looms over the hemophilic child.

Our experience with a group of parents of hemophilic boys resulted from many years of observations of young and adult hemophiliacs at University Hospitals in Cleveland, Ohio. Our medical colleagues had asked us to evaluate a number of bleeders because psychological problems complicated their physical illness. In some of these patients emotional stress seems to influence the frequency and severity of bleeding episodes (Agle, 1964; Mattsson and Gross, 1966a). We also reported other psychiatric syndromes, which in some patients directly affected the course of the illness (Agle, 1964). The counter-phobic or "daredevil" hemophiliac, for instance, repeatedly exposes himself to dangerous activities in order to deny his fears of injury. The opposite extreme is the markedly passive-dependent patient, who hardly dares to walk outside without crutches, lest he might injure himself. We also confirmed evidence that excessive overprotection of the child by his parents can be detrimental to his personality development, and that the mother's guilt concerning the genetic transmission often seems to be involved in causing her overprotectiveness (Alby et al., 1962; Browne et al., 1960; Mattsson and Gross, 1966a).

Subsequent long-term observations of a subgroup of 35 hemophilic children and adolescents led us to describe a variety of mental mechanisms used by these patients which promote realistic adjustments to their illness

Reprinted by permission from the *Journal of Child Psychiatry* 11 (3): 558–571, 1972. Copyright 1972, Pergamon Press, Ltd.

(Mattsson and Gross, 1966b). Included among these coping mechanisms of the ego (Lazarus, 1966; Murphy, 1962) are: cognitive functions, emotional expression, motor activity, and certain psychological defenses. The appropriate use of such mechanisms provides a more comfortable mental equilibrium. This in turn facilitates the child's independent functioning, his cooperation in medical management, and possibly a decrease in frequency of bleeding episodes.

The importance of promoting such healthful mental mechanisms was clear (Agle and Mattsson, 1968). Yet the restriction of our attention to the young patient ignored a vital factor in his adjustment, namely, the interaction with his family. All too often, brief counseling of parents of hemophiliacs seemed to have little effect. We concluded that other methods of counseling should be explored and that our knowledge of the methods of parental adaptation was insufficient. The tendency of parents of hemophiliacs to band together for mutual support suggested that the group process might be a useful vehicle for our observations and for the promotion of effective child-rearing practices.

METHOD

A group of 10 parents of young hemophiliacs was obtained through volunteers from the many families of hemophiliacs in the Cleveland area. Four married couples and 2 mothers constituted the group. Their hemophilic sons ranged in age from 3 to 19. The group was clearly not representative of the hemophilia parent population. It contained motivated, verbal parents of the middle socioeconomic class, who were not necessarily those parents most in need of assistance. We met with the 10 parents for a total of 25 weekly meetings, each meeting lasting 1½ hours. The meetings were conducted in a nondirective manner, and every effort was made to let the parents reach their own answers to questions raised in the group. All meetings were tape-recorded, and in addition each therapist noted his perception of the major contents and dynamics of each session. A 2-year follow-up was provided by two further group meetings and several individual interviews.

RESULTS

OBSERVATIONS OF PARENTAL ADAPTATION

The early group meetings were filled with the parents' sharing a variety of distressing events regarding their hemophilic sons. They vented feelings about common hardships such as overwhelming hospital bills, precautions against physical trauma, and unceasing attendance to their children when they were bleeding. The difference between adequate supervision and overprotection was debated, and the parents acknowledged the difficulties of providing normal rearing for children who do require special care. They expressed sadness at watching their sons being left behind in a variety of ways by their healthy peers and reminded each other not to ignore their healthy children lest they feel left out and unloved. The mother's feelings about having transmitted this affliction to her child were discussed, as well as the need to prepare their daughters for the possibility that they might be carriers. In short, the parents all felt that having a hemophilic son had suddenly and irrevocably changed many aspects of their life and ambitions. Feelings of anxiety, helplessness, sadness, guilt, and anger were reported as responses to these ongoing stresses.

Within 2 months the group began to recognize common methods used to deal with these uncomfortable feelings. We have chosen to present the parents' methods of adaptation by way of some well-known tension-relieving mechanisms of the ego, namely, the psychological defenses of isolation, denial, rationalization, control through thinking (related to intellectualization), reaction formation, and identification (Bibring et al., 1961).

By *isolation* we refer to the separation of an idea or an activity from the affects that would normally accompany it. This technique seemed to be particularly useful for parents in dealing with acute emergencies. Many of the group members described becoming almost unfeeling toward their children during a bleeding crisis. As one mother said, "A curtain goes up between my son and me." This provided a detachment from painful emotions such as anxiety and helplessness and promoted the mother's ability to function effectively. Her remaining calm also seemed to help her child to maintain his own controls. When the crisis was passed, a rebound phenomenon of a few hours to a few days often occurred. Paradoxically, at this time the parents might feel depressed, irritable, and "of no use to anyone." This indicates that certain affects had been repressed or suppressed and deferred to a time when it was safer to experience them. Medical staff may be deceived by a parent who through isolation seems to be in perfect control during crisis situations. Such a person may be in danger of becoming overwhelmed by the blocked emotions and would benefit from the opportunity to vent them appropriately. The parents in our group told how helpful it was to be able to share emerging anxieties and other feelings with the physicians and the nursing staff during their children's hemorrhagic crises. This sharing permitted the parents to remain calm and reassuring at their son's bedside.

The defensive mechanism of *denial* aims at a disavowal of certain facts, or of their significance, or of affects that may accompany them. Denial was frequently employed by the group members to avoid distressing aspects of both acute situations and the constant strain of raising a hemophiliac. The parents might refuse to hear or quickly forget crucial information about the illness, including realistic precautions against future problems. Several parents mentioned how important repeated instructions were, particularly during the months following the frightening information that their child was a hemophiliac.

A striking example of refusal to acknowledge a painful emotion was given by a devoted mother of an adolescent hemophiliac. For months she sharply criticized the idea expressed by some group participants that mothers of hemophiliacs universally experience guilt related to their carrier state. Far from feeling guilty, she claimed that she always felt honored with this God-given responsibility. She had answered her son's questions as to why he was so afflicted with the reply that God had given him this cross to bear so that he could be an inspiration to others. Repeatedly she reported that a surgeon had complimented her on the excellent condition of her son's knees. After several months she recalled and shared with the group her emotional turmoil when the diagnosis of hemophilia was made. At this time she had urged her husband to divorce her, providing only enough money to maintain care for her son. Fortunately, her husband did not satisfy her request for punishment.

A sense of helplessness may also be warded off by denial. The group often exhibited a marked attitude of superiority toward physicians, particularly toward house officers. The parents were convinced that they knew more about hemophilia and criticized their doctors for certain alleged errors. Some of their criticisms seemed valid, but we sensed that the parents were also trying to master some of their helpless feelings in this manner. This denial of their feelings of helplessness was often associated with displacement and projection onto others, pediatricians, hematologists, and the group therapists included. All physicians could be blamed for some mistakes in diagnosis and treatment and for "being poorly informed about the psychological aspects of hemophilia" and "not providing helpful counseling." The parents' sense of superiority usually would change at times of clinical exacerbations when their physicians were turned to as all-powerful and incapable of errors.

Subsequent to several weeks of venting anger and criticism toward the medical staff, the group turned to constructive suggestions for improving the hemophiliac's medicosocial situation, such as better training for the physicians, adequate outpatient treatment facilities during bleeding crises, and stepped-up education of school personnel and lay public.

Some of the parents gave evidence of transient, extreme use of denial of the realistic dangers inherent in hemophilia, a denial that seemed to have pathological consequences for their children. For example, some parents had not used reasonable restraints on their child's activity, hence exposing him to unnecessary physical danger.

Denial is closely associated with *rationalization,* i.e., the defensive use of "rational" explanations, valid or fallacious, in an attempt to hide true emotions or real motives for certain behaviors. We heard repeatedly from many of the parents, "What a wonderful thing it is to have a hemophilic child." We were told that it provided a special maturity for the whole family, including the young bleeder, had "emotionally sharpened" the parents, and made life "spiritually richer." While indeed there may be some truth in such statements, these attitudes also assisted the parents in hiding from themselves and their children sad, angry, and helpless states related to their unique burden.

In addition to their employment of denial and rationalization, all group members had frequently used intellectual processes to defend against emergent emotions, i.e., relied on the cognitive, defensive strategy of *"control through thinking."* Bibring et al. (1961) distinguished between this mechanism and the one of intellectualization. These authors emphasized that through the use of control through thinking, "The content of the frightening situation is not primarily drained of anxieties, but through extended anticipatory familiarization with the danger, an attempt is made to prepare oneself and thus lessen the anxiety" (p. 65). (This is in contrast to intellectualization, which "is a systematic overdoing of thinking, deprived of its affect.") Like our group members, many hemophilic parents make it a point to learn all they can about the medical, physiological, and even the psychological aspects of hemophilia. Obviously, this reliance on "control through thinking" was a strong motive for the parents of our group and appeared to be a useful mechanism for them in order to master their anxiety and sense of helplessness. It seemed useful, that is, if it did not lead to the parent playing physician to a dangerous degree. Many of the parents confessed to having done so at times, only to regret it later. All parents expressed their gratitude to those physicians who had provided them with repeated dosages of factual information regarding the disease and the treatment procedures. Such information helped the parents to prepare themselves for future changes in their son's condition.

The use of *reaction formation* refers to the mental mechanisms by which an individual turns unacceptable impulses or feelings into their opposites which become permissible to express. This mechanism may be helpful for any parents of chronically ill children who harbor affects of anger, guilt, and sadness regarding their child. It allows them to reverse these feelings and devote their energy to care for him. Reaction formation may become detrimental to the parents' adaptation, however, if it is employed to such a degree that no knowledge of their painful feelings is possible. Such parents often develop martyr-like attitudes and direct their whole life to caring for their "sufferers." The group members referred to such a maladaptation as a danger facing all parents of handicapped children and reported periods during which they had felt like martyrs, isolated from friends and social life. At these times bitterness and resentment about their fate had often been close to the surface. As group leaders we wondered if the extreme behavior of being a devoted martyr was not an effort to block an opposite wish toward the chronically ill child, that is, the desire to be completely free of parental responsibilities. No parent in the group vented such wishes.

Excessive degrees of overprotection of a young hemophiliac often appear to be related to the mother's guilt over the genetic transmission (Agle, 1964; Alby et al., 1962; Mattsson and Gross, 1966a). In addition, anger toward the sick child may, through the process of reaction formation, lead to parental overaffection and overprotection. This anger is an understandable response to the marked hardships that the child's disorder has imposed. Guilt and shame at the recognition of this anger would be too uncomfortable, hence the reaction formation leading to overprotection. Among the group members the fathers were better able to verbalize their anger and disappointment regarding their boys' disease. Several fathers described "furiously looking for some reason to blame" their sons for individual hemorrhagic episodes. They also admitted to more impatient and resentful feelings toward the doctors "in charge of our sons during bleeding crises"; the fathers wanted their sons out of the hospital as soon as possible, "back to a normal life," under the father's direction.

Identification with other parents of hemophiliacs was an essential adaptational mechanism of our group members. This has already been implied by the earlier references to the parents' high motivation to learn more about themselves so as to care better for their sons and also pass on some of their own experience to other parents of hemophiliacs. Imitative processes, facilitating identification, were readily observable during many group sessions as some parents began to model themselves upon attitudes of other group members. For example, they adopted more realistic and relaxed attitudes toward supervising their sons' physical activities, and became more open in discussing the genetic factors of hemophilia with both their sick and healthy children.

In addition to identification among the group members, the parents of the adolescent hemophiliacs at times seemed to gain strength by identifying with their sons' stoic and hopeful attitudes in the face of repeated bleeding episodes. Illustrative comments were, "Now when we feel frustrated, we can learn from him; he accepts setbacks and interrupted plans better than we do." Their growing son's effective adaptation to his chronic illness had become a helpful source of strength for his parents to imitate and identify with. Behind this recognition also was the awareness that they had "done a good job" in raising their hemophilic son and that their long-standing ordeal had "paid off."

THERAPEUTIC PROCESS

The venting of common hardships, at times sounding like abreacting "horror stories," was particularly frequent at the first meetings of the group. The discovery that others shared their experiences and painful thoughts brought relief to most of the parents. For one young couple with a 3-year-old hemophiliac, however, the detailed description of past bleeding crises by parents of older children became overwhelming and led them to leave the group after 8 meetings. In retrospect, this error in the use of the group process might have been avoided if the leaders had been more alert to this couple's anxiety and had mustered some reassuring and constructive resources in the group.

After the first 6 weeks, the group developed a strong cohesiveness (Yalom, 1970) which allowed for a freer expression of negative, resentful, and hostile feelings often displaced onto the therapists as "experts" and outsiders. We were presumed to have healthy children and hence to be unable to understand the plight of parents of chronically ill boys. The emergence of some group members as positive role models aided the supportive, confronting, and insight-giving processes of the sessions. After about 2 months the parents themselves began to recognize common aspects of their unique adaptational behavior prompted by raising a hemophiliac. This recognition also included their gradual awareness of each other's strengths.

Toward the end of the series of meetings, the group members uniformly reported a marked increase in self-esteem and a decrease in their frightened sense of isolation in dealing with an overwhelming problem. Such remarks as, "It's great to see that other people have these problems and feelings and it's not just that I am such a bad parent," illustrated their view of these positive changes. As they gained in self-awareness, the parents seemed to use more appropriate child-rearing practices, e.g., regarding healthful physical activities and a minimum of supervision. More realistic assessments of their own abilities and limitations also resulted from the increased mastery of distressing feelings.

One striking example of behavioral change was seen in a mother of two children, one hemophilic and one healthy, who had a marked fear of future pregnancies. Because of a physiological intolerance to contraceptive pills, this fear was strongly affecting her marital life. During several group sessions she expressed a desire for a tubal ligation, but was convinced that her respected family physician would be angry with her and refuse to help. It soon became clear that underlying this concern was her own guilt. She felt that the request for tubal ligation was the same as saying she did not want her hemophilic son. When these feelings were understood, she went to her physician, who calmly agreed with her request.

A 2-year follow-up, based on both individual and group meetings with the 10 parents, showed a continued improvement in their self-confidence as parents of chronically ill children. For the most part they were effectively promoting their son's acceptance of realistic limitations and his pursuit of appropriate physical and intellectual activities. Such group members had become engaged in counseling younger parents regarding practical aspects of raising a young hemophiliac. These nonprofessional counselors frequently consulted with the group therapists and referred families with more complicated medical and psychological problems to professional sources.

DISCUSSION

Our purpose for the series of group meetings with parents of young hemophiliacs was twofold: (1) to promote the parents' understanding and mastery of distressing emotions related to their sons' disease, hence improving the parent-child relationship; and (2) to gain information about common methods of adaptation used by parents to cope with the problems of raising a chronically ill child.

Similar therapeutic and investigative aims have prompted other pediatric and psychiatric workers to use the group process with parents of disabled children (Korsch, 1968; Korsch et al., 1954; Luzzatti and Dittmann, 1954; Mandelbaum, 1967; Milman, 1952). The early reports by Milman (1952), Korsch et al. (1954), and Luzzatti and Dittmann (1954) described group sessions with parents of children with neurological handicaps, nephrosis, and diabetes. Milman's (1952) therapeutic approach and ours seem to resemble each other in their emphasis on a nondirective group leadership. This technique caused some early sessions of frustrated parents, who resented the therapists' refusal to educate and give directions. As these initial reactions were understood, both Milman's and our group developed a strong cohesiveness which secured goal-directed work and good attendance.

Korsch and associates (1954) emphasized that their "pediatric discussion groups" should not be viewed as "group psychotherapy" and that much medical information and explanation was given to the parents. A similar approach was used by Luzzatti and Dittmann (1954), who assigned discussion topics for most of their meetings with parents of diabetic children. These authors concluded that their didactic material "would have reached a more receptive audience, had the discussion leaders allowed the questions of the group to lead to it, rather than presenting it as a planned outline" (p. 271). Our own experience suggests that such didactic material can only be used effectively by some parents after interfering feelings are verbalized and mastered.

Despite varying group techniques and disease entities of the children, the findings of Korsch and co-workers (1954) and Luzzatti and Dittmann (1954) parellel Milman's (1952) and ours in many respects. Thus, the parents of the chronically disabled children related painful feelings of isolation, fears, guilt, and self-blame. Overprotective attitudes toward their children were commonly shown, as well as considerable hostility and criticism toward the healing professions. Confused, unrealistic expectations regarding their children's future constituted an additional central discussion theme.

In her résumé of parent groups in pediatric practice, Korsch (1968) highlighted some of the hazards of group discussion. For instance, she described highly disturbed or manipulative parents who preclude group cohesiveness and identification, and inexperienced parents whose anxieties about their children often mount as they listen to other parents' dramatic accounts of their children crises. The latter hazard was exemplified in our group by the parents of a 3-year-old hemophiliac who left the group prematurely because intolerable anxiety had been produced by other members' disclosure of frightening hemorrhagic episodes.

Mandelbaum's report (1967) on group therapy with parents of retarded children gave a vivid account of all the distressing feelings that parents of a defective child try to master. Particularly illuminating were the parents' descriptions of mourning the "loss" of a desired normal child and their feelings of angry frustration, which in some instances led to an expression of veiled death wishes toward the retarded child. Such strongly negative attitudes became briefly apparent among our group as some parents related their martyrlike, isolated periods of life centering around caring for their hemophilic sons.

The major therapeutic factors operating in our parent group can briefly be described in terms of Yalom's (1970) recent outline of the primary curative factors in group therapy. Thus, both the parents and the therapists imparted information about the many hardships facing the family of a hemophiliac, the associated distressing feelings, and the common reactive attitudes of various family members. The beneficial cathartic effect of sharing these hardships and fearful, sad, helpless, and angry feelings was particularly evident during the first 6 meetings. Later, considerable explanation and clarification of hidden feelings and motives for certain behavior could take place. The group process facilitated the instillation of hope among the parents for becoming more knowledgeable, patient, and realistic in raising their sons. The universality of the members' experiences with their ill children was probably the key factor in binding the group together and maintaining its cohesiveness. The parents quickly accepted one another and came to accept the therapists as nonjudgmental and helpful in calling attention to both adaptive and maladaptive ways of parental coping with their stressful life situation. Imitative processes, facilitating identification, were common as some group members adopted positive attitudes of more experienced parents in regard to raising a hemophiliac. (Recently Guttmacher and Birk [1971] emphasized the *in vivo* expression of maladaptive social response patterns in group therapy and the importance of role modeling among group members.)

After the parents experienced frustration of their wishes to obtain psychological advice and medical information from the sessions, their habitual modes of coping with the many problems and disruptive affects related to raising a handicapped child emerged as part of the group interaction. The parents achieved considerable insight into both their adaptive and maladaptive use of some common psychological defenses such as isolation of painful feelings, denial of stark realities (including guilt feelings), rationalization of certain behavior, extensive use of intellectual processes, and reactive attitudes of overprotection and martyrlike devotion to their ill children. Our decision to conceptualize the parental methods of adaptation within the framework of ego coping mechanisms (Lazarus, 1966; Mattsson and Gross, 1966b; Murphy, 1962) was greatly influenced by the relative ease with which the parents recognized in themselves and described in nontechnical language the cited characteristic defensive processes.

The group members also became aware of situations in which their use of these coping strategies had ceased to be effective and beneficial for both parent and child. In retrospect, they were able to determine when marked reliance on various defenses precluded their awareness of potentially disruptive affects and hampered their ability to function effectively as parents. These situations illustrate Hartmann's (1939) statement that, "A 'successful' defense may amount to a 'failure' in achievement" (p. 12). The fact that a psychic defense can successfully spare an individual from consciously experiencing affective arousal, yet impair his adaptive, social functioning, has been emphasized in other studies of young patients' and their parents' adaptation to life-threatening illness (Mattsson and Gross, 1966b; Mattsson et al., 1971; Wolff et al., 1964).

We conclude that the group process is an effective vehicle whereby appropriate child-rearing practices may be promoted in parents of chronically ill children. It is particularly helpful for those parents whose ability to learn and use instruction is crippled by a lack of awareness of their affective responses and methods of adaptation.

SUMMARY

Ten parents of young hemophiliacs participated in a series of 25 weekly group meetings led by a general and a child psychiatrist. The therapeutic goal was to aid the parents' understanding and mastery of distressing affects related to their sons' serious disorder, hence to promote the parent-child relationship. The investigative purpose of the meetings was to gain information about common methods of mental adaptation used by parents of chronically ill children. The group process facilitated much ventilation of painful, sometimes incapacitating, affects of fear, sadness, anger, and guilt, all caused by the repeated hardships imposed on a hemophiliac's family. Guilt-laden doubts about their ability to foster independent and reality-oriented strivings of their sons constituted additional emotional strain. Considerable criticism and hostility toward medical staff were also vented. The sharing of these common experiences and feelings brought relief to most of the parents and furthered the development of a strong group cohesiveness. Gradually the parents began to recognize their unique ways of coping with their chronic stressful situation and periods of disruptive affects. These adaptational methods included many well-known psychological defenses such as isolation of painful affects, denial of frightening realities and a sense of guilt and helplessness, rationalization of certain behavior, extensive use of intellectual processes (control through thinking), reaction formation leading to a smothering overprotection, and identification with other parents of hemophiliacs and also, as their son got older, with his positive, hopeful outlook.

A 2-year follow-up showed a continued improvement in their self-confidence as parents of chronically ill children. They promoted their son's acceptance of the realistic limitations imposed by the disease and his pursuit of healthful physical and intellectual activities. For a few parents the group experience had stimulated them to serve as "lay counselors" to inexperienced parents of hemophiliacs. In this valuable counseling role these parents received professional supervision.

REFERENCES

Dr. Mattsson was Assistant Professor of Child Psychiatry at Case Western Reserve University School of Medicine in Cleveland, Ohio. He is now Professor of Psychiatry and Pediatrics at the University of Virginia Medical Center in Charlottesville, Virginia. Dr. Agle is Associate Professor of Psychiatry at Case Western Reserve University School of Medicine in Cleveland, Ohio.

This paper was presented in part at the annual meeting of the American Association of Psychiatric Services for Children in Philadelphia, November, 1970.

Agle, D. P. (1964), Psychiatric studies of patients with hemophilia and related states. *Arch. Intern. Med.*, 114:76–82.

—— and Mattsson, A. (1968), Psychiatric and social care of patients with hereditary hemorrhagic disease. *Modern Treatment*, 5:111–124.

Alby, J. M.; Alby, N.; and Caen, J. (1962), Psychological problems of the hemophiliac. *Nouv. Rev. Franc. Hemat.*, 2:119–130.

Bibring, G. L.; Dwyer, T. F.; Huntington, D. S.; and Valenstein, A. F. (1961), A study of the psychological processes in pregnancy and of the earliest mother-child relationship. Appendix B: glossary of defenses. *The Psychoanalytic Study of the Child*, 16:62–72. New York: International Universities Press.

Browne, W. J.; Mally, M. A.; and Kane, R. P. (1960) Psychosocial aspects of hemophilia: a study of twenty-eight hemophilic children and their families. *Amer. J. Orthopsychiat.*, 30:730–740.

Guttmacher, J. A. and Birk, L. (1971), Group therapy: what specific therapeutic advantages? *Compr. Psychiat.*, 12:546–556.

Hartmann, H. (1939), *Ego Psychology and the Problem of Adaptation*. New York: International Universities Press, 1958, p. 12.

Korsch, B. C. (1968), Parent groups. In: *Ambulatory Pediatrics*, ed. M. Green and R. J. Haggerty. Philadelphia: Saunders, pp. 156–158.

—— Fraad, L., and Barnett, H. L. (1954), Pediatric discussions with parent groups. *J. Pediat.*, 44:703–717.

Lazarus, R. S. (1966), *Psychological Stress and the Coping Process*. New York: McGraw-Hill.

Luzzatti, L. and Dittmann, B. (1954), Group discussions with parents of ill children. *Pediatrics*, 13:269–273.

Mandelbaum, A. (1967), The group process in helping parents of retarded children. *Children*, 14:227–232.

Mattsson, A. and Gross, S. (1966a), Social and behavioral studies on hemophilic children and their families. *J. Pediat.*, 68:952–964.

—— (1966b), Adaptational and defensive behavior in young hemophiliacs and their parents. *Amer. J. Psychiat.*, 122:1349–1356.

—— and Hall, T. W. (1971), Psychoendocrine study of adaptation in young hemophiliacs. *Psychosom. Med.*, 33:215–225.

Milman, D. H. (1952), Group therapy with parents: an approach to the rehabilitation of physically disabled children. *J. Pediat.*, 41:113–116.

Murphy, L. B. (1962), *The Widening World of Childhood*. New York: Basic Books.

Wolff, C. T.; Friedman, S. B.; Hofer, M. A.; and Mason, J. W. (1964), Relationship between psychological defenses and mean urinary 17-OHCS excretion rates: I. A predictive study of parents of fatally ill children. *Psychosom. Med.*, 26:576–591.

Yalom, I. D. (1970), *The Theory and Practice of Group Psychotherapy*. New York: Basic Books.

35

Group Treatment of Families of Burn-Injured Patients —MARCIA ABRAMSON

PROBABLY no injury causes more physical and psychological trauma than a severe burn. Both the injury and the treatment that follows are frightening and painful, and the patient is often left with residual deformities that can radically alter his life. Varying degrees of fear, depression, grief, loss of hope, and psychotic reactions during the course of the treatment and during the long recovery period have been reported. In addition, the burn-injured person and his family are faced with the prospect of enormous medical costs and extensive hospitalizations that mean long separations from home and community. It is no wonder that a severe burn creates a severe crisis situation for patients and their families.

Interest in the psychological reactions of burn patients was first aroused at the time of the Cocoanut Grove fire in Boston in 1942. It was found that many of the persons burned at that time suffered from persistent and serious emotional problems.[1] Subsequent literature on the subject has supported these earlier findings.[2] One of the significant outcomes of a study at the University of Iowa Hospitals and Clinics, previously reported in SOCIAL CASEWORK, was that the relatives of burn patients undergo many of the same stresses as do the patients.[3]

During the early, acute stages of treatment, when the patient is faced with the initial physical and psychological shock to his system, the relative is often stunned and depressed. As the patient begins to cope with the active demands of the convalescence and the rehabilitation processes, the relative must also adjust to these changes. Because the focus of the medical staff must be on the patient, the relative often faces his anxieties about death and deformity and his boredom with a prolonged hospital stay without the active support of the professional staff. In addition, the families are faced with the trauma of watching a loved one suffer, often without being able to intervene in a meaningful way.

As a result of these findings,[4] it was recommended that a group be organized at the burn unit of the University of Iowa Hospitals and Clinics to help relatives cope with the stresses of being supportive to a seriously burned patient. It was apparent that relatives who remain for long periods of time with their burned family member form a natural group on the ward. They orient one another to procedure, offer each other support at times of stress, and develop an informal grapevine to disseminate information. It

Reprinted by permission of the Family Service Association of America from *Social Casework* 1975 (April): 235–241.

was anticipated that with the added leadership and participation of a social worker and a nurse to help focus the group's attitudes, feelings, and beliefs, the natural group could be utilized to achieve certain educational and counseling goals.

The original plan was to include only those persons who planned to remain with their relatives for the duration of the hospitalization and who would therefore be available to come to weekly meetings on a regular basis. It soon became apparent, however, that relatives who are not able to stay for the duration of the hospitalization are equally in need of support from the group and can contribute to the other members. It was also decided to include the relatives of patients who were returning for follow-up checks or reconstructive surgery. Recovery from a severe burn takes two years or more; the relatives can benefit from the continued support of the group and can help those persons whose relatives are still hospitalized to appreciate the problems that occur after discharge.

GROUP STRUCTURE

Initially, a sign was posted just outside the nurses' station announcing a weekly meeting and asking relatives to sign up if they were interested in attending. Subsequently, during the week following each patient's admission to the burn unit, the relatives were approached and asked whether they would like to attend the group.

The meetings were co-chaired by a social worker who was knowledgeable about the problems of families of seriously ill patients and a nurse who was familiar with the burn unit's medical and nursing procedures. The physical therapist and chaplain from the unit attended a few meetings in which the focus of group concern was on issues relevant to their services.

At the beginning of each group meeting, the purpose of the group was reiterated by the social worker: to help orient the relatives to the burn unit and give them the opportunity to share common concerns and questions with others undergoing similar stresses and to help the burn unit staff better understand these problems in order to be more helpful to them and to other families in the future. Although group members often already knew one another and were familiar with the patients, the social worker usually asked each member to introduce himself and describe the circumstances of the burn and the patient's current condition. Coffee was served, and group members were encouraged to talk with each other about their experiences in the hospital.

A notebook was kept on nursing care issues and made available to the rest of the unit nursing staff. Periodic meetings of nursing staff and the group leaders were held to share information and help the nursing staff understand and deal with the emotional reactions of family members. During a two-year period, meetings were held at weekly intervals, whenever there were two or more relatives present on the burn unit who wished to attend. In all, thirty-eight group meetings were held.

INITIAL REACTIONS

It was found that at meetings in which there was a preponderance of relatives of newly admitted patients, there were many specific questions about the medical and nursing care. Questions relating to shock, intravenous medications, diet, debridement, burn rounds, the use of silver nitrate, and the timing of procedures were raised, and relatives of patients who had been in the hospital longer were encouraged to share their relevant experiences. Only when the emotional implications of the procedures had been discussed did the nurse answer the specific question. If more experienced relatives were not present, the social worker would attempt to have the group members discuss the psychological implications of the various procedures before specific responses were given.

The need for specific information about procedures seemed to be closely related to the initial shock the relatives suffered during the early weeks of the hospitalization. At the same time that he had to begin to face the severity of the injury that had occurred to the patient, the family member had to get used to the sights, smells, sounds, and procedures of the unit. Explanations about the procedures often were not understood and had to be repeated; the relatives had to be helped to know what and whom to ask when they had questions. The group acted as a forum and catalyst for this procedure.

> Mrs. L's husband was injured after suffering a seizure while burning trash. Mrs. L complained at the meeting that she never had an opportunity to talk with the doctor about her husband's condition. As she spoke to the group about her husband, it became clear that she had many misconceptions about his condition and his need for posthospital care. Underlying her inability to formulate questions for the medical staff was the fear that they would tell her that he was in an even worse condition than she imagined. The group helped her to talk about her fear that her husband had suffered permanent mental deterioration from a recent seizure and would therefore require twenty-four-hour supervision upon discharge from the hospital. She responded well to the group's suggestion that she talk with the unit social worker about these fears and enlist her aid in formulating the questions to ask of the medical staff.

GROUP SUPPORT

More experienced members of the group have been able to share their experiences and solutions to problems with newer members in a way that can be highly supportive to the new members, as well as therapeutic to themselves.

> At the first meeting he attended, Mr. P, whose two children were burned in a house fire two weeks earlier, spoke of how other persons who had relatives on the burn unit had welcomed him to the unit, informed him about procedures, helped him to ask questions and understand what the doctors and nurses were telling him, and encouraged him to attend the group for

further support and clarification. He discussed his children's different reactions to their burns. The group began to prepare him for the fact that his daughter, who was the more badly burned of the two but much more stoical than her brother, would probably begin to feel more pain and become increasingly depressed as treatment progressed. In later meetings, Mr. P spoke of how this discussion had helped him to understand his daughter's withdrawal and depression when it did occur and to deal with it as part of the normal reaction to a severe burn.

Among the problems discussed in the early stages of hospitalization were the primary relative's discomfort at being torn between the patient and the family at home, his need for support from other family and friends, and the visits from other family members, especially small children whose imagination about the burn was often much worse than the actual injury.

A phenomenon that occurred in the group was the mobilization of group effort to help a particular relative or patient. Sometimes it was a person like Mr. P, who needed information and support during the early stages of hospitalization. Other times it was someone who needed help in coping with the demands of a patient and could accept advice from the group more easily than from the staff.

Mrs. K, whose fifteen-year-old son was hospitalized with severe burns for several months, had promised her son at the time of his admission to the unit that she would remain with him throughout his hospitalization. After many weeks of constant attendance at his bedside, she was becoming emotionally and physically exhausted by the strain, and it was clear that she would end up a patient herself if she did not leave. All the encouragement, direction, and advice of the medical and nursing staff was to no avail until other members of the group decided that it was time for her to take a few days of rest away from the hospital. They convinced her, and then her son, who later believed that it had been his idea to send his mother home.

Sometimes the group served as surrogate family for a patient who had no relatives available.

Carl, a fifteen-year-old who had been burned in a gasoline explosion, had no relationship with his family. As his sixteenth birthday approached, different members of the group expressed concern that the day not go uncelebrated. They spent part of two group sessions planning a party and delegated a group member to involve the staff and take up a collection. The party turned into a gala event for staff, patients, and relatives and clearly demonstrated the burn unit group's interest in one another.

Often relatives who were having difficulty coping with the patients, procedures, or staff were able to express some of their own feelings by focusing on the problems of others.

Mrs. D, whose husband was burned in a farming accident while working as a migrant laborer, came a great distance to stay with him. She spoke little English, had few financial resources, and had much concern about her two small children who had been left at home with relatives. The usual problems experienced on the unit were compounded by her inability to communicate and her resulting isolation. The group spent several meetings giving her practical advice about financial resources and emotional support to cope with her husband's demands. The group also suggested ways to communicate better with the staff and activities that could help her become more involved with other people. Other patients who were having problems with finances and communication difficulties with staff and were also suffering from isolation were able to express their own needs indirectly while they were helping Mrs. D.

FROM ACUTE CARE TO REHABILITATION

One of the most stressful periods for burn patients and their relatives seems to occur when the focus changes from acute care to rehabilitation efforts. From being immobilized for days at a time, dependent, cared for by staff and relatives, and encouraged to express his feelings freely when in pain, the patient is suddenly faced with new instructions to be independent, take care of his own eating or toileting needs, do a prescribed number of exercises a day, and control his expression of negative feelings. The relative who has been so important in feeding, entertaining, and encouraging is often asked to leave if the patient continues to ask for assistance with tasks the patient is expected to do himself. For many patients, especially children, who have felt that the family member will stay only as long as he participates actively in the treatment process, and for their relatives, who suddenly seem to have no purpose, rehabilitation can be an anxious time. Patients complain about the nurses and physical therapists who are pushing them, or else they cooperate with staff instructions and take their frustrations out on the family member. Relatives find themselves caught between concern for the patient and fear of alienating the staff.

> Mrs. R, whose ten-year-old daughter, Marie, was burned when her dress caught on fire, found herself distressed by her daughter's expression of pain and the staff's expectations that Marie exercise control over her screaming. Believing that Marie's extreme fear increased her inability to cope with the pain of the exercises, Mrs. R became overwhelmed with the strain of being supportive while trying to keep Marie and herself from alienating the staff by too much expression of concern. She expressed to the group her feelings that the staff wanted her to leave the burn unit.
> The group was able to be helpful in a number of ways. It provided a place for Mrs. R to express her anger, not only toward the staff but also toward Marie for putting her in such an uncomfortable position. She continued to receive support and acceptance from the group despite her expression of angry feelings. She was able to express her anger directly to staff in the persons of the co-leaders without fear of retaliation. The co-leaders and group were able to help her examine and better understand her daughter's behavior and her own and the staff's reactions to it in a way that lent itself to the formulation of new solutions to the problems.

Relatives often use the group to express their pleasure in the fact that the burn crisis had made them appreciate strengths in themselves, the patient, and other family members that they did not know existed. A wife who had thought of herself as the dependent, helpless partner found she could assume the role of caring for the family farm and operating the machinery. She amazed the male members of the group when she described how she had changed the clutch on a tractor. One mother was delighted at the way her burn-injured adolescent boy, who previously had expressed a great deal of dissatisfaction with school and family life and had threatened to drop out of school, seemed to be able to redirect his energies toward finishing high school. Other mothers found that their teen-age children at home were willing and able to assume new responsibilities for themselves and younger children when a burned sibling kept the mother away from home for long periods of time. The expression of these strengths in the group and their positive reinforcement by other group members encouraged the participants to continue their efforts to cope effectively with the crisis.

PREPARATION FOR DISCHARGE

As the time for discharge from the hospital draws near, family members experience anxiety about how they will manage the patient at home. While the patient becomes increasingly concerned about returning to home, school, work, and other activities, the relatives begin to realize that at home they will be responsible, without the help of the physicians, nurses, and physical therapists, for exercises, wrappings, and dressing changes. The group experience permits the family member to express a natural ambivalence about taking on this responsibility alone. Returning relatives can share experiences and solutions to problems with those who are about to face them.

EVALUATION OF THE GROUP BY PARTICIPANTS

A few weeks after the patient's discharge from the hospital, every relative who attended two or more meetings was sent a questionnaire asking for his evaluation of the burn unit's relatives' group. Of the thirty-three letters sent out, twenty-three were returned. These relatives had participated in from two to twelve meetings of the group, with an average of four meetings per person.

When asked to indicate how helpful they found the group sessions, seventeen checked "very helpful," four "helpful," and two "not too helpful." When asked to comment on the ways in which they found the group helpful, many said the group meeting was a place to share problems with others who understood—both relatives and staff. One wife commented, "It was good to just be able to discuss some of my fears regarding my husband's condition with people who understood so well because they were going through the same ordeal." A mother added, "The nurse and social worker listened to everything I had to say. They were very reassuring when I needed it. I felt I could talk about any problem." Relatives indicated that they had come away with increased understanding of what patients go through physically and psychologically and had a better understanding of procedures and staff problems. The group meetings had helped them feel closer to one another and had relieved some of their tensions. Several commented that it was good for both the relative and patient for the family member to get away from the burn unit to talk. A husband commented, "I was able to release tension and ask questions about my wife's case without feeling like a nuisance."

When asked to comment on how the group failed to be helpful to them and what could be done to make it more valuable for relatives in the future, most replied that the group had fulfilled all their expectations, although there were some comments about the fact that a few relatives monopolized the conversation. Suggestions were made about timing, including making the meetings longer, scheduling them at a time when more relatives could attend, having more frequent meetings, and involving relatives as soon as the patient is admitted to the unit.

Relatives were also asked to comment on the problems that they and the patient faced on return home for which they had not been prepared. A number said that the most difficult adjustment was to the patient's moods and irritability. According to one mother, it was "mostly the change in personality which lasted—stubbornness." A wife said, "The only problem we had was getting adjusted to his moods, because mentally he was very unstable and at times he is very despondent." Another mother commented, "I didn't realize the full strain I was under. I did a lot of worrying and wondering if I was doing all of it right—the wrapping and such of my son."

OBSERVATIONS FROM THE WARD

In addition to what happened within the group and the reported benefits from group members after discharge, certain observations were made about the effect on the ward of the establishment of the relatives' groups. In the past, when many severely ill patients required much staff attention, relatives often reacted to the feeling that their patient was being neglected by expressing hostility toward one another or toward the staff. Cliques would form and one or two relatives or staff would become recipients of all the hostile feelings. With the advent of the group, the scapegoating of one another diminished. The relatives appear to have gained a greater understanding of why nursing and medical efforts need to be concentrated on certain sicker patients. The family members fill in with care and support for patients who do not need as much nursing attention, patients who would previously have felt neglected and uncared for. Furthermore, group meetings provided an opportunity for members to examine the emotional forces operating within the close-knit family of burn patients and their families. Some scapegoating of staff continued, but the group leaders were much better able to offer the relatives the opportunity to handle their anger and complaints in a manner conducive to productive change.

The group meetings also gave one member of the nursing staff the opportunity to share nursing concerns with the relatives, and other nurses were able to share their concerns with the nurse leader who brought them to the group. The group's reactions could then be conveyed to the rest of the nurses individually, by means of the group notebook and in staff meetings. The periodic meetings that the social worker and nurse co-leader held with the nursing staff permitted the sharing of information about patients' and relatives' psychosocial problems and needs and how these could best be met by nursing staff. As a result of these meetings, the nursing staff expressed a desire for more social work coverage so that they could have a better understanding of the patients and families as early as possible in the hospitalization.

The use of a nurse who was part of the burn unit staff and a social worker who had no direct responsibility on the ward seemed to be particularly effective. The nurse was knowledgeable about patients, procedures, and individual problems and in continuous communication with the rest of the staff. She demonstrated to the relatives the interest and concern that the staff must have for them, as shown by sending her. The social worker, on the other hand, because she was not identified as a member of the burn unit, could ask questions about issues that others took for granted and could focus primarily on the needs of the relatives, unlike other professional staff for whom the patient is the primary person. Thus, she brought a different point of view.

RECOMMENDATIONS

Although burn injuries are particularly stressful because of their suddenness, intensity, painfulness, and duration, there are many other medical problems that create significant stress for patients and families. Any illness that results in drastically altered life-styles or that causes temporary alteration in the patient's ability to cope can produce stress and crisis for the patient and his family. Cancer, chronic renal disease, cardiac illnesses, neurological problems, and birth defects are just a few of the medical problems that cause significant stress for patients and relatives. Relatives as well as patients need support from others who understand and who can provide some relief from the demands of the illness and treatment process. A group especially designed to provide such support for family members can ultimately help the patients and the medical and nursing staffs responsible for the care of such seriously ill patients.

REFERENCES

Marcia Abramson is associate director of the Department of Social Services at the University of Iowa Hospitals and Clinics in Iowa City, Iowa.

1. Stanley Cobb and Erich Lindeman. Neuropsychiatric observations, *Annals of Surgery,* 117:814–24 (June 1943): and Alendra Adler, Neuropsychiatric complications in victims of Boston's Cocoanut Grove disaster, *Journal of the American Medical Association,* 123:1098–1101 (December 1943).
2. David A. Hamburg et al., Clinical importance of emotional problems in the care of patients with burns, *New England Journal of Medicine,* 248:355–59 (February 26, 1953); David A. Hamburg, Beatrice Hamburg, and Sydney DeGoze, Adaptive problems and mechanisms in severely burned patients, *Psychiatry,* 16:1–20

(February 1953); Helen L. Martin, J. H. Lawrie, and A. W. Wilkinson, The family of the fatally burned child, *Lancet,* 295:628–29 (September 14, 1968); Helen L. Martin, Antecedents of burns and scalds in children, *British Journal of Medical Psychology,* 43:39–47 (March 1970); idem, Parents' and children's reactions to burns and scalds in children, *British Journal of Medical Psychology,* 43:183–91 (June 1970); and N. J. C. Andreasen et al., Management of emotional problems in seriously burned adults, *New England Journal of Medicine,* 286:65–69 (January 13, 1972).

3. Gene A. Brodland and N. J. C. Andreasen. Adjustment problems of the family of the burn patient, Social Casework, 55:13–18 (January 1974).
4. Ibid.

36

Rehabilitating the Stroke Patient through Patient-Family Groups
—JUDITH GREGORIE D'AFFLITTI, M.S.N., and
G. WAYNE WEITZ, M.S.W.

THE intermediate service of the West Haven Veterans Administration Hospital is designed as a rehabilitative setting for medical patients who have completed the phase of diagnosis and early treatment. In our nursing and social work with recuperating stroke patients and their families on this service, we noticed that although many patients were engaged in a program of physical, occupational, and speech therapy, they and their family members were frequently having great difficulty with the emotional acceptance of the patients' disabilities. This was clear from the patients' depressive affect and inability to express their feelings about their illness, with the concurrent inability of families to exchange reactions with the patients about the stroke and the ways in which this was going to affect their family life. For example, patients were often very frightened that any disability would mean that they could not function at home again. Family members sometimes shared this fear, and families and patients could not communicate their concerns. Because of this poor communication, there often was a strained relationship between patient and family, and realistic discharge plans could not be made. In addition, the patients did not use the appropriate community supports that would have allowed the most effective community adjustment, i.e., rehabilitation centers, visiting nurse associations, and vocational retraining centers.

The importance of interpersonal relationships in the rehabilitation of chronic disease patients is noted in the medical and psychiatric literature. Litman (1964) reported that 75 per cent of his patients looked first to their

Reprinted by permission of the American Group Psychotherapy Association from the *International Journal of Group Psychotherapy* 24: 323–332, 1974.

families for support and encouragement and second to the hospital staff. Also, there are some indications that if patients can anticipate re-entry into a functioning family unit, this influences their decision to engage themselves in a therapy program. Bruetman and Gordon (1971) discuss rehabilitation in terms of a concurrent restoring of the patient's physiologic and environmental equilibrium. They see the family's having great impact on the patient's motivations and expectations. Robertson and Suinn (1968) state that there is a relationship between the stroke patient's rate of progress toward recovery and the degree of empathy between the patient and his family members. Specifically, they indicate that stroke patients improve more rapidly when there is predictive empathy, i.e., the ability of patients and family members to foresee each other's attitudes. Finally, Millen (1970) states that optimum rehabilitation of stroke patients occurs only when there is physical and psychological stimulation. Frequently, stroke patients grouped together can influence one another toward working out problems, while providing a mutual source of encouragement as well.

With these ideas in mind, we believed that we might be helpful to our patients and their families by having them participate in a patient-family group. It was hoped that the group process would facilitate communication so that the illness and feelings about it could be discussed more freely and that this would lead to a more realistic perception by the patient and his family of the amount of disability and the limitations imposed by it. Plans could then be initiated and implemented that would be consistent with these limitations, and the group could support individual members toward more independent functioning.

We began our group with two major goals: first, to encourage patients and families to talk and to share their feelings about the stroke in order to promote a constructive adjustment to the illness; second, to encourage the patient and his family to use the appropriate community resources and supports available to them. From our experience, it seemed that patients who had contacts outside the family after discharge were less likely to become depressed and regress in their physical and social functioning.

In order for the group to be viewed as part of the total rehabilitation effort of the Intermediate Service, our project needed the support of the director of the service and of the staff members. This was accomplished through our joint contact with the director, followed by his introduction and our presentation of the purposes and goals of the planned group at a staff meeting. This presentation enabled the staff to understand how the group would be structured and how its activities would complement rather than subvert or interfere with those of the medical, nursing, and rehabilitation staff.

There were four criteria for participation in the group:

1. The patient had to have had a stroke, although he might have additional medical problems.
2. He had to be competent mentally and verbally to participate in a group.

3. He had to have a family member who was willing to participate.

4. His final destination from the hospital had to be his home.

These strictures were not intended to imply that the needs of the severely damaged patient or the patient without a family or the patient who would have to be placed out of a home setting were any less important than those of the group selected, only that the problems of such patients cannot be dealt with appropriately in a patient-family group and need to be approached by other methods of intervention.

The group met for an hour and a half weekly for three months. Members were to participate for this time even if they were discharged. To date, four consecutive groups have been conducted. The authors worked as co-leaders for the group sessions and shared the outside administrative responsibilities, i.e., referrals and contacts with community agencies, preadmission interviews, and contacts with staff members. Each group had three to five patients, each with his accompanying family participants. These included spouses, brothers, sisters, children, and sometimes friends. The selected patients were predominately male because the agency is a Veterans Administration Hospital. A variety of ethnic and cultural backgrounds were represented. There was a wide patient age range, 34 to 76 years. Most of the patients and family members approached the group with interest and enthusiasm; however, the group was not appropriate for all situations. For example, Mr. A. discontinued attending because no family member would join him, and he felt anxious and uncomfortable without family support. Mrs. C. showed her resistance by attending sporadically and arriving late; soon it became clear that she and her husband had marital problems which predated his stroke, and because she covertly planned placement of her husband in a nursing home, she had difficulty identifying with the other group members. Mr. C. felt uncomfortable about attending without her.

PROBLEMS OF GROUP ORGANIZATION

We encountered some unique problems organizing the patient-family group in a medical setting. Routine issues, such as selection of a meeting place and the physical preparation of the patients for the meetings, required special effort. We finally obtained the use of a quiet classroom. We needed the cooperation of the nursing staff on the units to have the patients up, fed, and toileted in time for the meeting. Although the staff verbalized interest in the group and a desire to help with it, their behavior sometimes indicated difficulty in accepting this new program. On some units, staff members continually forgot which patients needed to be ready and at what time. We tried to minimize this problem by keeping staff informed of the patients' group participation and progress. However, our patient-family group seemed to raise questions for staff members about their own involvement and competence with the patients. Since general medical ward atmosphere is often geared to the suppression of uncomfortable emotions, it was difficult for patients and staff members to accept such a group.

Another difficult organizational problem was the establishment of a contract with the patient and his family. Through trial and error, we learned that the patient should be approached first with an explanation and an invitation to join the group. Then if he expressed interest, permission to contact a family member was given to one of us or the patient would make the contact himself. If the patient was not first consulted and given the opportunity to be in control of the decision, he would be resentful and resistive to participating in one more thing being imposed upon him.

In meeting with the patient and his family to discuss the group contract, we discovered that they could not accept the view that the illness produced a family problem. This seemed too frightening at a time when the family was mourning and shifting roles. Their anxiety was bearable only if the patient's *stroke* was seen as the focal problem. Most people were willing to participate in a group which had as its purpose the sharing of problems and ideas related to the stroke and to the home care of the person with the stroke. The following is the statement of contract we found most successful in the initial meeting with patient and family, and in the initial group meeting:

> It is often difficult for patients and their families to adjust their lives to a chronic disability, especially when it's time for the patient to come home from the hospital. We've found it can be helpful if people with these kinds of problems talk together about them. The purpose of this group is for discussion of the concerns you are and will be facing.

We experimented with an open and closed group structure, and found the latter more comfortable and apparently more productive. In the open group, as people left we replaced them with new members. This meant that the group was often disrupted by comings and goings and the issues of getting to know new members. Consequently, establishing a sense of group stability was particularly difficult. A cohesion developed in the closed group that allowed us to go further in the work of facing and living with the losses produced by the stroke.

In both types of group, we attempted to have patients continue participating in the group after discharge from the hospital. In most cases, however, people did not continue after discharge. They said it was too difficult physically to get the patient from home to the hospital. One patient did tell us he felt that "everything would be all right" once he got home, and he did not want to come back and tell us if things were not going well. We can only speculate that those first weeks at home are very difficult for the patient and family to face and share. Perhaps it is the first real confrontation with the change in physical and family functioning and the realization that everything is not "all right" in the sense that it is not the same as it was before the stroke. Additionally, the patients viewed the return to the hospital after discharge as a threat which seemed to heighten their fears and desires of being an inpatient again.

One last problem was in establishing a meeting time that was convenient for family participation. This varied with the composition of the group. If the participating family members did not work, they preferred meeting in the afternoon. If they worked, a time following the patient's evening meal seemed preferable.

GROUP ISSUES AND REACTIONS

Once the group was organized and group work begun, it became clear that the group members were mourning and trying to learn to live with their losses. The patient had lost some parts of bodily control and functioning. This resulted in loss of some independence, a change in self-concept, and a consequent loss of self-esteem. The patient feared total loss of control over himself, loss of his family because they might regard him, as he regarded himself, as an inadequate and useless burden, and the ultimate loss, death. The family also feared the total loss of a loved one as they had once known him and as he had once functioned in the family. The changes in the patient forced changes in the functioning of the rest of the family as they attempted to fill the places left vacant by the patient.

The patients and families struggled with their grief in the group, and this struggle can be seen in the framework of Engel's (1964) process of grieving.

1. SHOCK AND DENIAL

In every meeting the group members expressed their disbelief and wished the loss away. "How could something like this happen so fast? What caused it? It can't be real. Some nights I'm sure when I awaken in the morning it will be gone as quickly as it came. I just can't believe it!"

"I'm getting better every day. Soon I'll be good as new. This arm will be fine if I just exercise it enough. You can do anything with will power, you know. I'll be back working and fishing in a few weeks."

"My husband's going to be fine, no problems. They're holding his job for him and he'll be back at work soon. I was worried when it first happened, but I'm not worried anymore."

2. DEVELOPING AWARENESS

Although it did not often appear overtly, anger was expressed by the group members. "Why did this happen to me? What did I do to deserve it? Hospital staff don't take good care of me. The physical therapists don't tell me how to get this arm moving. The nurses wake me too early in the morning. The doctor never comes to check me." Occasionally, a patient would cry for the limbs that wouldn't move or the job he'd never work at again.

The family members felt resentment toward the patient for being ill and thus a burden, but guilt over this resentment prevented its direct expression. Instead, the family was often overprotective of the patient. "I wouldn't think of leaving him at home alone . . ." "It took me three hours to get him dressed this morning" (patient able to dress himself on the unit in the hospital).

3. RESTITUTION AND RESOLUTION

A great deal of group time was spent sharing together what life used to be like. This is the way in which they began to resolve the losses. The men shared tales of their military experiences, of their work and pastime activities. The family members talked of the things they used to enjoy together and do for each other. There was a feeling of trying to recapture the "good old days." Sometimes this reminiscing led to an attempt to reconcile the past and present. "I know we won't be able to go out as much, but do you think we could go out to dinner sometimes?"

"Maybe I can't do my old job, but there are some things around the house I could manage."

"I can't fish anymore, but the boys could put me in the boat and take me with them anyway."

In the first stage, reminiscing can be seen as part of avoidance and denial; in this stage, it is adaptive and part of the resolution of the loss. The patients and their families moved in and out of these phases and feelings of grief throughout the three months of group participation. Although phases exist concurrently, the overall movement is toward resolution. Engel says that successful mourning takes a year or more; however, in these three months, the work was well begun.

The group members also spent a lot of time discussing the more concrete aspects of being at home again. What kind of equipment was needed in the house for the patient to live comfortably? Could he get up a flight of stairs to the only bathroom? How do you manage to get the patient in and out of a car? Can the patient be left alone in the house at any time? The group supported one another in facing problems, and such focusing on concrete details served the function of decreasing anxiety and allowing families to deal with the emotional aspects of restructuring their lives.

PROBLEMS AND REACTIONS OF LEADERS

It was difficult to lead a new kind of group in a somewhat nonsupportive setting. Although the literature reports a few group experiences with medical patients *or* their families (Strauss et al., 1967; Piskor and Paleos, 1968; Bardach, 1969; Heller, 1970), we could find no precedent for a patient-family group of this nature.

We had the supervision of a psychiatrist whose expertise is group work and this was most useful. He helped us examine our structure and process, and encouraged us to experiment with new tactics when necessary. Most importantly, he supported us in our reactions to the helpless-hopeless feelings of our patients. A stroke is a catastrophe. The damage is highly visible. We found that we had strong wishes to "do something" for these patients and their families in a concrete way. These wishes made us vulnerable to their complaints that we were not doing enough and susceptible to their feelings of helplessness. In the beginning we tried to compensate for these problems by being active and directive leaders. We initiated conversation in most silences and often focused on individuals instead of allowing group involvement with issues raised by individuals. Both of these techniques served to suppress anger from group members about not being helped to recover permanent losses. Also, we often responded directly to questions for which there was no answer that could resolve the real issue for the patient. For example, members repeatedly asked for information about the specific causes of a stroke and specific cures. Our concrete answers seemed unsatisfactory because the real questions were: "Why me? What did I do to deserve this? Am I going to have to live this way?" With experience and supervisory support, we came to understand that the real work of the group was in the patients' experiencing these hopeless-helpless feelings. Our role was to be less directive and more supportive of the group members so that, through our empathy and acceptance, they could express their feelings and work with them toward a more productive and independent emotional state.

OUTCOMES

There were several important outcomes of the group meetings. First, to a greater or lesser extent, nearly all patients and their families shared difficult feelings. Through such openness, the participants often recognized that negative feelings about the stroke were not so frightening or threatening. For example, Mr. J. often felt depressed about his damaged body and inability to work at his former place of employment. At times, he started to cry, but his wife became anxious and made statements such as, "We can only think cheery thoughts." When Mr. J. was encouraged to express more of what he really felt to the group, he experienced a sense of relief, and the group helped his wife to tolerate her husband's tears and depression.

As the lines of communication became more open, families and patients began to be more realistic about their expectations. For example, Mrs. R. was secretly frightened that she would be tied to a life of drudgery once her husband was discharged from the hospital because she thought he would need constant supervision and care. When Mr. R. began to plan rehabilitation activities for discharge, she saw that he was not as helpless as she had thought. Other wives supported this idea through their experiences.

At other times, the outcomes were much more concrete and often revolved around decision making. Mr. and Mrs. L. had a two-level house which was inconvenient for Mr. L. because his wife worked and the facilities he needed were on both floors. After several group discussions, they were able to make the decision that they no longer needed the large house. They sold it and rented a ground-level apartment before Mr. L. was discharged.

As medical and rehabilitation evaluations became known to the patients and their families, they often shared the information with the group. From these discussions came the guidelines for using community supports. Mr. and Mrs. W. had lived a life of near isolation for eight years after Mr. W.'s first stroke. Both were unrealistically frightened of the stroke and remained in their third floor flat almost constantly. Although they were never able to resolve their fears completely in the group, this time they were able to make more realistic community plans for discharge. Mr. W. was able to involve himself for several hours weekly in a work activities program of the local rehabilitation center, thus allowing Mrs. W. some time of her own.

A final outcome was perhaps less tangible, but certainly no less important. This was the increased knowledge and sensitivity of ourselves and floor staff to the reactions of stroke patients and their families to this illness. Althouth the floor staff were sometimes resistive to our group, they could see that there were changes in patients and families which could be related to their involvement in the group. For example, some patients were less withdrawn on the units and some families were more willing to accept the patients on weekend pass. We saw directly the negative and positive influences a family can have on the acceptance and adjustment a stroke patient makes to his limitations.

CONCLUSION

We have described a group method for helping stroke patients and their families adjust to this chronic disability through a shared mourning of their losses. The purpose of the article is to describe the methodology and technique of such a group so that others might be encouraged in similar endeavors. Although research needs to be done to evaluate such groups, we feel that the patient-family group described has been a positive force in the rehabilitation of stroke patients and their families toward a more independent and satisfying adjustment.

REFERENCES

Ms. D'Afflitti is a Clinical Nurse Specialist in Liaison Psychiatry at the Veterans Administration Hospital in West Haven, Conn. Mr. Weitz was a medical social worker with the West Haven Veterans Hospital, and is presently a psychiatric social work supervisor with the Brooklyn State Hospital, Division V Outpatient Services, in Brooklyn, New York.

The authors wish to thank Dr. Walter Igersheimer for his guidance and support.

Bardach, J. L. (1969). Group sessions with wives of aphasic patients. *This Journal.* 19:361–365.

Bruetman, M. E., and Gordon, E. E. (1971). Rehabilitating the stroke patient at general hospitals. *Postgraduate Med.,* 49:211–215.

Engel, G. L. (1964). Grief and grieving. *Amer. J. Nursing,* 64:93–98.

Heller, V. (1970). Handicapped patients talk together. *Amer. J. Nursing,* 70:332–335.

Litman, T. J. (1964). An analysis of the sociologic factors affecting the rehabilitation of physically handicapped patients. *Arch. Physical Med. & Rehab.,* 45:9–16.

Millen, H. M. (1970). The positive approach to the care of the stroke patients. *Michigan Med.,* 69:887–890.

Piskor, B. K., and Paleos, S. (1968). The group way to banish after-stroke blues. *Amer. J. Nursing,* 68:1500–1503.

Robertson, E. K., and Suinn, R. M. (1968). The determination of rate of progress of stroke patients through empathy measures of patient and family. *J. Psychosomatic Res.,* 12:189–191.

Strauss, A. B., Burrucker, J. D., Cicero, J. A., and Edwards, R. C. (1967). Group work with stroke patients. *Rehab. Rec.,* Nov.–Dec. 30–32.

37

Dynamic Group Psychotherapy with Parents of Cerebral Palsied Children
—VERDA HEISLER, Ph.D.

CLINICAL psychology and rehabilitation psychology have in common a humanistic orientation toward serving human needs. Since for each of these the life adjustment of the individual is a central concern, some degree of overlap between them would seem to be inevitable, and yet it has been minimal.

Needs and possibilities exist for the application of psychotherapeutic knowledge and skills to the adjustment problems of the handicapped and their families. Reasons for the current insufficiency of such application stem from both areas of psychology. Developing out of social psychology, rehabilitation psychology has emphasized the mobilization of environmental resources. The problems of handicap are such that environmental support is essential for meeting primary needs. Only when the challenges of helping the handicapped to cope with the outer world have been met can attention be given to their inner world. And yet, so long as the inner resources of the handicapped person are not actualized, his place in the outer world will remain more limited than it need be.

Psychotherapists as a group have not felt any special responsibility toward the physically handicapped. A tenet of successful psychotherapy is that it must be self-initiated. Also, many handicapped people do not have the necessary financial resources. Parents of handicapped children seem to have been less motivated than the general population toward therapeutic help and this seems related to the rationalization provided them by the externally visible problem of the child's handicap. It is a misconception that

Reprinted by permission from *Rehabilitation Literature* 35 (11): 329–330, 1974.

the existence of a reality problem beyond a person's control contraindicates a need for psychotherapy. The question most relevant to the psychological health of a person is that of how well he adjusts to that which is not within his control. The challenge is to find the inner means of adjustment that are most conducive to the fullest actualization of the people involved.

A N attempt to meet this challenge was made through the author's study, "The Applicability of Principles of Dynamic Group Psychotherapy to the Adjustment Problems of Parents of Children with Cerebral Palsy." Supported by two grants from United Cerebral Palsy Research and Educational Foundation, Inc., the study came about initially through the efforts of the president of a local United Cerebral Palsy agency, himself the father of a 5-year-old cerebral palsied child. His request to the author for psychological work with a group of parents led to a search of the literature that indicated that group work with parents of cerebral palsied children had been limited to parent education and counseling at a strictly behavioral level. The closest approach to dynamic psychotherapy had been made by Justin Call,[1] who regarded his work as experimental so far as the applicability of this method to this population was concerned. He definitely concluded a need for it, stating

> . . . this study reveals that reality factors alone are quite insufficient to account for the gamut of perceptions and feelings which parents show . . . their attitudes and behavior, often unconsciously determined, influence . . . the psychological development of their children . . . The parent of the child with cerebral palsy has a vast array of external circumstances upon which to project and rationalize almost all of his feelings and behavior and it is probably for this reason that individual help is so infrequently sought. [p. 14]

Dr. Call's conclusions were consistent with the author's basic premise that parental adjustment to a child's handicap is rooted within the deeper dynamics of the parent's personality. Based on this premise, a therapy group was set up and conducted according to principles of dynamic group psychotherapy over a period of 66 2-hour sessions on a frequency of once a week. All the sessions were tape-recorded, and some of the material was used in a book written with the purpose of moving parents toward a quest for deeper understanding of the problem of handicap in which life has involved them and of stimulating interest on the part of agencies and professional personnel toward the provision of therapeutic services to parents.[2]

T HE remainder of this paper presents the meaning and significance of such therapeutic work. The condition of cerebral palsy—or of any physical handicap—imposes certain limitations upon the functioning and life experiences of the person so impaired. Thus, in addition to the challenges to psychological adjustment met by nonhandicapped people, the handicapped person must achieve personal reconciliation to this special deprivation and frustration and must maximize his potential for living within this framework of limitations. In the case of one handicapped from childhood, the extent to which he is able to do this will be a function of all those factors that influence and determine the development of his personality and his level of personal actualization.

Psychologists have long recognized the crucial importance of the parent-child relationship in the development of the child. Parents, in ways of which they are most often unconscious, are involved in the creation of their child's formative experiences, and the significant interchanges are more often covert than overt. What kind of person the parent is will constitute a more powerful influence than what he does.

Underlying the therapeutic approach in this project was the assumption that the child's adjustment to his handicap is facilitated or limited by the parents' reactions to and ways of coping with the problem and that these are, in turn, a function of the parents' own psychological dynamics, life orientation, and level of actualization as individuals. The problem of the child's handicap calls forth his parents' characteristic ways of functioning just as does any life problem.

From these basic assumptions came the decision to orient the therapeutic work toward the goal of promoting the actualization of the parents as individuals, with the expectation that this would enable them to relate to the problem of their child's handicap in healthier and more constructive ways. The parent who is involved in a process of inner growth is better able to respond to the inner life of the child with empathy and understanding. While all children need this from their parents, it is a special need of the handicapped child because of the isolating effect of his handicap. The isolation of necessary exclusion from certain physical and social activities is obvious. Not so obvious are the feelings this may evoke in the child and the isolating effect of having to cope with experiences that are significantly different from those of other people. If the parent has established a conscious relationship to his own inner world, he is better able to connect with the inner world of his handicapped child and thus break through the wall of isolation that encapsulates the child.

IN these days of increasing emphasis on the behavioral level, there is grave danger of the loss of attention to the inner world of the human being. In the case of the handicapped child, this is particularly damaging. Communication of the inner being is always a problem area for the handicapped person for two reasons. First, he is limited in his means of self-expression. Whatever the locus of his handicap, in some way it limits the implementation of the expression and communication of his inner being. Second, those around him may have difficulty in seeing beyond the handicap to the person. People may relate more to his handicap than to him. This is a frequent problem among parents of handicapped children—that they do not reach through and beyond the handicap to the inner being of their child. The depersonalizing effect of this may be disastrous. When a depersonalizing approach from the parents is added to all the problems intrinsic to the handicap, the child is in great danger of withdrawal into a state of alienation that prohibits the actualization of his inner resources.

This is all the more tragic because it is in the inner world of the handicapped person that his greatest resources reside. These are of two kinds. The first kind is in the area of ego-strength and includes such attributes as frustration-tolerance, patience, persistence, and courage, which must be developed to an exceptional degree if the handicapped child is to achieve active involvement in living. The second kind of inner resource potential in the handicapped child is that creativity which evolves from a deepening awareness of life as a function of his enforced introversion. It is paradoxical but true that the limitations on extraverted activity that carry a danger of alienation also carry a potential for creative depth. In order for these potential resources of the handicapped child to be actualized, he needs from his parents a sensitive recognition and support of his developing identity. Such sensitivity on the part of the parent is born of his own self-awareness.

Toward these ends, further attempts toward humanistic depth therapy with parents of handicapped children is encouraged.

REFERENCES

Dr. Heisler is a Diplomate in Clinical Psychology of the American Board of Professional Psychology and is state licensed in California.

This article is adopted from a paper presented as part of a symposium, Bridging the Gap Between Rehabilitation Psychology and Psychotherapy, at the American Psychological Association convention in Montreal.

1. Call, Justin D. Psychological problems of the cerebral palsied child, his parents and siblings as revealed by dynamically oriented small group discussions with parents. *Cerebral Palsy Rev.* Sept.-Oct., 1958. 10:5:3–5, 11–15.
2. Heisler, Verda. *A handicapped child in the family: A guide for parents.* New York: Grune & Stratton, 1972.

38

Management of Family Emotion Stress: Family Group Therapy in a Private Oncology Practice — DAVID K. WELLISCH, Ph.D., MICHAEL B. MOSHER, M.D., and CHERYLE VAN SCOY, R.N., M.N.

THIS paper describes the structure and psychological issues in a multiple family therapy group which has functioned for eleven months. The group is supported by and derives its patients from a three-man private practice of medical oncology. The purpose of the group is to aid the cancer patients and their families in coping with the difficult and unique psychosocial problems presented by having a cancer diagnosis. The basic aims of the group from its inception have been: (1) enhancing communication between cancer patients and their family and friends, (2) enabling both the patients and family members to deal with the inevitable intrapsychic conflicts concerning serious and often terminal illness, (3) working toward more direct and complete communication between patients/family members and the physicians, (4) providing input to the physicians and office staff to help them in the care of the patients, and (5) working toward "appropriate deaths" as defined by Weisman (1972) in terms of the psychological states of the terminal patients.

STRUCTURE OF THE GROUP

The group has met for eleven months, one evening per week for two-hour sessions, always in the waiting room of the group practice. The group has been led by a clinical psychologist with special training in both family therapy and in psychological treatment of the terminally ill. The psychologist works in a team-therapy approach with members of the office staff including a nurse-oncologist and several office personnel. Although the psychologist is the designated group leader, the other office staff participate fully in the psychological work. The physicians have never attended the group sessions. This was purposefully structured to facilitate maximal openness in terms of patients' and family members' feelings about their involvements with the doctors.

For the first seven months, only members of the cancer patients' families were invited and not the cancer patients themselves. It was felt that such a group would be too psychologically threatening and emotionally

Reprinted by permission of the American Group Psychotherapy Association from the *International Journal of Group Psychotherapy* 28 (2):225–231, 1978.

overwhelming for the patients. Interestingly, after a change was made and the cancer patients as well as family members were invited, attendance increased markedly. The reality of the group experience has been the opposite of what the therapy team and physicians had imagined and feared. The cancer patients have been significantly more open about issues than other family members and have felt supported and reassured by the group rather than threatened or overwhelmed. We have felt, in retrospect, that this is an excellent example of how not only family fears but also health-care professionals' fears can be easily projected onto the cancer patient.

The major responsibility for contacting the families and patients about attending the group was assumed by the office staff. This was done by mailing a description of the group to each patient in the practice; notices were posted in the office and verbal descriptions of the group were given to patients and families during regular office visits. The physicians have recommended group attendance if psychological and family communication problems were noted during contacts with patients and family members. At no time was a fee charged for attending the group.

PHILOSOPHY OF THERAPY AND THERAPIST ISSUES

The general philosophy of the group has been oriented around a crisis-intervention model as described by Caplan (1964). The emphasis has been on strengthening existing defenses and developing coping strategies to deal with the terrific stresses exerted upon the families by the impact of living with cancer. Little therapeutic energy has been devoted toward insight-oriented psychodynamic work. The therapist team agrees with Kubler-Ross (1975) that the terminal stage of life can also be the final stage of psychological growth. Thus, an attempt to focus on how the family can work toward maximal intimacy, sharing, and support as well as deal with the oncoming death and separation during the terminal period has been the major goal. It follows that the group has not been "thanatological" or death-focused as much as focused on maximal utilization of life. The issue of death is never denied or avoided in the group, but it has also not been an obsessive or singular focus.

THE PATIENTS AND FAMILIES

The patients and family members have utilized the group on an "as needed" basis. The usual number of attendees has been six per session, with a range of from four to sixteen. Above twelve the group cannot work effectively, and below four the same has been true. Approximately forty different family units have utilized the group. Families may attend for as short a period as one session or for as long a period as the entire eleven months of the group's existence. No commitment has been asked of group members, and attendees have tended to utilize the group during crisis periods.

Families and patients attend the group at all stages of the disease process. This often includes families of patients who have died in the recent past. We originally were concerned that the cancer patients would be disturbed by being in group sessions with families in mourning. This, too, was not the case in fact. The cancer patients have felt reassured and encouraged by viewing the other families' feelings and remembrances of their dead members. It is as if the message is transmitted that: "You will not be forgotten; you will survive with us."

CLINICAL ISSUES

The families function in a perpetual psychological limbo in relation to the cancer. As the articulate wife of one patient stated, "Cancer is like another member of our family, an unwelcome member." These families have had to adjust to a new psychological "family homeostasis" (Jackson, 1959) which includes this new member. It has been the repeated observation of the therapist-team that those families who experience the greatest difficulties in coping with cancer and who are most prone to develop serious psychosomatic or psychological symptomatology are those in which one of its members has had significant psychological difficulties previously. These difficulties have included such events or patterns as psychiatric hospitalizations, drug abuse in adolescents, suicide attempts, serious depressive episodes requiring treatment, and manic-depressive illnesses. Thus, inability to adjust emotionally to cancer is not a unitary phenomenon but the latest example of long-term difficulties in the family system, especially in adjusting to life changes. When families state that, "Cancer is the only thing we cannot talk about," closer probing of the family relational history and observation of current communication patterns has usually proven such assertions to be untrue. What these families cannot talk about is not "cancer" but their feelings in regard to the suffering they are experiencing and their fears about the impending separation of one of their members.

Cancer in a family member dramatically alters the social patterns of the family system. Often, attending the weekly group meeting is the only social event for the family member of a very ill patient. Guilt in the attending member is inevitable because of the feeling that every moment should be spent with the ill family member. Generally these isolated family members experience relief and much-needed support during encounters with group members in the same position. The characteristic interactions of this subset of group members involves mutual sharing of information on coping with daily problems of feeding the cancer patient, living with frequent vomiting due to chemotherapy, maintaining reasonable sleep patterns, and dealing with the deep depressions accompanying such restricted states of living. The physicians cannot reduce the weight of isolation for these family members, but the mutual support in the group does help to alleviate this stress.

The process of the group resembles that described by Blinder et al. (1965) and by Laquer et al. (1964) in their respective papers on multiple conjoint family therapy in psychiatric settings. The focus is on one family at a time, with the observing families drawing inferences about their own processes. The families have often tended to be more confrontive of each other, with less tolerance of resistance to change, than are the therapists. The teamwork approach has been essential in enabling the therapists to avoid the pitfall of becoming enmeshed in the families' defenses. Were this to happen, the therapist would begin to behave like a family member, avoid dealing with anxiety-inducing issues, and treat the cancer patient in a deferential, infantilized fashion. The tendency to avoid dealing with the anxiety-laden issues surrounding terminal illness is strong for family members and therapists alike, and both groups need a wide base of support to do so effectively.

The group is a safe arena for the expression of powerful emotions such as fear, rage, and sadness. Prohibitions against expression of these emotions have frequently been set up by family and friends, usually out of fears not adaptively dealt with by these individuals but maintained with the rationalization that expression of such feelings would surely make the cancer patient worse. The group deals with these rationalizations and gives permission to vent these feelings. Dealing with anger toward the physicians is a task of the group. The group reinforces the notion that patients and family members are persons of equal stature with the physicians and will not face revenge (psychologically experienced as fears of lack of treatment) if honest emotions are expressed toward them. A special subgroup of families, the survivors of concentration camps, have had particular difficulties in dealing with anger and harbor extreme suspiciousness toward the physicians. For this group, the development of trust is a critical treatment problem, and it appears that being out of control and in a state of helpless dependency is particularly difficult.

Children of the cancer patients have frequently attended the group sessions. They have been very reactive to cancer in a parent, but usually in less verbal ways than adults. Rather than becoming depressed, younger children will regress, lose bladder control, become temperamental, and draw very aggressive pictures, and have school problems. Adolescents have also had school problems and increased drug use in a seemingly unconscious attempt to deflect the attention of the family from the cancer and onto their own problems. Children in their late teens and early twenties have found themselves parentified in that they are placed in the role of emotionally parenting their frightened and regressed parents before they feel adequate to do so.

Husbands and wives coping with the effects of mastectomy have occupied a significant segment of the group's time. These couples have not necessarily been facing the issues of potential terminality but are trying to deal with the assault on the woman's self-image and the subsequent stress on the marital relationship. It has been the experience of the group and that of recent studies (Jamison et al., in press; Wellisch et al., in press) that most husbands are very concerned and troubled by mastectomy in their spouses, but a significant subgroup of husbands deny any problem and are unable to cope with their wives' conflicts and problems. Such men have found themselves to be the target of much group hostility, particularly from the female members. The women who have undergone mastectomy describe difficulties in coping with the continued potential disruption to their self-image by the effects of post-mastectomy adjuvant chemotherapy.

The feedback from the physicians has been extremely positive, as is perhaps best demonstrated by their commitment to continue and finance the group in the future. They report a striking increase in the level of intimacy between themselves and the group attendees which has greatly facilitated communication with these families and has made the medical care of the patients more efficient and individualized. The physicians also report that the mere availability of such a group has improved relationships even with families who do not attend, as if such families take the offering of the group as a demonstration of concern for them by the practice.

REFERENCES

Dr. Wellisch is Assistant Professor of Medical Psychology at the UCLA Neuropsychiatric Institute in Los Angeles, California. Dr. Mosher is Assistant Clinical Professor of Medical Oncology at the UCLA School of Medicine in Los Angeles, California. Ms. Van Scoy is a nurse in private practise in Los Angeles, California.

Blinder, M.; Colman, A.; Curry, A.; and Kessler, D. (1965). Multiple conjoint family therapy: Simultaneous treatment of several families. *Amer. J. Psychother.,* 19:559–569.

Caplan, G. (1964). *Principles of preventative psychiatry.* New York: Basic Books.

Jackson, D. D. (1959). Family interaction, family homeostasis, and some implications for conjoint family psychotherapy. In : *Individual and familial dynamics,* ed. J. Masserman. New York: Grune & Stratton.

Jamison, K.; Wellisch, D.; and Pasnau, R. (in press). I. Psychosocial aspects of mastectomy: The man's perspective. *Amer. J. Psychiat.*

Kubler-Ross, E. (1975). *Death, the final stage of growth.* Englewood Cliffs, N.J.: Prentice-Hall.

Laquer, P.; La Burt, H.; and Morong, E. (1964). Multiple family therapy: Further developments. *Internat. J. Soc. Psychiat.,* 2: 70–80.

Weisman, A. (1972). *On dying and denying.* New York: Behavioral Publications.

Wellisch, D.; Jamison, K.; and Pasnau, R. (in press). II. Psychosocial aspects of mastectomy: The man's perspective. *Amer. J. Psychiat.*

Personal Awareness: Individual Exercises

1. You are informed you can never have a child. You accept a child for adoption and later discover it is physically disabled. How would you respond? What would be the best and the worst effects of your response?

2. After being a widow(er) for two years, you make the acquaintance of a woman/man to whom you are attracted. After forming a relationship and becoming serious, you decide to marry. At this point, the person tells you she/he has a physically disabled, institutionalized child (cerebral palsy, age nine) who comes home once a month and is to be discharged in one year. Knowledge of the child was kept from you because of the fear of how you would react. Any comments?

3. Volunteer at a children's hospital for one month. Record your reactions.

4. Many people express interest and concern with rehabilitation issues. What have you and/or your family actually done to make such concerns an active part in your lives? If little, are there rehabilitation related activities with which you and your family might become involved?

5. Visit a nursing home and interview residents and staff on the topic of family involvement in residents' rehabilitation planning. Discuss your findings, implications, and recommendations.

6. Meet with parents whose children have disabilities and discuss the problems encountered. Explore the concerns expressed and determine what you might do to improve the situation(s).

7. Select three disabilities; (a) one which you consider to be *mildly* severe, (b) one which is *moderately* severe and (c) one which you

consider to be extremely severe. Would your feelings and/or behaviors toward the people you love change if one of them were disabled by any of the disabilities you selected? If so, how? Discuss your reaction. Does this awareness suggest any changes you might consider for interacting with these people? Discuss any changes and be specific.

Structured Group Experience in Disability
—Return Unopened*

The parents of disabled children face difficult situations for which they are often not prepared and which they must frequently resolve alone. The process of problem resolution can be stressful, painful, and destructive to the family system as well as to the marital relationship. A disabled child might become a source of conflict between the parents regarding the best approach to the child's future care.

GOALS

1. To present the potential impact of a disabled child upon selected aspects of the marital relationship.

2. To involve participants in the exploration of their personal reaction to a specific situation.

PRELIMINARY CONSIDERATIONS

1. *Level of Intensity:* High

2. *Group Size:* Six to ten

3. *Time:* Two to three hours

4. *Materials:* Role card

5. *Physical Setting:* Comfortable room

PROCEDURE

1. Participants read the following role description: "You are the parent of a two-week-old hospitalized child who is severely handicapped. You have not had the child home from the hospital.

---

*See Appendices A and B for detailed information on use of the structured group experiences in disability.

One spouse wants to put the child in an institution, while the other wants to bring her home."

2. When this is read, all members write their response concerning which position they would take and what they would do.

3. Having written the response, group members explore their reactions to this situation.

LEADERSHIP SUGGESTION

1. Focus on differences between parents and nonparents.

2. Look for cognitive styles (e.g., rigid beliefs, masking of anxiety) related to the situation.

3. Attend to differences between men and women.

VARIATIONS

1. Have child spend time at home—one year, two years, five years.

2. Introduce concepts of negative and positive impact on other children in the home.

3. Explore alternative solutions.

CHAPTER SEVEN

Structured
Experiential
Training (SET)

*A Group Designed
for the Rehabilitation and
Health Care Process*

Overview

Group counseling is rapidly emerging as a vital rehabilitation resource. The articles that have been presented in this book attest to the expanding use of group approaches in rehabilitation and health care settings. More importantly, the use of group approaches has been shown to be a valuable and therapeutic experience for participants as well as group leaders. The group experience gives participants the opportunity to share their aspirations and concerns by providing them with a supportive milieu within which group members can help each other cope with the challenges posed by a physical disability. For group leaders the value is found in learning more about the unique needs of group members, which can result in appropriate interventions.

However, while the trend toward increasing the use of group approaches is encouraging, there were several factors, suggested by the articles, that are important to explore. First, there appears to be an overreliance on insight-oriented group approaches in rehabilitation and health care settings. While such approaches have been shown to be meaningful in helping disabled persons to better understand their disabilities, insight alone is seldom sufficient to promote the development of skills required to participate successfully in the rehabilitation process. Secondly, there are few group approaches that include persons having various disabilities in the same group. While a homogeneous disability grouping has certain advantages, heterogeneous groupings can be advantageous when group members are attempting to cope with issues that transcend the uniqueness of their differences and to focus upon common problems of life and living that are shared by persons who are disabled. Thirdly, there is a lack of a systematic model that capitalizes upon the skills and resources of group participants. Too often traditional group counseling approaches focus primarily on deficits, do not provide the structure for participants to learn and practice specific skills in preparation for community re-entry, nor do they provide long-term support following discharge from the hospital or rehabilitation center. Lastly, some group approaches exclude significant others from the group rehabilitation process. This could be a hindrance to maximized client functioning considering that significant others may represent an important rehabilitation resource that can be developed by the group counseling process.

The following chapter is the presentation of a group model, Structured Experiential Training (SET), which is an attempt to respond to these concerns. SET is timely for rehabilitation, since it focuses on the development of resources and skills for those persons who are experiencing the rehabilitation and health care process. In addition, it is a model that (a) systematizes group counseling; (b) stresses active involvement by group members and leaders; (c) challenges both members and leaders to be accountable for their actions; (d) provides a structure that can be adapted to a variety of populations and settings; and (e) can be experienced by people with and without disabilities who are coping with problems of life and living. The SET model enables the group members to explore their personal frontiers, and it provides a platform for personal, interpersonal, and environmental evaluation and change. The combination of these elements enhances the viability of the SET process as a resource that can be used to supplement other group approaches that have recently been developed and applied to the disabled (Roessler, Milligan and Ohlson, 1976; Roessler, 1978; Roessler, Cook, and Lillard, 1977). Chapter 7 presents a detailed description of the SET Model and is followed by several appendices related to the SET group process.

39

Structured Experiential Training (SET):
A Group Rehabilitation Model*
—ROBERT G. LASKY, ARTHUR E. DELL ORTO,
and ROBERT P. MARINELLI

STRUCTURED Experiential Training (SET) is a group rehabilitation approach that was developed to respond to the needs of persons with physical disabilities through the implementation of an eclectic and systematic group approach. Disabled persons frequently share common concerns, such as adjustment to the personal impact of disability (Kerr, 1961; Wright, 1964), as well as interpersonal stress and stigma often imposed upon disabled persons by nondisabled persons (English, 1971; Ladieu-Levitan, Adler & Dembo, 1948). In an effort to help both physically disabled and nondisabled persons to overcome these and related difficulties the authors felt the need for a group counseling model which went beyond the verbalization of problems.

When disabled persons share their concerns in a group format they often capitalize on each others' strengths and benefit from the role models in the group. Additionally, they often feel a heightened awareness and sensitivity toward one another that communicates trust and understanding. This awareness highlighted the importance of including a major focus on *Mutual Concern,* or interpersonal caring, in the SET group model. It was apparent that if group member sharing and caring could be stressed, the constructive impact of the group would be intensified. In addition, uncertainty of future goals often adversely affects the disabled person's ability to meaningfully plan for the future. This realization indicated the need for a second major focus on *Goal Involvement* which could be personalized and developed within the SET model. Action in implementing goals and related behaviors is another important component of SET which is referred to as *Accountability.* This third major factor was emphasized considering that physically disabled persons often do not become actively involved with rehabilitation planning because of the lack of a system which stresses personal responsibility in the rehabilitation process. These three major emphases are developed more fully later in this chapter.

Structured Experiential Training (SET) attempts to combine the positive aspects of currently utilized group approaches within a systematic framework to benefit persons who are being rehabilitated. A key compo-

---

*Portions of this chapter are reprinted from Robert P. Marinelli and Arthur E. Dell Orto, Editors, *The Psychological and Social Impact of Physical Disability,* pp. 321–324. Copyright © 1977 by Springer Publishing Company, Inc., New York. Used by permission.

nent in the SET model is the utilization of structured experiential learning and the use of a variety of structured experiences related to group and personal functioning.

In recent years, structured experiences have been used to facilitate many types of goal-oriented group processes (Danish & Zelenski, 1972; Kaplan & Sadock, 1971; Pfeiffer & Jones, 1972), although such experiences have not, to the knowledge of the authors, been systematically implemented with persons having disabilities. The term "structured experiences" refers to "an intervention in a group's process that involves a set of specific instructions for participants to follow" (Kurtz, 1975, p. 167). Such an intervention ,then develops through five experiential steps described by Pfeiffer & Jones (1975): (1) *Experiencing*—the participant becomes involved in an activity; (2) *Publishing*—following the experience, the participant shares or publishes reactions and observations with others; (3) *Processing*—the dynamics that emerge in the activity are explored, discussed, and evaluated with other participants; (4) *Generalizing*—this involves developing principles or extracting generalization from the experience; and (5) *Applying*—using new learnings behaviorally. After reviewing the results of research related to structured experiences in groups, Kurtz (1975) found that such interventions led to (1) more cohesive groups, (2) participants who are more involved in the group activities, (3) participants who perceive their leaders in a more favorable light, and (4) participants who report that they learned more from the group experiences.

The SET group procedure is viewed as applicable to a wide range of persons having problems with life and living although its use with persons having disabilities has been a primary thrust. This current model represents the culmination of the developmental changes that have taken place since SET originated as a group treatment approach for rehabilitating substance abusers (Dell Orto, 1975) to its recent application with physically disabled persons (Lasky, Dell Orto & Marinelli, 1976; Pelletier, 1978; Marinelli, Dell Orto & Lasky, 1976). SET has also been used with physically disabled and nondisabled persons within the same group (Dell Orto, Lasky & Marinelli, 1979) and with female alcoholics (Trudel, 1977).

Structured Experiential Training (SET) utilizes structured experiential learning, the power of the group process, and an explicit goal orientation. Its focus is on skill acquisition and related therapeutic issues that are significant in the rehabilitation process. It is presented as a mode that can provide an alternative group approach that can be applied to a variety of populations and settings.

PRELIMINARY CONSIDERATIONS

Certain factors must be considered to maximize the potential effectiveness of the SET group experience.

1. Selection of Members. Potential SET group members are individually screened by the SET group leaders. Group candidates have an opportunity to view a SET group in action on a videotape and are given a written and verbal description of the SET group in addition to the SET group written contract. Such activities help potential group members obtain a better grasp of their responsibilities in the SET group experience and help to increase their expectations of what they stand to gain from the experience. Prospective group participants are encouraged to ask questions and voice concerns. Rather than automatically screening out potential members on the basis of physical disability or psychodiagnostic labeling, such as brain damage, sociopath, drug abuser, (Yalom, 1975) members are selected on an individual basis, focusing not on apparent deficits, but on potential to benefit from the SET group experience. A primary selection concern, determined on the basis of the interview, is a member's commitment to become goal-involved, accountable for his or her goal-directed behavior, and his/her agreement with the goals outlined in the SET group contract. Members who express a commitment to these principles and appear able to benefit from the group are invited to become a part of the SET group.

2. Group Size. The SET group is usually composed of six to ten participants. This size is consistent with recommended guidelines from a variety of research studies and practical experiences relating group size to time demands, group interaction, and participant satisfaction with the group process (Castore, 1962; Yalom, 1975). However, in certain settings the SET group may be larger or smaller dependent on how the number of members would affect the optimal potential functioning of the group.

3. Group Composition. The SET group has usually been composed of members who are interested in and capable of working toward personally relevant goals. SET groups have been conducted with groups of (1) drug abusers (Dell Orto, 1975); (2) female alcoholics (Trudel, 1977); and (3) physically disabled persons (Marinelli, Dell Orto & Lasky, 1975). SET groups have also been used with mixed groups of disabled and nondisabled persons (Dell Orto, Lasky & Marinelli, 1979). At this point, SET groups are especially useful when the participants are physically disabled and are grouped on the basis of their unique needs, regardless of homogeneity or heterogeneity concerning disability grouping or related factors. A primary concern is that participants have the potential for a cohesive group experience and the opportunity to observe, model, and learn a wide variety of alternative behaviors and skills.

4. Frequency of Meetings. The SET group usually meets once per week for approximately three consecutive hours. This time frame gives each member the opportunity to share his or her personal concerns and/or to report on significant experiences which occurred since the previous meeting. Also, due to the mobility problems of some members, it is more viable to have one longer meeting than two shorter ones. However, meeting times are flexible and may occur more or less frequently depending on the unique considerations of the setting or group member characteristics.

5. Written Contract. A written contract is given to the potential members prior to their inclusion in the SET group process. Subsequently, a mutual agreement is made between the leaders and the prospective group members concerning responsibilities in the SET group. This contract contains information on the goals and general expectations of the SET experience. Contracts have been shown to be highly effective in providing individuals with clearly defined expectations, goals, and interpersonal guidelines, and in enhancing the effectiveness of the therapeutic process (Haimowitz, 1973; Mallucio & Marlow, 1974; Montgomery & Montgomery, 1975; Steiner, 1971). Furthermore, the emphasis on individual and group goals, and mutuality of group members is highlighted as soon as possible, rather than by chance. Participants also have the opportunity to focus on the impact of their signatures on the contract in the initial SET group, and the importance of both personal and interpersonal responsibilities within an agreed-upon framework of interactions.

6. SET Workbook. SET group members are expected to record their perceptions of the group process and to keep notes outside the group on influences relating to their goal-seeking. In addition, participants are frequently given systematic directions to follow both within and external to the SET group experience. These personal notes, assigned structured experiences, and related SET information develop into a personalized SET Workbook that helps participants to: (1) become aware, during the group interaction, of various aspects of themselves and others that may otherwise be only indirectly focused on; (2) determine personally meaningful goals and appropriate group goals; and (3) become a more cohesive group. The workbook provides a uniform direction that facilitates the group process.

7. Group Leadership. It is advisable that SET groups be led by persons who have at least: (1) obtained their professional entry degree or have related academic experience; (2) had at least two academic group counseling courses; and (3) had supervised practice and experience in using group approaches. However, when used as a part of a group counseling course, graduate students may conduct the SET group with competent supervision. Rather than an informal structure and limited involvement of the leader, SET stresses using the specialized skills, techniques, and experiences of the leaders as well as their function as role models and facilitators. Guidance of the leaders develops group cohesiveness and mutual concern. Whenever possible, co-leaders share the responsibilities and direction of the SET. Pfeiffer and Jones (1975) have discussed several advantages of using co-leaders in groups, including providing alternative models for group members, complementing styles, and increasing ability to deal with heightened affect. The use of co-leaders in group practice has also been shown to be useful in training experienced group leaders (McGee and Schuman, 1970).

8. Structured Experiential Techniques. A key practice in SET is the use of structured experiential techniques to help participants more quickly attain their own goals and the mutually agreed-upon goals of the group contract. Group goals focus upon learning to identify, explore, evaluate, and respond to specific problem areas shared among group members. By providing a guided, relatively nonthreatening here-and-now focus, structured experiences give group participants a unique opportunity to discover the individuality and commonality of group members. Such awarenesses and perceived similarities are usually important factors in achieving group cohesiveness and personal and interpersonal growth. SET groups make frequent use of structured experiences designed to enhance personal and group goal acquisition.

THE SET MODEL

The SET group model is multi-dimensional and has identifiable phases and stages.

SET PHASE DEVELOPMENT

SET groups have three sequential phases which develop from a personal to a more broadly defined life perspective. These three SET phases are shown in figure 1.

The phases in figure 1 indicate SET participant involvement beginning with a focus on individual concerns, strengths, and problems brought by members to the SET group (Personal Phase), continuing through a focus on

FIGURE 1. *The Phases of the SET Model*

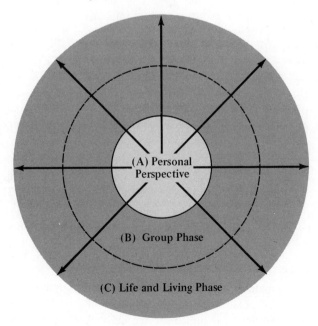

(A) Personal Perspective

(B) Group Phase

(C) Life and Living Phase

the functioning of the group itself as a goal-directed unit (Group Phase) and, ultimately, concluding with an emphasis on developing group resources to help SET participants use the newly acquired skills in their everyday lives (Life and Living Phase).

PHASE A—Personal.   Phase A focuses on the early development of a SET group and the encouragement of personal responsibility in the group. Structured experiences are used to help individuals to: (1) identify personal goals; (2) clarify these goals using descriptive behavioral language; (3) take responsibility for the excessive or deficient maladaptive behavioral difficulties which have led to problems in living; (4) develop a strategy to attain goals and become accountable for goal-directed behavior; and (5) develop the resources of the group to help group members succeed in reaching their goals.

PHASE B—Group.   In Phase B, the focus of the SET group is on helping the group to work together in a cohesive manner toward some relevant group-determined goals. Group leaders place increasing emphasis on demonstrated mutual concern and interpersonal sharing. Specific goals for Phase B include: (1) encouraging group members to work together toward some mutually determined purpose; (2) helping participants experience the constructive power the group has on all group members; (3) experiencing the effects of facilitative sharing of a common goal; (4) experiencing how to contribute to and benefit from teamwork; and (5) internalizing the values related to goal-directed activities.

PHASE C—Life and Living.   Phase C of the SET group is oriented toward helping group members internalize the knowledge, skills, and experiences that were attained in Phases A and B. Participants are given the opportunity to develop, work toward, and receive feedback on individual and/or social concerns related to functioning outside of the group. One specific emphasis in Phase C for persons who are physically disabled is to begin active involvement in self-help groups related to physical disability that are designed to: (1) provide a supportive outlet for group members following the termination of the SET group; (2) develop community action plans to serve the needs of persons with physical disabilities; and (3) become active providers of rehabilitation services using various strategies inherent in or consistent with the concept of self-help (Anthony, 1972; Anthony and Cannon, 1969; English and Oberle, 1971; Jaques and Patterson, 1974; Merlin and Kauppi, 1973; Siller and Chipman, 1965). If documented prejudice and negative attitudes by nondisabled toward disabled persons are to be overcome, active and organized consumer involvement is essential. Gartner and Riessman (1977, p. 107) suggest that "the essence of the human services depends on the involvement and motivation of the consumer." There is a need for a self-help consumer organization composed of persons who have a variety of physical disabilities who are working together to enhance service delivery systems and overcome prejudicial attitudes by nondisabled persons. Individual SET group members present and discuss long- or short-term personal concerns which may adversely affect their adaptation to life and living. The group focus is then channeled toward helping each person continue to progress through the SET stages toward a purposeful transition to the world beyond the group. Representative Phase C goals for all SET group members include: (1) demonstrating a transfer of the learned goal-involvement to long-range real world concerns; (2) skillfully applying significant experiences from the group activities to everyday living; (3) challenging participants to demonstrate consistent behaviors, affect, and cognitions, i.e., being congruent; and (4) evaluating the gains experienced by the SET group experience relative to the everyday process of life and living.

SET STAGE DEVELOPMENT

Within the SET phases there are twelve progressive stages which are shown in figure 2.

FIGURE 2. *The Stages in the SET Model*

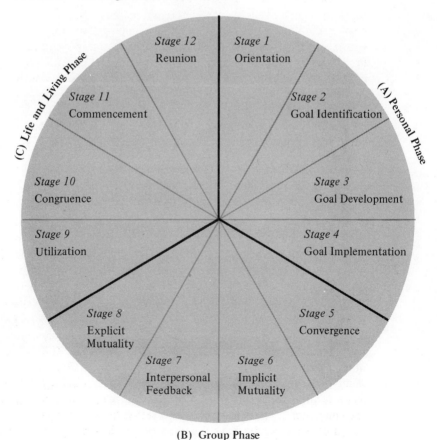

(B) Group Phase

These twelve SET stages are directly related to the three previously described SET phases. This relationship is shown by figure 3.

FIGURE 3.   *The Phases and Stages in SET Model*

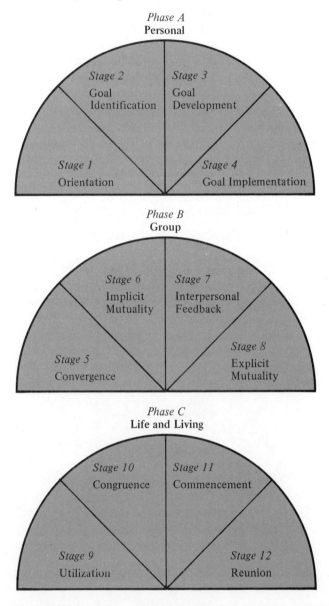

As shown in figure 3, in Phase A (Personal) there are four stages beginning with Orientation (Stage 1) and ending with Goal Implementation
(Stage 4). A major emphasis in Phase A is personal learning concerning
goal planning and involvement. In Phase B (Group) there are also four
stages, beginning with Convergence (Stage 5) and concluding with Explicit

Mutuality (Stage 8). A primary focus in this phase is the development of constructive group involvement and demonstrated mutual concern between group members. In the last phase, Life and Living (Phase C), there are also four stages, the first of which is Utilization (Stage 9) and the final stage, Reunion (Stage 12). Phase C stresses the utilization of significant learnings from the SET group experience to generalized concerns in ever-expanding areas of life and living. Each of the twelve SET stages is more fully described in table 1.

TABLE 1. *Description of the SET Stages*
PHASE A—Personal

Stage	Focus	Description
1. Orientation	Clarifying the purpose of the SET group and becoming acquainted.	Group members become acquainted with each other and share their feelings about beginning a group experience. Group participants are introduced to the SET group contract, which describes the SET group, responsibilities of group members and leaders, and ground rules.
2. Goal Identification	Selecting and exploring a personally relevant goal.	Group members become better acquainted by sharing their self-selected goals. By sharing their goals, participants have the opportunity to know each other in a nonthreatening, and facilitative manner. Group members also have the opportunity to explore significant aspects of selected goals.
3. Goal Development	Operationalizing and developing a plan to reach the goal.	A sequential plan of action is developed with a step-by-step process toward the goal. Each step in the process must be operationalized (i.e., behavioral, attainable, understandable, relevant, measurable, time limited). The goal cannot be meaningfully implemented until each step toward the goal is operationalized, with the last step in the process being the ultimate goal itself.
4. Goal Implementation	Actively pursuing the goal.	With the help and consent of the group, the participant is ready for active involvement with the goal, in accordance with stage 3 guidelines. Additionally, group members provide feedback on goal seeking, citing strengths and limitations in the process. Group members are encouraged to share comments and concerns to facilitate each others' goal involvement.

PHASE B—Group

5. Convergence	The group works together to formulate a goal which requires total group effort to accomplish.	The Convergence stage emphasizes the SET group coming together to work on a goal which is relevant for all group members. Structured experiences are designed to encourage maximum participation of group members and to apply goal development strategies, learned previously, to the group goal.

PHASE B—Group (continued)

6. Implicit Mutuality	Assessing interpersonal relationships and implications of various relationships.	As the group begins to work together, there are varying degrees of involvement in the goal-seeking process. Implications of divergent involvement are explored with a specific focus on acquainting group members with the concept of mutuality in relation to successful group goal involvement.
7. Interpersonal Feedback	Providing open, honest and direct feedback concerning group member involvement in the group task.	Continuing involvement related to the goal-seeking behaviors and attitudes of group members often brings some members together while alienating others. Interpersonal relationships and goal involvement are explored, with continued emphasis on the importance of mutual concern among group members.
8. Explicit Mutuality	Demonstrating genuine interpersonal concern between group members.	Explicit mutuality refers to demonstrated concern, respect and caring between group members. Participants share their thoughts and feelings concerning their giving and receiving mutual concern and how such actions have influenced their beliefs and values.

PHASE C—Life and Living

9. Utilization	Expanding significant learnings from the SET group experience to everyday living.	Group members are encouraged to apply significant SET group experiences (e.g., goal development, mutual concern) to their daily lives. This includes establishment of short- and long-term goals, involvement with other people, and movement away from group dependence to independence in coping with real world concerns.
10. Congruence	Demonstration of consistent thoughts, feelings, and actions.	Congruence in the SET model refers to a consistent integration of participants' thoughts, feelings, and actions with a special emphasis on constructively channeling these focal points towards growth-enhancing involvements. Group members share perceptions about each others' congruence, giving feedback concerning how congruence might be enhanced.
11. Commencement	Sharing SET group experiences and projected perspectives on future accomplishments.	The group discusses their SET experience, focusing on significant group experiences that have had impact on their lives. An important emphasis is on the solidarity of the group, continued goal-directed activities and demonstrated mutual concern in ongoing life and living situations.
12. Reunion	Coming together to share personal growth experiences and exploring further, needs for helping SET members.	The Reunion is held to reinforce significant learnings from the SET group experience and to determine if any members could benefit from further group or other forms of therapeutic involvement. It provides an opportunity to share success as well as to re-evaluate disappointments.

THE SET GROUP PROCESS

There are three primary emphases in the SET group model: (1) Goal-Involvement; (2) Mutual Concern; and (3) Accountability. These three emphases are augmented throughout the SET group process by the SET group contract, the SET workbook, leadership influence, and structured experiential interventions.

Goal-Involvement. SET stresses the importance of group members working on two levels of goal-directed behavior. On the most obvious level, each group participant works toward self-determined goals that are personally relevant, understandable, behavioral, measurable, attainable and time limited. A second level of goal-directed involvement pertains to the developmental process of the SET group, which progresses through three general phases and twelve distinctive stages. Ultimately, the SET group is concerned with goals related to increased intra- and inter-personal awareness, and acquisition of both enhanced interpersonal skills and values that are behaviorally, cognitively, and affectively congruent and that allow the individual increased functional capabilities.

Mutual Concern. Another emphasis in the SET group is on mutual concern, demonstrated respect, and interpersonal responsibility. Much of this focus is based on valuing principles accentuated in experiential and existential therapeutic practices (Barrett-Leonard, 1974; Gibb, 1971). Members are encouraged to become increasingly aware of their contractual obligation to extend themselves by demonstrating explicit concern for one another. While most group models do not encourage participants to be in contact with each other outside of the group, SET reserves the right to prompt external contact and involvement among members whenever there is potential for personal and interpersonal growth. Only by such structured and reinforced external group contact can members begin to transfer skills, behaviors, and values to real world situations. The emphasis on group support and guided external involvement helps to facilitate the seemingly difficult transitions necessary for the generalization of growth experiences.

Accountability. A major focus in the SET group process is on personal and interpersonal responsibility. This includes involvement in constructive activities within and external to SET group experiences. Group members are perceived as being responsible for their behavior rather than attributing behavioral difficulties to external forces beyond their control. This concept of internalizing rather than externalizing personal responsibility has been viewed as a primary factor related to emotional stability and constructive interpersonal relationships (Ellis, 1962; Rotter, et al, 1972). While some problems may be related to forces beyond the control of the individual (e.g., prejudice and negative attitudes by nondisabled toward disabled persons) it is important that group members take appropriate action on such problems rather than passively accept aversive situations, such as those that violate human rights.

Any one of the three primary factors of Goal-Involvement, Mutual Concern, and Accountability may be emphasized in a particular SET group. The determination of which aspect to emphasize is made by a close evaluation of the previous SET group and clinical judgement concerning the logical focus of the subsequent SET group. For example, the last SET group meeting may have been highly oriented towards goal-involvement with little or no emphasis on mutual concern or accountability. If these omissions adversely affected the functioning of the group, the group leaders might decide to emphasize mutual concern or accountability and de-emphasize goal-involvement. The process of determining tentative structured experiences is illustrated in figure 4.

In order to facilitate the development of the SET group and to maximize its potential effectiveness, structured experiential tasks are included in the SET model. Structured experiences are viewed as important to help

FIGURE 4.   *The Process of SET Group.*

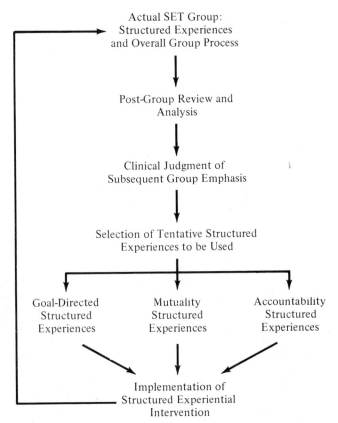

group members integrate, internalize, and relate to the SET model. Such experiences place greater emphasis on the experiential process and dynamics of the group, together with the cognitive aspects of goal involvement. Too often the latter are overemphasized, with the effect of reducing attractiveness of the group to group members. Conversely, groups emphasizing the processing of group dynamics often lack the structure needed to keep group activities focused.

To help the reader obtain a better appreciation for structured experiential interventions, representative structured experiences are described in table 2. The primary criterion for whether a structured experience should be used is the potential effectiveness of the experience to facilitate group or personal growth and development.

TABLE 2.   *Representative Structured Experiential Interventions Used in SET[1]*
PHASE A—Personal

Stage	Focus	Title and Description
1. Orientation	a. Goal Involvement	*Why Am I Here?* In this structured experience, group members are asked to write down their reason(s) for choosing to participate in the SET group. These reasons are read to the group and discussed as necessary.
	b. Mutual Concern	*The Gift.* This structured experience directs participants to pause and reflect on two questions: (1) How can I help others in this group? (2) How can the group help me? Reactions to these questions are shared with the group.
	c. Accountability	*The Signature.* Group members receive a copy of the SET group contract, which describes the group, states group member and leader responsibilities, and gives a listing of ground rules. After a discussion of issues related to the contract, members are asked to sign their contract. Implications of their signature are explored and discussed.
2. Goal Identification	a. Goal Involvement	*Pick a Goal.* Group members individually list three personal goals they would like to work on in the SET group. Participants then rank-order these goals from most to least meaningful. Dyads are formed with directions to take turns interviewing each other about their goal choices. Dyads are instructed to identify at least one way their goals are similar and dissimilar. Partners share this information with the group; the group's task is to determine relevant similarities and dissimilarities of selected goals.

[1]*The structured experiences included in table 2 are brief descriptions.*
A representative structured experience is presented in Appendix C.

PHASE A—Personal (continued)

Stage	Focus	Title and Description
	b. Mutual Concern	*Spotlight.* This structured experience is designed to help group members select a personally meaningful goal. Group member(s) who have difficulty determining a goal are asked to sit in the center of the group. Remaining group members are asked to list questions which will help the member in the center explore potentially meaningful goals. Each member then asks his or her question in turn, with the person in the "spotlight" giving a response. After each round, the spotlighted person summarizes any goal-directed learnings obtained from the questioning.
	c. Accountability	*Be Real.* Occasionally, group members may not take the group process seriously and/or identify irrelevant or innane goals. It is important that selected goals are personally meaningful if participants are expected to grow from the group experience. In this structured experience, group members are asked to reflect on each person's goal. Group members are then asked to: (1) select the one goal that was most "real" or relevant to be worked on, (2) give reasons for this selection, and (3) compare the choice with their stated goal. The same process takes place for the least "real" goal. For the latter, group members are challenged to help the person selected to modify the goal in a more personally relevant direction.
3. Goal Development	a. Goal Involvement	*RUMBAT.* This structured experience is designed to operationalize each SET member's selected goal. The group leaders describe RUMBAT,[2] an acronym relating to a goal which is Relevant, Understandable, Measurable, Behaviorable, Attainable, and Time-limited. Examples of how a goal is operationalized are given, followed by one member stating his or her goal and the SET group helping the member to operationalize the goal using RUMBAT criteria. Other SET group members are given a homework assignment to operationalize their goal prior to the subsequent SET group meeting.
	b. Mutual Concern	*Pairs.* Goal development may be difficult for some group members and may require time and effort between group meetings. In this structured experience, the group is broken into dyads with least known partners being paired. Each dyad is given approximately 30 minutes to help each other operationalize their goals. Subsequently, the large group reconvenes and discusses their task and how working in pairs was experienced. Any unfinished task or personal business is given to be completed as a homework assignment.

[2]*Developed by Douglas L. Mace, Ph.D., Director of Education & Training, V.A. Hospital, Syracuse, New York.*

PHASE A—Personal (continued)

Stage	Focus	Title and Description
	c. Accountability	*Responsibility Pie.*[3] In order to move the group members toward goal-directed activities, each member in the group must take some personal responsibility. Each group participant is given a sheet of paper with a circle drawn on it (all the same size). Members are instructed to individually draw a slice within the circle, to demonstrate how much responsibility they plan to take in working toward the group goal. All drawings are collected and pinned on a wall for all to see. A discussion of the drawings and related personal responsibility follows.
4. Goal Implementation	a. Goal Involvement	*Winners/Losers.* Group members are asked to name the two members who are perceived to be making the most progress toward their goals. Each choice is given on a 3 x 5 index card. These "votes" are then tallied. The winner(s) and loser(s) are discussed in terms of how each is different from the other in relation to their goal seeking and/or group behavior.
	b. Mutual Concern	*Helping Hand.* The focus of this structured experience is to encourage group members who are succeeding at accomplishing their goals to actively help others who are having difficulty. Group members are asked to rate their success in accomplishing their goal on a 100 point scale (0=totally unsuccessful to 100=extremely successful). After each has made his or her rating, group members are asked to rate all other group members on the same questions. Often, members will have difficulty doing this which presents the opportunity to challenge the group to involve themselves with others in their goal implementation, outside of the group. Reports of such involvement may be given in subsequent groups.
	c. Accountability	*The Payoff.* SET group members are given envelopes containing identical and progressive denominations of money (i.e., penny through dollar). Then each member is directed to consider who in the group is most productive, and so on to least productive in working on the group goal, and pay each person accordingly (i.e., dollar for most productive, etc.). This symbolic feedback is then discussed with a focus on perceptions of who gave what to whom.

PHASE B—Group

5. Convergence	a. Goal Involvement	*The Team.* Group members are instructed to pause and reflect on their SET group, and consider in what

[3]*Developed by Douglas L. Mace, Ph.D., Director of Education & Training, V.A. Hospital, Syracuse, New York.*

PHASE B—Group (continued)

Stage	Focus	Title and Description
		way the group might best work together. Participants individually select two goals external to the group, which the SET group could meaningfully attain. All goals are recorded on a poster board, group members discuss each goal and a consensus is reached as to the group's selected goal.
	b. Mutual Concern	*The Project.* This structured experience is designed to assess how group members will work together on their group project. A box of materials such as tinker toys, is placed in the middle of the group. The group is challenged to construct something worthwhile. (This is the only direction given.) After 30 minutes or more, the Project is discussed, with a focus on who were the doers and the do nothings. Implications for working as a group are explored, as are suggestions to overcome any problems experienced by participating in The Project.
	c. Accountability	*The Crew.* Usually the more the group works together as a unit, the faster and better their goal will be accomplished. Group members are directed to set their chairs in a straight line, to imagine the chairs are seats in a boat, and then to select the seat, from No. 1 rower to the last rower, which symbolizes how much each perceives he or she has contributed to the group goal. After this has been done and discussed, chairs are reversed. A second discussion takes place concerning how participants feel about their new responsibility, or lack of it.
6. Implicit Mutuality	a. Goal Involvement	*Partners.* The SET group is randomly divided into dyads, with partners selecting stages of the selected group goal for which they would like to take responsibility. Partners are given twenty minutes to meet and draw up a contract pertaining to their involvement. Each contract should state stage involvement according to RUMBAT criteria or be operationalized in some similar fashion.
	b. Mutual Concern	*Helping Hand.* In this structured experience, a survey is taken to explore who in the group went above and beyond their personal responsibility in working on the group goal. The rationale behind such action is processed in the group. Focus is also shifted to contractual obligations that were not met and reasons behind such lack of involvement.
	c. Accountability	*My Contribution.* After group members have developed their goal in a sequential fashion as in Step-by-Step, each member is asked to select the three sub-goals which he or she would like to take personal responsibility for, and to briefly give a

PHASE B—*Group (continued)*

Stage	Focus	Title and Description
		rationale for each. This information is shared with the group, discussed and agreed upon by all.
7. Interpersonal Feedback	a. Goal Involvement	*The Unforeseen.* Group members are asked to reflect on their goal involvement related to the group goal. Each is then asked to write down any problems being experienced in accomplishing the group goal. These problems are then expressed, discussed, and written down on a poster board. The group then determines, by consensus, the three most significant problems, and how each might be overcome, with an emphasis on determining who will have responsibility for implementing selected solutions.
	b. Mutual Concern	*Thanks, I Needed That.* Group members are asked to reflect on who in the group has been the most helpful, regarding the goal-seeking process. Each is then asked to bring an inexpensive (less than $5) gift for this person to the subsequent group meeting (a poem may be substituted). Gifts are exchanged, and group members asked to focus on the feelings behind getting and giving tangible feedback.
	c. Accountability	*Guilty as Charged.* Occasionally, one or more group members are deficient in carrying out their designated responsibilities. Group members are asked to select the one member who is seen as least responsible in working toward the group goal. These selections are written on 3 x 5 index cards and placed in a hat. Prior to examining the results, open-ended discussion takes place with a focus on who the group contributors are, and specifically what they have done to be considered contributors. The vote is then tallied and the least contributing member focused on only in terms of what might be helpful to motivate this person to be more contributing.
8. Explicit Mutuality	a. Goal Involvement	*The Call of Caring.* By the time the SET group reaches this stage, increasingly explicit mutual concern is usually being demonstrated. In this structured experience the focus is on how members can help each other attain their group goals. Each member is asked to repeat his or her group sub-goal. After everyone has done this, each member lists two people in the group who he/she can help in some way to reach their sub-goal. For each person chosen, the group member also indicates in *what* way help is planned, *where* the help will be given, and *when* the chosen member will be helped.
	b. Mutual Concern	*Beyond.* If mutual concern is being realized by group members, there will be indications of this

PHASE B—Group (continued)

Stage	Focus	Title and Description
		beyond the group experience. In this structured experience, group members are challenged to develop a plan of action whereby they will have the opportunity to facilitate the growth of others outside of the SET group. Plans are first shared and discussed in triads, then shared within the larger group. Important components of this experience include a follow-up feedback session and similar unplanned feedback sessions.
	c. Accountability	*The Guest.* This structured experience is an extension of "Beyond," previously described. SET group members are asked to bring into the group persons who were directly affected by the planned or unplanned demonstration of explicit mutuality. Guests may be asked to form a separate group to discuss their experiences as recipients of explicit mutuality before sharing these with SET group members.

PHASE C—Life and Living

Stage	Focus	Title and Description
9. Utilization	a. Goal Involvement	*Living Goal.* In this structured experience triads are formed. Triads are directed to select one goal which will help the participants to function more effectively in their everyday lives. Group members are then asked to present a role-play depicting important aspects of the goal. After each triad has performed a role-play, in the large group, group members explore relevant aspects of the goal which may not be clear. The goal may be changed to better represent the participants' more relevant concerns.
	b. Mutual Concern	*The Volunteer.* This structured experience is designed to give SET group members the opportunity to share their learnings from the group with friends, or family. From these categories group members are to select one person and try to help that person to become goal-directed. Results of attempts are discussed in subsequent groups.
	c. Accountability	*Lights, Camera, Action.* In this structured experience, group members give a verbal report of how they are utilizing their SET group experiences. Following this, a group member is selected to stage a role-play of the described situation. Group members are encouraged to provide feedback concerning the SET group member's performance, with opportunities to replay the situation to improve members' skills in the selected situation.
10. Congruence	a. Goal Involvement	*Leaders.* This structured experience is designed to explore the extent to which group members are actively involved with goal-seeking behaviors. Group

PHASE C—_Life and Living (continued)_

Stage	_Focus_	_Title and Description_
		members are given the task of directing the group themselves for the next sessions (the actual group leaders may choose not to be present). The group continues in this way, followed by a report with group leaders facilitating the discussion on how the group was experienced without intervention by the group leaders. A special focus is whether or not goal-directed group involvement was continued and reasons for such inclusion or exclusion.
	b. Mutual Concern	_Production_ In this structured experience, group members are given written tasks which they are expected to perform outside of the group before the next group meeting. These tasks will be straightforward, such as developing a plan to help a group member most in need. How these tasks were experienced is the focus of the subsequent group. This is a good test to see if group members have actually owned their avowed commitment to mutual concern. Emphasis should be placed on the creativity and quality of the help.
	c. Accountability	_Evidence._ Group members are given the homework assignment of examining their SET logs closely for signs of progress. A handout, with columns headed (1) Thoughts, (2) Feelings, and (3) Actions, may be used to help give group members a method of organizing the evidence of self-perceived change. Then, group members are asked to cite the most significant thought, feeling, and action which affected their SET experience. Members are asked to predict how each other would respond to these questions.
11. Commencement	a. Goal Involvement	_I've Only Just Begun._ As in the song, SET group members have often only recently started to apply their SET experiences in their everyday lives. Group members are asked _how_ they are using their SET group experiences, _with whom, where, how often,_ etc. This helps provide specific interpersonal feedback on the effectiveness of the group experiences.
	b. Mutual Concern	_The Letter._ Group members are asked to write a farewell letter to the group, keeping in mind that this group is ending. No specific structure is necessary; group members who have difficulty expressing themselves may request help from another group member. Letters are read aloud in the final group meeting and explored for future implications.
	c. Accountability	_Commandments._ Group members are asked to make a list of how they might hold themselves ac-

PHASE C—Life and Living (continued)

Stage	Focus	Title and Description
		countable for future constructive activities. Contingency contracts, aversive procedures, positive reinforcers, etc. are shared among group members to give all members insight concerning how to keep straight and involved in purposeful goal activities. Individual lists are revised following the sharing of ways to help members continue their goal-seeking.
12. Reunion	a. Goal Involvement	*Time Tunnel.* The group is asked to visualize the entire group going on a train ride through a time tunnel. Their task is to select a time when they would like the train to stop so the group could step into the future and examine where they are and what they've been doing; this will be their reunion. Members individually choose a time period from one month to five years. Reactions are discussed with a group focus on selecting a future time for the next SET group meeting.
	b. Mutual Concern	*Impact.* Group members are directed to pause and reflect on what they have experienced in and outside of the SET group since the group began. Members are asked to select one person, either within or external to the SET group, who had the most impact on them. This experience is shared with group members with a focus on how each member might have as much impact on other persons.
	c. Accountability	*Action Speaks.* This structured experience highlights the accomplishments of group members since leaving the group. Each member is asked to list his accomplishments since the previous group. This information is shared with the group, with a subsequent focus on how group members can be of further help to one another. Interpersonal helping contracts (implicit or explicit) may be designed in dyads or triads and shared with the entire group.

SUMMARY

SET is an eclectic group rehabilitation model which is especially designed to meet the needs of persons with physical disabilities and emphasizes group member goal-involvement, mutual concern, and accountability. These emphases are incorporated throughout the SET model, which is composed of three sequential phases and twelve developmental stages. Structured experiential tasks are frequently used in SET to help group members to: (1) achieve their self-selected goals, (2) become more concerned with the welfare of other persons, and (3) take personal responsibility for their lives. While the SET model is systematic and developmental, flexibility is stressed by encouraging personal goal development, the implementation of many different kinds of structured experiential interventions, and the frequent use of the resources of group members. Most importantly, the SET group is designed to help participants experience and acquire generalizable skills (e.g., goal development, genuine concern for others, responsible social action) which can be utilized throughout their lives.

SET groups are applicable to rehabilitating persons who are interested in and capable of working toward meaningful personal and interpersonal goals. While goal-involvement is stressed in SET groups, it is the importance of people working together for common concerns which is most strongly emphasized. The unique aspect of goal-involvement, highlighted in the SET model, is that the process of working toward a goal is in the context of interpersonal sharing and caring. This has been shown by the planning and development of a self-help organization for people having various disabilities by a group of SET group graduates.

Within a SET format, people have the opportunity to be themselves, to explore their functional freedom, to develop skills, to receive feedback from others, to express their aspirations and to share their joy, sorrow, elation, and pain. Through involvement with others, their peers and allies, the sense of isolation and loneliness is alleviated. These concerns during the process of rehabilitation can intensify the smallest discomfort and distort the most relevant aspiration. Seen as a means to transcend the barrenness of despair, powerlessness, and hopelessness, the SET procedures introduce a shared experience that may not make the long journey of rehabilitation shorter, but frequently makes it more bearable.

REFERENCES

Dr. Lasky is Director of Graduate Studies, and Dr. Dell Orto is Chairman, Department of Rehabilitation Counseling, Sargent College of Allied Health Professions, Boston University. Dr. Marinelli is Associate Professor, Department of Counselor Education and Rehabilitation, College of Human Resources and Education of West Virginia University, Morgantown, West Virginia.

Anthony, W. A. Societal rehabilitation: Changing society's attitudes toward the physically and mentally disabled. *Rehabilitation Psychology,* 1972, 19: 117–126.

Anthony, W. A. and Cannon, J. A. A pilot study on the effects of involuntary integration on children's attitudes. *Rehabilitation Counseling Bulletin,* 1969, 12: 239–240.

Barrett-Leonard, G. T. Experiential learning groups. *Psychotherapy: Theory, Research and Practice,* 1974, 11 (1): 71–75.

Castore, G. F. Number of verbal inter-relationships as a determinant of group size. *Journal of Abnormal Social Psychology,* 1962, 64: 456–457.

Danish, S. J. and Zelenski, J. R. Structured group interaction. *The Journal of College Student Personnel,* 1972, 13 (1): 53–56.

Dell Orto, A. E. Goal group therapy. A structured group experience applied to drug treatment and rehabilitation. *Journal of Psychedelic Drugs,* 1975, 7: 363–371.

Dell Orto, A. E.; Lasky, R. G. and Marinelli, R. P. *Structured experiential therapy: Theory, model and application.* Framingham, Mass.: E.R.A., P.C., 1978. (In press.)

Ellis, A. *Reason and emotion in psychotherapy.* New York: Lyle Stuart, 1962.

English, R. W. Correlates of stigma toward physically disabled persons. *Rehabilitation Research and Practice Review,* 1971, 2: 1–17.

English, R. W. and Oberle, J. B. Toward the development of new methodology for examining attitudes toward disabled persons. *Rehabilitation Counseling Bulletin,* 1971, 15 (2): 88–96.

Gartner, A. and Riessman, R. *Self-help in the human services.* San Francisco: Jossey-Bass, 1977.

Gibb, J. R. The effects of human relations training. In *Handbook of psychotherapy and behavior change,* eds., A. E. Bergin and S. L. Garfield, pp. 839–862, New York: Wiley, 1971.

Goffman, E. *Stigma.* Englewood Cliffs, N.J. Prentice Hall, 1963.

Haimowitz, M. Short-term contracts. *Transactional Analysis Journal,* 1973, 3 (2): 34.

Herman, S. Some observations on group therapy with the blind. *International Journal of Group Psychotherapy,* 1966, 16 (3): 367–372.

Jaques, M. E. and Patterson, K. M. The selfhelp group model: a review. *Rehabilitation Counseling Bulletin,* 1974, (18): 48–58.

Kaplan, H. J. and Sadock, B. J. Structured interactions: A new technique in group psychotherapy. *American Journal of Psychotherapy,* 1971, 25 (3): 418–427.

Kerr, N. Understanding the process of adjustment to disability. *Journal of Rehabilitation,* 1961, 27 (6): 16–18.

Kurtz, R. R. Structured experience in groups: A theoretical and research discussion. In *The 1975 Annual Handbook for Group Facilitators,* eds., J. E. Jones and J. W. Pfeiffer, pp. 167–172. LaJolla, California: University Assoc., 1975.

Ladieu-Leviton, G.; Adler, D. and Dembo, T. Studies in adjustment to visible injuries: Social acceptance of the injured. *Journal of Social Issues,* 1948, 4 (14): 55–61.

Lasky, R. G.; Dell Orto, A.E. and Marinelli, R.P. Structured experiential therapy (SET-R): A group approach to rehabilitation. Paper presented at the Northeast Regional Conference of the National Rehabilitation Association, Cherry Hill, New Jersey, 1976.

Mallucio, A. N. and Marlow, W. D. The case for the contract. *Social Work,* 1974, 19: 28–36.

Marinelli, R. P. and Dell Orto, A. E. *The Psychological and social impact of physical disability.* New York: Springer, 1977.

Marinelli, R. P.; Dell Orto, A. E. and Lasky, R. G. Integrating rehabilitation consumers and providers: A structured experiential approach. Unpublished presentation at the New Hampshire Division of Vocational Rehabilitation. Manchester, New Hampshire, May, 1976.

Means, B. L. and Roessler, R. T. *Personal achievement skills leader's manual and participant's workbook.* Fayetteville, Ark.: Arkansas Rehabilitation Research and Training Center, 1976.

Merlin, J. S. and Kauppi, D. R. Occupational application and attitudes toward the physically disabled. *Rehabilitation Counseling Bulletin,* 1973, 16 (3): 173–179.

Montgomery, A. G. and Montgomery, D. J. Contractual psychotherapy: Guidelines and strategies for change. *Psychotherapy: Theory, Research and Practice,* 1975, 12 (4): 348–352.

Pelletier, J. *Group work in Quincy: A program update.* Unpublished paper. Quincy, Mass.: Massachusetts Rehabilitation Commission, 1978.

Pfeiffer, J. W. and Jones, J. E. *The annual yearbook for group facilitators.* LaJolla, California: University Associates, 1972–1976.

Roessler, R. An evaluation of Personal Achievement Skills training with the visually handicapped. *Rehabilitation Counseling Bulletin,* 1978, 21: 300–305.

Roessler, R.; Cook, D. and Lillard, D. The effects of systematic group counseling with work adjustment clients. *Journal of Counseling Psychology,* 1977, 24, 313–317.

Roessler, R.; Milligan, T. and Ohlson, A. Personal Achievement Training for the spinal cord injured. *Rehabilitation Counseling Bulletin,* 1976, 19: 544–550.

Rotter, J.; Chance, J. and Phares, J. *Applications of a social learning theory of personality.* New York: Holt, Rinehart & Winston, 1972.

Siller, J. and Chipman, A. *Personality determinants of reaction to the physically handicapped. II. Projective techniques.* Alberston, New York. Unpublished manuscript, Human Resources Library, 1965.

Steiner, C. Contractual problem-solving groups. *Radical Therapist,* 1971.

Trudel, R. *Structured experiential therapy for alcoholics (SET-A) versus assertive training: A comparison of two structured group formats for helping female alcoholics.* Unpublished doctoral dissertation, Boston University, 1977.

Wright, B. Spread in adjustment to disability. *Bulletin of the Menninger Clinic,* 1964, 28: 198–208.

Yalom, I. D. *The theory and practice of group psychotherapy* 2nd Ed. New York: Basic Books, 1975.

_____ **Personal Awareness:**
Individual Exercises

1. How are goals important in your life? Have you set immediate and long-term goals for yourself? If so, write them down and process them using the RUMBAT format described in this chapter. If you became disabled, how would they change?

2. Assume you are planning to be the group leader with a group of disabled persons. What would be the most difficult issues for you to deal with? Develop an approach which would help you deal with these issues more effectively.

3. Imagine that you are disabled (if you are, select another disability). List those elements you would like to see included in a group counseling model which would be part of your rehabilitation program.

4. If you were a member of a group which included both physically disabled and nondisabled persons, what would be the most difficult issues for you to share with the group.

5. Imagine you are contacted by a local chapter of an organization of disabled consumers and asked if you would like to be a member of a group counseling experience designed to explore prejudice between disabled and nondisabled persons. What would you do and why?

Structured Group Experience in Disability
—Building a Better Mousetrap*

After having experienced several structured group experiences in disability as a group leader and participant, people often get innovative ideas for creative structured group experiences. In this structured group experience in disability, group participants have the opportunity to develop a structured group experience.

GOALS

1. To discover how to develop a structured group experience in disability.

2. To share creative ideas with other persons in a group.

3. To develop specific goals and strategies for structured group interventions.

4. To experience how cooperative group efforts lead to task accomplishment.

5. To experience how structured guidelines may enhance or detract from task and interpersonal functioning.

PRELIMINARY CONSIDERATIONS

1. *Level of Intensity:* Low to Moderate

2. *Group Size:* Any number of groups of four to six persons

3. *Time Required:* 3 hours

4. *Materials:* Paper and pencils for each participant

5. *Physical Setting:* Comfortable room with moveable chairs

---

*See Appendices A and B for detailed information on use of the structured group experiences in disability.

PROCEDURE

1. The group leader introduces the structured group experience by briefly discussing the above goals. Participants are also told that they will have the opportunity to develop a creative structured group experience in disability.

2. Small groups are formed.

3. The group leader distributes copies of the "Guidelines for Developing Structured Group Experiences in Disability" (see Appendix D) to half of the groups, with all members in these groups getting a copy of the handout. The remaining groups each get a copy of the Structured Group Experience in Disability, "Welcome Back," from chapter one to serve as a model.

4. Group members are directed to begin working on the development of a structured group experience in disability with a 1½ hour time limit.

5. The group leader helps to process what took place in each of the groups focusing on issues such as task versus person orientation by members, disability groups selected and how and why the disability was selected, and related group process issues.

6. One group is asked to conduct their structured group experience in disability by selecting two co-leaders and having them select a small group of members.

7. The structured group experience in disability is conducted with remaining group members being process observers.

VARIATIONS

1. The group leader can select the disability group to be used in the structured experience.

2. All group members can use the model structured group experience in disability or the "Guidelines for Developing Structured Group Experience in Disability" form.

3. One group can be selected to develop the structured experience while other persons become observers and recorders of the group process.

APPENDIX A

Group Leader
Feedback Guide

The Group Leader Feedback Guide is a structured questionnaire which has been developed to give group members the opportunity to provide constructive feedback regarding the group process and to facilitate group leadership skills. This questionnaire is completed by group members subsequent to their participation in a Structured Group Experience in Disability. There are three primary components in this questionnaire: (1) Goals, (2) Mutual Concern, and (3) Accountability. These primary areas are major focal points of the Structured Experiential Therapy (SET) group model. Within each of these components is a focus on critical incidents* which may be experienced in the group. Critical incidents are recorded by group participants on the questionnaire. Such reactions serve as feedback for group leaders regarding their leadership skills and related issues. Specific critical incidents may be replayed to allow group leaders the opportunity to acquire more effective group leadership skills.

GOALS

1. To allow group members to provide constructive feedback to the group leader(s) following a group experience.

2. To allow group leaders and members to react to and process issues regarding physical disability.

3. To provide group leaders with systematic, purposeful feedback regarding their group leadership skills.

4. To acquaint group leaders and participants with the strengths and limitations of conducting structured group interventions.

5. To provide group members and leaders with a greater awareness of issues regarding physical disability through structured experiential interventions.

6. To provide group leaders with the opportunity to learn and apply alternative behaviors to facilitatively lead a group.

---

*Cohen and Smith (1976) define a critical incident as "the confrontation of a group leader by one or more members, in which an explicit or implicit opinion, decision or action is demanded of him. It may also be an observed conversation, a confrontation among members, an event taking place, or a period of silence in which an expectation or demand is made of the leader" (p. 114). Cohen, A. and Smith, R. *The critical incident in growth groups: Theory and technique.* LaJolla, Calif.: University Assoc., 1976.

HOW TO USE

1. The group leader(s) select a relevant structured group experience in disability from those given at the end of each chapter in this book.

2. The group experience is conducted by the group leader(s) as described.

3. Group members complete the group leadership feedback guide following the group experience.

4. The group members provide feedback to the group leaders as directed (e.g., page by page, open-ended).

5. Critical incidents which are agreed with by group members are discussed, with specific attention formed on how the leaders might have better reacted to the critical incident(s).

6. After there is a basic agreement about alternative strategies which could be used to better react to the critical incident, the group replays the critical incident.

7. The original group leaders use the newly agreed-upon strategy to better react to the critical incident.

8. Group members and leaders share feedback about the differences which are experienced in the replay. An emphasis on positive changes (i.e., improvements in group leadership) is recommended.

9. Other critical incidents can be discussed and role-played as time permits.

GROUP LEADER FEEDBACK GUIDE

Leaders: 1 _____

          2 _____

Rater _____

Date _____

Group Phase _____
  (Place (✔) on line) Beginning   Middle   End

Group Number _____

Title of Structured Experience _____

Disability Population Focus: _____

Directions: In order to become an effective group leader it is important for leader–trainees to receive feedback from observers and/or group members. Please take some time to respond to the following questions. Refer to the directions for using this questionnaire to facilitate learning group leadership skills.

A.   Significant Positive Aspects of the Group Leadership _____

_____

_____

B.   Suggested Areas for Leadership Improvement _____

_____

_____

C.   Goals for the Session
    1.   Stated _____

    2.   Implied _____

D.   Primary Emphasis Related Questions

    1.   *Goals*
       a. Did the leader(s) present an overview of the group session, including mention of the goal(s)?

       Yes _____   No _____   Unsure _____

       Comments _____

b. Did the leader(s) encourage members to react to the goal(s) which were stated?

Yes _____ No _____ Unsure _____

Comments _____

c. Did group members agree with the stated goals verbally and/or nonverbally?

Yes _____ No _____ Unsure _____

Comments _____

d. Were there any critical incidents in the group which were related to the stated or implied goals?

Yes _____ No _____

If yes, please describe the situational context of the critical incident _____

_____

   i. What events preceded this critical incident? _____

_____

  ii. What did you see as the surface *and* underlying issues related to this critical incident?

_____

 iii. How did the group leaders react to this critical incident? _____

_____

 iv. Describe any suggestions, and give your rationale, to more facilitatively cope with this critical incident _____

_____

2. *Mutual Concern*
   a. Were the leaders sensitive to the feelings and concerns of the group members?

   Yes _____ No _____ Unsure _____

   Comments _____

   b. Did the group leaders attempt to facilitate appropriate *group* communication versus dyadic discussion?

   Yes _____ No _____ Unsure _____

   Comments _____

   c. Did the leaders provide a favorable balance between task-orientation and people-concern in this session?

   Yes _____ No _____ Unsure _____

   Comments _____

d. Were there any critical incidents in the group which were related to the concept of mutual concern?

Yes _____   No _____   Unsure _____

Please describe the situational context of a critical incident _____

_____

   i. What events preceded this critical incident? _____

      _____

   ii. What did you see as the surface *and* underlying issues related to this critical incident? _____

      _____

   iii. How did the group leaders react to this critical incident? _____

      _____

   iv. Describe any suggestions you would make, and give your rationale, to facilitatively cope with this critical incident _____

      _____

3. *Accountability*
   a. Did the group leader(s) act responsibly in their roles as leaders in the group?

   Yes _____   No _____   Unsure _____

   Comments _____

   b. Did the leaders encourage the group members to be accountable for their actions within the group (e.g., encouraging members to be congruent with their feelings and actions) and between group sessions (e.g., doing relevant homework assignments)?

   Yes _____   No _____   Unsure _____

   Please describe _____

   _____

   c. Were there any critical incidents in the group which were related to the concept of accountability?

   Yes _____   No _____   Unsure _____

   Please describe the situational context of a critical incident _____

   _____

      i. What events preceded this critical incident? _____

         _____

    ii. What did you see as the surface *and* underlying issues related to this critical incident? _____

    _____

    iii. How did the group leaders react to this critical incident? _____

    _____

    iv. Describe any suggestions you would make, to more facilitatively react to this critical incident _____

    _____

4. Discuss any other aspects of this session which you observed that would serve as helpful feedback for the group leaders _____

  _____

5. List and briefly describe any significant learnings which you experienced from this session _____

6. Other comments _____

  _____

7. Overall Leadership Rating for this Session (Circle the word which most closely applies to your impressions of group leadership skills shown in this session.)

    Poor   Fair   Good   Very Good   Excellent

APPENDIX B

Guidelines for Using Structured Group Experiences in Disability

Prior to conducting a Structured Group Experience in Disability, group leaders should be familiar with the following:

Goals of Structured Group Experiences in Disability are to help participants to:

1. become more sensitive to the potential impact of physical disability on their lives.

2. facilitate self-disclosure and interpersonal feedback regarding disability related concerns.

3. explore their attitudes and values regarding the impact of physical disability.

4. better understand how disability affects their lives and the lives of persons with disabilities.

5. live more congruent lives by better integrating their thoughts, feelings and actions regarding physical disability and related issues and concerns.

6. become better group leaders by providing a structure for group process and a format for systematic feedback regarding group leadership skills.

Considerations in Conducting Structured Group Experiences in Disability

1. Group Leadership: Structured Group Experiences in Disability are designed for use by leaders who have had training and experience in group practices. However, when used as part of a group counseling course, undergraduate or graduate students may conduct these experiences with supervision from the instructor. When student group leaders conduct the experiences it is recommended that systematic feedback on their group leadership skills be provided by group members, observers and the instructor; the Group Leadership Feedback Guideline has been developed for such feedback procedures.

2. Group Membership: Structured Group Experiences in Disability have been designed for students in rehabilitation and health fields to help them attain the aforementioned goals. However, these experiences may also be used with people in general who are interested and potentially capable of reaching one or more of the aforementioned goals.

3. Introducing Structured Group Experiences in Disability: Prior to involv-

ing a group in Structured Group Experience in Disability the group leader(s) should present a rationale and related information to substantiate the potential usefulness of participating in the experience. Of course, the group leader(s) should be thoroughly knowledgeable about the structured experience which is selected, e.g., procedures, variations, etc.

4. Process of Structured Group Experiences in Disability: It is extremely important that the group leader(s) encourage group participants to relate how they experienced the Structured Group Experience in Disability; develop major themes which emerge from participants sharing the experience; discuss how major themes which emerge from the experience affect each participants' past, present, and future life and living; and help each participant to apply significant learnings from the experience to their daily lives.

5. Integrating Knowledge, Values, and Skills: Perhaps the most desirable way to use a Structured Group Experience in Disability is to sequentially (a) develop meaningful reading assignments related to the disability area focused upon in the structured experience, (b) encourage participants to become actively involved with one or more Personal Awareness Individual Exercises, (c) discuss issues and concerns related to a and b, and (d) allow selected student co-leaders to conduct the Structured Group Experience in Disability using the Group Leadership Feedback Guideline to promote group leadership skills.

Representative Structured Group Experience:
—Pick a Goal

SET Phase: Personal (A)
SET Stage: Goal Identification (Stage 2)
SET Focus: Goal Involvement

SET group members are often unaware of the importance of having goals to work toward. People often have difficulty when asked to state their goals. Goals are often vaguely stated necessitating the presentation of a framework for group members to assist them to identify meaningful goals. In order to facilitate this process the following structured experience was developed.

GOALS

1. To encourage participants to become goal-focused

2. To help participants to prioritize their goals

3. To promote interpersonal sharing of goal related ideas

4. To become better acquainted with other group members

PRELIMINARY CONSIDERATIONS:

Level of Intensity: Low

Group Size: Small groups of no more than 8 persons

Time Required: Two hours

Materials: Paper and pencils for each participant
Felt tip marker and large poster paper

Physical Setting: Comfortable room with moveable chairs

PROCEDURE:

1. The group leader presents a brief overview concerning the importance of selecting and working towards goals.

2. Group members are asked to select three goals for themselves on which they might work in the group and to write these down.

3. In rotating order, each member states one goal which he or she has written. Stop after one round.

4. Participants are asked to share any perceptions regarding the goals which were presented. The leader might focus on similarities and dis-similarities between goals.

5. Repeat steps 3 and 4 for two more rounds.

6. The group leader presents a brief talk on additional ways to determine goals (e.g. identifying problems, making wishes, focusing on key areas in life, using a time-frame).

7. Participants are regrouped into dyads with each person conducting a five minute interview with a partner to help to identify additional goals using the strategies described by the group leader.

8. Group members return to the larger group and each person describes his or her partner's new goals and results from the interview.

9. The group leader presents a brief talk on prioritizing goals. One person's goals may serve as a model or a prepared written model of goal prioritization may be distributed and discussed.

10. Group members are asked to begin prioritizing their goals from 1 (most important) to 10 (least important).

11. After the initial prioritization, dyads may again be formed to discuss the results of goal prioritization.

12. A list of common problems in social, family, work and personal life areas may be given to group members to take home and review to determine if relevant goals may have been omitted. Group members are encouraged to have three priority goals determined before the next group convenes.

LEADERSHIP SUGGESTIONS:

1. Some members may find it difficult to select meaningful goals using an open-ended method. The leader might assist such a person using an interview or problem checklist format.

2. Questions should be encouraged and models of goals developed by other persons shown to the group.

3. Occasionally a group member may deny the need to work toward a relevant goal. The leader may want to discuss the relationship between such defenses and their adverse affect on goal selection.

VARIATIONS:

1. Have group members complete a problem checklist prior to discussing goals.

2. Triads may be used, rather than dyads, with one member acting as observer.

3. One group member's goals can be determined with the leader as the interviewer while other members observe the goal selection interview process.

4. Relevant goal themes might be prompted by the leader, such as disability related goals, achievement related goals, or personality change goals.

Guidelines for Developing Structured Group Experiences in Disability

When developing Structured Group Experiences in Disability there are many questions which need to be considered if the experience is to be meaningful. Listed below are a variety of representative questions:

GOALS

— Who is the structured experience designed for?

— What specific aspects of the experience would you like participants to learn?

— Are there differences between the knowledge, feelings, and cognitive processes which you would like the experience to convey?

— Have you considered the balance between the structured experiential task and the interpersonal dimensions involved in the experience?

— Are the expectations of the participants and your intentions congruent?

— Is disability a major thrust of the experience?

PRELIMINARY CONSIDERATIONS

Level of Intensity:

— Is the experience too easy or too difficult for group members?

— Is there a fragile group member who might be adversely affected by the experience?

— Could the experience be modified to reflect greater or lesser intensity?

— Are you prepared to deal with critical incidents which the experience might evoke?

Group Size:

— How large a group should you have?

— How many groups can be run simultaneously?

— Do you have at least two methods ready to break the group into smaller groups?

Time Required:

— What time constraints affect your experience?

— Which aspects of your experience should be stressed or limited?

— Is your introduction to the experience too long or too short?

Materials:

— What materials will participants need to comlete the experience?

— Have you considered when the materials should best be disseminated?

— Are there disabled group members who might not be able to use certain materials?

Physical Setting:

— Are there any architectural barriers in the location where the experience will be conducted?

— Is the room well lit and comfortable?

PROCEDURE

— Is the experience described in a step-by-step sequential fashion?

— Could the process be replicated by others in a similar manner?

— Do participants know what is expected of them at each step in the process?

— Are there potential critical incidents to be aware of that could disrupt or change the focus of the experience?

— How is feedback to be provided to members?

VARIATIONS

— What could be done to emphasize other aspects of the experience?

— Will a variation significantly change any of the preliminary considerations?